Imaging of Paranasal Sinuses

Editor

VARSHA M. JOSHI

NEUROIMAGING CLINICS OF NORTH AMERICA

www.neuroimaging.theclinics.com

Consulting Editor
SURESH K. MUKHERJI

November 2015 • Volume 25 • Number 4

ELSEVIER

1600 John F. Kennedy Boulevard • Suite 1800 • Philadelphia, Pennsylvania, 19103-2899

http://www.neuroimaging.theclinics.com

NEUROIMAGING CLINICS OF NORTH AMERICA Volume 25, Number 4
November 2015 ISSN 1052-5149, ISBN 13: 978-0-323-41342-8

Editor: John Vassallo (j.vassallo@elsevier.com)
Developmental Editor: Casey Jackson

Neuroimaging Clinics of North America (ISSN 1052-5149) is published quarterly by Elsevier Inc., 360 Park Avenue South, New York, NY 10010-1710. Months of issue are February, May, August, and November. Business and editorial offices: 1600 John F. Kennedy Blvd., Suite 1800, Philadelphia, PA 19103-2899. Business and editorial offices: 6277 Sea Harbor Drive, Orlando, FL 32887-4800. Periodicals postage paid at New York, NY, and additional mailing offices. Subscription prices are USD 360 per year for US individuals, USD 514 per year for US institutions, USD 180 per year for US students and residents, USD 415 per year for Canadian individuals, USD 655 per year for Canadian institutions, USD 525 per year for international individuals, USD 655 per year for international institutions and USD 260 per year for Canadian and foreign students and residents. To receive student/resident rate, orders must be accompanied by name of affiliated institution, date of term, and the *signature* of program/residency coordinator on institution letterhead. Orders will be billed at individual rate until proof of status is received. Foreign air speed delivery is included in all *Clinics* subscription prices. All prices are subject to change without notice. POSTMASTER: Send address changes to *Neuroimaging Clinics of North America*, Elsevier Health Sciences Division, Subscription **Customer Service, 3251 Riverport Lane, Maryland Heights, MO 63043. Telephone: 1-800-654-2452 (U.S. and Canada); 314-447-8871 (outside U.S. and Canada). Fax: 314-447-8029. E-mail:** journalscustomerservice-usa@elsevier.com **(for print support);** journalsonlinesupport-usa@elsevier.com **(for online support).**

Reprints. For copies of 100 or more of articles in this publication, please contact the Commercial Reprints Department, Elsevier Inc., 360 Park Avenue South, New York, NY 10010-1710. Tel.: 212-633-3874; Fax: 212-633-3820; E-mail: reprints@elsevier.com.

Neuroimaging Clinics of North America is covered by *Excerpta Medical/EMBASE,* the RSNA Index of Imaging Literature, *MEDLINE/PubMed (Index Medicus),* MEDLINE/MEDLARS, SciSearch, Research Alert, and Neuroscience Citation Index.

PROGRAM OBJECTIVE

The goal of *Neuroimaging Clinics of North America* is to keep practicing radiologists and radiology residents up to date with current clinical practice in radiology by providing timely articles reviewing the state of the art in patient care.

TARGET AUDIENCE

Practicing radiologists, radiology residents, and other healthcare professionals who utilize neuroimaging findings to provide patient care.

LEARNING OBJECTIVES

Upon completion of this activity, participants will be able to:
1. Review the normal anatomy and CT imaging techniques of the paranasal sinuses.
2. Discuss the role of imaging in the diagnosis and treatment of disorders of the paranasal sinuses, such as sinonasal inflammatory disease and fungal sinusitis.
3. Recognize post-treatment imaging and evaluation following paranasal sinus treatments and surgeries.

ACCREDITATION

The Elsevier Office of Continuing Medical Education (EOCME) is accredited by the Accreditation Council for Continuing Medical Education (ACCME) to provide continuing medical education for physicians.

The EOCME designates this enduring material for a maximum of 15 *AMA PRA Category 1 Credit*(s)™. Physicians should claim only the credit commensurate with the extent of their participation in the activity.

All other health care professionals requesting continuing education credit for this enduring material will be issued a certificate of participation.

DISCLOSURE OF CONFLICTS OF INTEREST

The EOCME assesses conflict of interest with its instructors, faculty, planners, and other individuals who are in a position to control the content of CME activities. All relevant conflicts of interest that are identified are thoroughly vetted by EOCME for fair balance, scientific objectivity, and patient care recommendations. EOCME is committed to providing its learners with CME activities that promote improvements or quality in healthcare and not a specific proprietary business or a commercial interest.

The planning committee, staff, authors and editors listed below have identified no financial relationships or relationships to products or devices they or their spouse/life partner have with commercial interest related to the content of this CME activity:

Mauricio Castillo, MD, FACR; Aditi Chandra, MD; Benjamin Cohen, MD; Steve E.J. Connor, FRCR; Girish M. Fatterpekar, MD; Anjali Fortna; Priya Ghosh, MD; Daniel Thomas Ginat, MD, MS; Mari Hagiwara, MD; Benjamin Y. Huang, MD, MPH; Varsha M. Joshi, DNB, DMRD; Yvonne W. Lui, MD; Suresh K. Mukherji, MD, MBA, FACR; Sumit Mukhopadhyay, MD; Eytan Raz, MD; Sansi Rima, DNB; Erin Scheckenbach; Saugata Sen, MD; Brent A. Senior, MD, FACS, FARS; Karthik Subramaniam; Sanjay Vaid, MD (Radiology); Neelam Vaid, MS, DNB (ENT); John Vassallo; William Win, MD.

UNAPPROVED/OFF-LABEL USE DISCLOSURE

The EOCME requires CME faculty to disclose to the participants:
1. When products or procedures being discussed are off-label, unlabelled, experimental, and/or investigational (not US Food and Drug Administration [FDA] approved); and
2. Any limitations on the information presented, such as data that are preliminary or that represent ongoing research, interim analyses, and/or unsupported opinions. Faculty may discuss information about pharmaceutical agents that is outside of FDA-approved labelling. This information is intended solely for CME and is not intended to promote off-label use of these medications. If you have any questions, contact the medical affairs department of the manufacturer for the most recent prescribing information.

TO ENROLL

To enroll in the *Neuroimaging Clinics of North America* Continuing Medical Education program, call customer service at 1-800-654-2452 or sign up online at http://www.theclinics.com/home/cme. The CME program is available to subscribers for an additional annual fee of USD 235.

METHOD OF PARTICIPATION

In order to claim credit, participants must complete the following:
1. Complete enrolment as indicated above.
2. Read the activity.
3. Complete the CME Test and Evaluation. Participants must achieve a score of 70% on the test. All CME Tests and Evaluations must be completed online.

CME INQUIRIES/SPECIAL NEEDS

For all CME inquiries or special needs, please contact elsevierCME@elsevier.com.

NEUROIMAGING CLINICS OF NORTH AMERICA

RELATED INTEREST

Radiologic Clinics of North America, January 2015 (Vol. 53, No. 1)
Head and Neck Imaging
Richard H. Wiggins III and Ashok Srinivasan, *Editors*
Available at: http://www.radiologic.theclinics.com/

THE CLINICS ARE AVAILABLE ONLINE!
Access your subscription at:
www.theclinics.com

Contributors

CONSULTING EDITOR

SURESH K. MUKHERJI, MD, MBA, FACR
Professor and Chairman, Walter F. Patenge
Endowed Chair, Department of Radiology,
Michigan State University; Chief Medical
Officer and Director of Health Care Delivery,
Michigan State University Health Team,
East Lansing, Michigan

EDITOR

VARSHA M. JOSHI, DNB, DMRD
Senior Consultant, Department of CT and MRI,
Vijaya Diagnostics, Hyderabad, Telangana;
Visiting Consultant, Department of Imaging,
Tata Medical Center, New Town, Kolkata,
India

AUTHORS

FRANCESCO BERTAGNA, MD
Staff Specialist, Nuclear Medicine, University
of Brescia, Brescia, Italy

MAURICIO CASTILLO, MD, FACR
Professor, Department of Radiology, University
of North Carolina, Chapel Hill, North Carolina

ADITI CHANDRA, MD
Senior Consultant, Department of Radiology
and Nuclear Medicine, Tata Medical Center,
New Town, Kolkata, India

BENJAMIN COHEN, MD
Department of Radiology, NYU School of
Medicine, New York, New York

STEVE E.J. CONNOR, FRCR
Neuroradiology Department, King's College
Hospital, London, United Kingdom

LUCA FACCHETTI, MD
Resident, Department of Radiology,
University of Brescia, Brescia, Italy

DAVIDE FARINA, MD
Professor, Department of Radiology,
University of Brescia, Brescia, Italy

GIRISH M. FATTERPEKAR, MD
Associate Professor, Department of
Radiology, NYU School of Medicine, New
York, New York

PRIYA GHOSH, MD
Senior Fellow, Department of
Radiology and Nuclear Medicine, Tata
Medical Center, New Town, Kolkata,
India

DANIEL THOMAS GINAT, MD, MS
Department of Radiology, University of
Chicago Medical Center, Pritzker Medical
School, Chicago, Illinois

MARI HAGIWARA, MD
Department of Radiology, NYU School of
Medicine, New York, New York

BENJAMIN Y. HUANG, MD, MPH
Clinical Associate Professor,
Department of Radiology, University
of North Carolina, Chapel Hill,
North Carolina

VARSHA M. JOSHI, DNB, DMRD
Senior Consultant, Department of CT and
MRI, Vijaya Diagnostics, Hyderabad,
Telangana; Visiting Consultant, Department of
Imaging, Tata Medical Center, New Town,
Kolkata, India

DAVIDE LOMBARDI, MD
Staff Specialist, Department of
Otorhinolaryngology, University of Brescia,
Brescia, Italy

YVONNE W. LUI, MD
Department of Radiology, NYU School of
Medicine, New York, New York

ROBERTO MAROLDI, MD
Professor, Department of Radiology, University
of Brescia, Brescia, Italy

SUMIT MUKHOPADHYAY, MD
Associate Consultant, Department of
Radiology and Nuclear Medicine,
Tata Medical Center, New Town,
Kolkata, India

PIERO NICOLAI, MD
Professor, Department of
Otorhinolaryngology, University of Brescia,
Brescia, Italy

MARCO RAVANELLI, MD
Staff Specialist, Department of Radiology,
University of Brescia, Brescia, Italy

EYTAN RAZ, MD
Department of Radiology, NYU School of
Medicine, New York, New York

RIMA SANSI, DNB
Consultant, Department of CT and MRI,
Vijaya Diagnostics, Hyderabad, Telangana,
India

SAUGATA SEN, MD
Senior Consultant, Department of Radiology
and Nuclear Medicine, Tata Medical Center,
New Town, Kolkata, India

BRENT A. SENIOR, MD, FACS, FARS
Professor, Department of
Otolaryngology-Head and Neck Surgery,
University of North Carolina, Chapel Hill,
North Carolina

NEELAM VAID, MS, DNB (ENT)
Consultant, Department of
Otorhinolaryngology, K.E.M. Hospital, Pune,
Maharashtra, India

SANJAY VAID, MD (Radiology)
Head Neck Imaging Division, Star Imaging
and Research Center, Pune, Maharashtra,
India

WILLIAM WIN, MD
Department of Radiology, NYU School of
Medicine, New York, New York

Contents

As endoscopic sinus surgery (ESS) has evolved since its introduction to the United States, so has technology for imaging the sinonasal cavities. Although imaging is most frequently performed for evaluating chronic sinusitis refractory to medical therapy, its uses have expanded beyond inflammatory sinus disease. Multidetector Computed Tomography is the current workhorse for both diagnosis and preoperative planning in prospective ESS patients, while MR imaging remains a complementary tool for evaluating suspected tumors or intracranial and orbital complications of rhinosinusitis. In this article, the authors review current trends and potential future directions in the use of these modalities for sinus imaging.

 A video showing a coronal CT depicting multiplanar attachments of the middle turbinate accompanies this article

It is imperative for all imaging specialists to be familiar with detailed multiplanar CT anatomy of the paranasal sinuses and adjacent structures. This article reviews the radiologically relevant embryology of this complex region and discusses the region-specific CT anatomy of the paranasal sinuses and surrounding structures. Radiologists also need to know the clinical implications of identifying preoperatively the numerous anatomic variations encountered in this region and prepare a structured report according to the expectations of the referring clinician.

While most patients with inflammatory rhinosinusitis are successfully diagnosed clinically, imaging is indicated in patients with recurrent or chronic sinusitis, atypical symptoms and complicated acute sinusitis. Non-enhanced high resolution, thin section computed tomography (CT) is the reference standard in evaluating such patients. It provides superb anatomical details and enables a fairly accurate diagnosis and delineation of the disease, addressing all concerns of the endoscopic surgeon prior to intervention. Contrast MR imaging is preferred for assessing intra-orbital or intracranial complications. The radiologist must have a systematic approach to sinonasal CT and generate a clinically relevant report that impacts patient management.

also a variety of complications that can result from endoscopic sinus surgery. Radiological imaging plays an important role in the evaluation of patients after endoscopic sinus surgery. Thus, it is important to be familiar with the expected and complicated imaging findings associated with endoscopic sinus surgery, which are reviewed in this article.

Roberto Maroldi, Marco Ravanelli, Davide Farina, Luca Facchetti, Francesco Bertagna, Davide Lombardi, and Piero Nicolai

The aim of imaging in the follow-up of asymptomatic patients treated for sinonasal neoplasms is to detect submucosal relapsing lesions. The challenge is to discriminate recurrent tissue within the changes resulting from unpredictable healing of tissue after surgery and radiotherapy. Scar, inflammation, and recurrence can be better separated with a multisequence MR imaging approach. The choice of the field of view should take into account the risk of in-field intracranial recurrences, craniofacial bone metastases, and perineural spread. Fluorodeoxyglucose-PET has a role in assessing distant metastasis. Its usefulness in local and regional surveillance has yet to be established.

Foreword
Imaging of Paranasal Sinuses

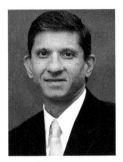

Suresh K. Mukherji, MD, MBA, FACR
Consulting Editor

I have the distinct pleasure to welcome and thank Dr Varsha Joshi for editing this issue of *Neuroimaging Clinics* on the paranasal sinuses. I have known Dr Joshi for over 15 years when she was a Visiting Research Fellow working under me at University of North Carolina. It has been very enjoyable to see her grow into an internationally recognized head and neck radiologist. She is one of the brightest minds in the field of Head and Neck Imaging and has established herself as one of the leaders of imaging in India.

The issue is a practical and concise monograph comprising eight articles covering topics ranging from anatomy, pathology, and to current trends in sinonasal imaging. There are separate articles covering the anterior skull base as well and posttreatment imaging. I congratulate the authors on their excellent articles and thank them for their efforts in contributing to such an outstanding issue.

Final thought...one of the greatest pleasures a mentor can have is seeing their mentees achieve excellence. But the greatest satisfaction is watching those you train surpass their own expectations and the talents of their mentors. Congratulations Varsha! It has been a privilege to play a small role in your success!

Suresh K. Mukherji, MD, MBA, FACR
Department of Radiology
Michigan State University
846 Service Road
160 Radiology Building
East Lansing, MI 48824, USA

E-mail address:
mukherji@rad.msu.edu

Neuroimag Clin N Am 25 (2015) xi
http://dx.doi.org/10.1016/j.nic.2015.08.002
1052-5149/15/$ – see front matter © 2015 Published by Elsevier Inc.

Neurosurg. Clin. N Am. 25 (2015) xi
http://dx.doi.org/10.1016/j.nec.2015.08.002
1042-3680/15/$ – see front matter © 2015 Published by Elsevier Inc.

Preface

Paranasal Sinuses— Decongested!

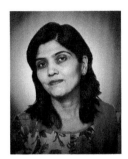

Varsha M. Joshi, DNB, DMRD
Editor

The last three decades have witnessed tremendous progress in the imaging evaluation of the paranasal sinuses. Driven by the introduction and numerous advances in endoscopic sinus surgery and management of sinonasal disease, there has been a parallel evolution from plain radiography to cross-sectional imaging of the sinuses with CT and MRI. These modalities provide better understanding of the anatomy and have made the diagnosis and disease mapping a far more exact process. These, in turn, enable a better and more intelligent dialogue between the radiologist and the endoscopic or head and neck surgeon prior to any form of intervention in such patients.

In this issue, we have put together all the relevant topics in sinonasal imaging under one cover. The issue comprises eight articles covering topics ranging from current trends in sinonasal imaging, anatomy, and imaging of the diverse spectrum of diseases that occur in the sinonasal cavities. A separate article describing the importance of imaging the anterior skull base in sinonasal diseases has been provided. The challenging area of post-treatment appearances of the sinuses has been dealt with by the authors in two dedicated articles.

All the authors have put in their best efforts to provide a descriptive text with numerous illustrations and high-quality images that have been reproduced beautifully by our publishing staff. Numerous highly detailed annotated images have been used; multiple tables and checklists have been provided wherever appropriate.

The intent has been to provide a simple, practical, one-stop-shop reference for sinus imaging that can be used by one and all during our day-to-day practice. Hopefully, with the help of all the authors, I have succeeded in this goal. I sincerely hope that like the title, the issue serves as an "effective decongestant" to simplify the interpretation of sinonasal imaging studies and further enhance our diagnostic skills to positively impact patient management. Feedback on the issue will be much appreciated. I can be reached at drjoshivarsha@gmail.com.

Varsha M. Joshi, DNB, DMRD
Department of CT and MRI
Vijaya Diagnostic Centers
Hyderabad 500034, India

Department of Imaging
Tata Medical Center
Kolkatta, India

E-mail address:
drjoshivarsha@gmail.com

Neuroimag Clin N Am 25 (2015) xiii
http://dx.doi.org/10.1016/j.nic.2015.08.001
1052-5149/15/$ – see front matter © 2015 Published by Elsevier Inc.

neuroimaging.theclinics.com

Current Trends in Sinonasal Imaging

Benjamin Y. Huang, MD, MPH[a],*, Brent A. Senior, MD[b], Mauricio Castillo, MD[a]

KEYWORDS

- Paranasal sinuses • Functional endoscopic surgery • Multidetector CT • Cone beam CT
- MR imaging • Image-guided surgery

KEY POINTS

- Multiplanar computed tomography (CT) imaging in the coronal, axial, and sagittal planes is now commonplace for the assessment of the paranasal sinuses. The addition of sagittal images is particularly helpful for assessing the frontal sinus outflow tract.
- Appropriate indications for CT imaging of the paranasal sinuses currently include chronic sinusitis refractory to appropriate medical therapy, recurrent acute or chronic sinusitis, complications of surgery or sinusitis, cerebrospinal fluid (CSF) rhinorrhea, suspicion of invasive fungal sinusitis in immunocompromised patients, tumor surveillance, or surgical planning for new or revision sinus surgery.
- In addition to standard radiation dose-reduction strategies, such as adjusting tube voltage, current, or scanner pitch, new techniques, including automated exposure control, automated tube voltage selection, and iterative reconstruction, are commonly used in sinus imaging to help reduce the effective dose while maintaining image quality.
- Cone beam CT (CBCT) is becoming increasingly popular for in-office point-of-care imaging of the sinuses and for intraoperative imaging and produces high-resolution images at a substantially reduced dose compared with multidetector CT (MDCT); however, current CBCT scanners still lag behind MDCT in image quality.
- MR imaging remains a complementary imaging tool to CT for sinonasal disease but is indicated and is particularly useful for characterizing sinonasal tumors and for suspected intracranial and orbital complications of rhinosinusitis.

INTRODUCTION

Advances in therapeutic and diagnostic technologies over the last 3 decades have fundamentally transformed the way we evaluate and treat diseases of the sinonasal cavities and skull base. Before the popularization of endoscopic sinus surgery (ESS), surgical management of sinus disease primarily focused on open approaches to the maxillary, ethmoid, and frontal sinuses with high complication rates and the possibility of facial incisions. The introduction and development of endoscopic techniques suddenly made it possible to explore and dissect areas in the sinonasal cavities that had been previously inaccessible using safe, minimally invasive approaches. As a result, in the roughly 30 years since it was first introduced in the United States, ESS has become one of the most common otolaryngologic surgical procedures, with an estimated 350,000 sinus surgeries now being performed in the United States annually; the application of endoscopic techniques now includes treatment of sinonasal and skull base tumors and repair of skull base defects.[1]

Disclosure: The authors have nothing to disclose.
[a] Department of Radiology, University of North Carolina, CB# 7510, 101 Manning Drive, Chapel Hill, NC 27599, USA; [b] Department of Otolaryngology-Head and Neck Surgery, University of North Carolina, CB# 7070, 170 Manning Drive, Chapel Hill, NC 27599, USA
* Corresponding author.
E-mail address: bhuang@med.unc.edu

Neuroimag Clin N Am 25 (2015) 507–525
http://dx.doi.org/10.1016/j.nic.2015.07.001

neuroimaging.theclinics.com

Over the same period of time, the evolution in imaging technology used for evaluating the sinonasal cavities has, in many ways, paralleled the development of ESS. Before the introduction of computed tomography (CT) for routine clinical imaging, the primary modalities available for visualizing the sinonasal cavities were plain radiography and polytomography.[2] The standard 4-view sinus series of the time was generally adequate for the purposes of depicting sinus size, assessing septal deviation, and demonstrating opacification and/or the presence of fluid levels in the sinuses.[3] However, these studies were actually fairly poor in their ability to accurately diagnose sinusitis and provided only limited anatomic information.[4]

For a short time, polytomography was popular for sinus imaging because of its improved ability, compared with plain radiography, to demonstrate fine bony architecture. Polytomography was actually the imaging technique used by Messerklinger and his colleagues in Europe in their initial descriptions of nasal endoscopy. However, background blurring from structures above and below the focal plane frequently prevented tomograms from being able to adequately depict small bony structures in the area of the ostiomeatal complex (OMC), which is the primary region of interest for practitioners of ESS.[5,6] At roughly the same time that ESS was taking root, CT was emerging as a fledgling clinical imaging technology and was quickly recognized as being an ideal planning tool for ESS.[7] As a result, over the last 30 years, CT and, more recently, MR imaging have come to play a key role not only in the diagnosis of sinonasal disease but also in its management. Otolaryngologists now routinely order imaging studies to aid in the diagnosis of rhinosinusitis, sinonasal tumors, and cerebrospinal fluid (CSF) leaks; for help with preoperative planning and intraoperative guidance during ESS; and for disease surveillance following surgical and nonsurgical treatment of skull base tumors.

The goal of this article is to discuss current trends in the use of imaging in the paranasal sinuses, including an overview of modern imaging techniques, such as CT, cone beam CT (CBCT), MR imaging; strategies for radiation dose reduction in sinus CT; indications for sinonasal imaging; image-guided surgery; and potential areas for future development in sinonasal imaging.

OVERVIEW OF MODALITIES USED IN MODERN SINUS IMAGING
Computed Tomography

Because of its high spatial resolution and ability to depict fine osseous detail, CT is the imaging test of choice for providing the necessary information for ESS planning, such as the presence of fluid and degree of mucosal thickening, the presence of bone dehiscence or osteitis, and the anatomy of the sinuses, including important sinonasal anatomic variants. In their initial description of CT imaging for ESS, Kennedy and colleagues[7] endorsed acquiring coronal and axial images; these continue to be the workhorse viewing planes for routine sinus imaging today. The coronal plane is generally the preferred orientation for viewing the OMC and other landmarks, such as the skull base, orbital laminae, and orbital floors, whereas the axial plane provides better characterization of the anterior and posterior walls of the frontal sinuses, the sphenoid ostia, and the anatomic relationships between the posterior ethmoid and sphenoid sinuses[8,9] (Fig. 1).

Early generation single-slice CT units required each acquisition plane to be obtained directly, meaning that if one needed images in both the coronal and axial planes, patients essentially had to undergo 2 separate scans, substantially increasing imaging time and doubling the radiation dose compared with a single-plane acquisition alone. In addition, acquisition of direct coronal images traditionally required patients to lie prone in the scanner with their head hyperextended and the scanner gantry angled perpendicular to the infraorbitomeatal line in order to best approximate the true coronal plane of the sinuses.[7] With the technology at that time, it took roughly 2 seconds to generate a single CT image; as a result, a complete coronal scan through the sinuses generally took several minutes to complete.[5] This position was often not well tolerated by patients with limited cervical motion; as a result of this and the long acquisition time, direct coronal scans were particularly susceptible to motion artifacts. In addition, amalgam from dental restoration could produce beam hardening artifacts, which had the potential to significantly obscure sinus anatomy[10] (Fig. 2).

The introduction of spiral CT in the late 1980s and multidetector CT (MDCT) roughly a decade later led to marked improvements in sinus imaging. The ability to perform helical acquisitions significantly decreased scan times and allowed one to acquire volumetric data without anatomic misregistration. This technology ultimately paved the way for the development of 3-dimensional (3D) image-processing techniques, such as multiplanar reformation (MPR) and volume rendering techniques (VRT), which are now commonly used in head and neck imaging.[11] The development of MDCT led to even further reductions in scan times and improvements in spatial resolution because of the increased tissue coverage and the use of

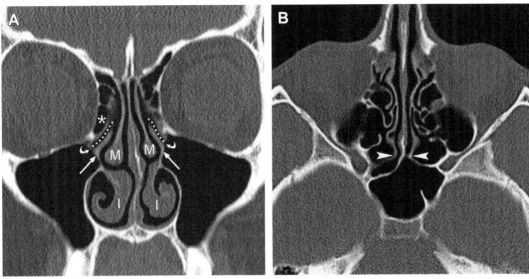

Fig. 1. Normal coronal (A) and axial (B) sinus anatomy. Coronal CT images (A) are ideal for demonstrating the normal anatomy of the OMC, which includes the maxillary ostium (*curved arrows*), ethmoidal infundibulum (*dotted lines*), ethmoidal bulla (*asterisk*), uncinate process (*arrows*), and hiatus semilunaris (located at the medial end of the ethmoidal infundibulum between the ethmoidal bulla and free edge of the uncinate process). The coronal plane is also excellent for visualizing the orbital lamina and anterior skull base. The axial CT plane (B) is better for evaluating the sphenoid ostia (*arrowheads*), the anatomic relationship between the posterior ethmoids and sphenoid sinus, and the posterior sphenoid sinus wall. It is also better than the coronal plane for demonstrating the anterior and posterior walls of the frontal sinuses (not shown). I, inferior turbinate; M, middle turbinate.

smaller detector collimators, which allowed for even higher-quality reformations.

In spite of these advances, as recently as a decade ago, many institutions, including the authors', were still using protocols that called for direct coronal scanning of the sinuses. Over the last decade, however, with MDCT scanners with 64 or more detector arrays becoming increasingly commonplace, many centers have abandoned the practice of obtaining separate coronal acquisitions.[10] Modern 64-slice MDCT systems can now acquire an entire sinus examination in roughly

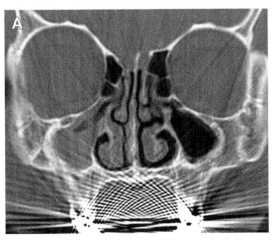
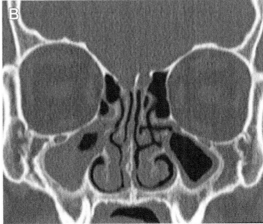

Fig. 2. Comparison of sequential direct coronal CT acquisition (A) and a coronal multiplanar reformation from an axial helical CT acquisition (B), performed in the same patient on different dates. On (A), there is significant beam hardening caused by dental amalgam fillings, which obscures some of the fine bony details. This problem is avoided by acquiring data in the axial plane then reconstructing the images in the coronal plane (B). With modern multidetector scanners, the resolution of reconstructed images is nearly equivalent to direct coronal images.

5 seconds while producing near isotropic submilli-meter voxels, which can be reconstructed at high resolution in any plane.[11] Although MDCT of the paranasal sinuses carries a higher radiation dose compared with the sequential single-slice CT scan obtained with otherwise similar parameters (roughly 20% higher[12]), with MDCT one need perform a single acquisition, which can be used to create any desired viewing plane, which ulti-mately translates to an overall radiation dose sav-ings over a traditional 2-plane coronal and axial acquisition.

The use of MPR has also led to an increase in use of sagittal reformations for routine viewing. For obvious reasons, direct sagittal imaging was not routinely performed with single-slice scanners, and early attempts at reconstructing nonaxial im-ages from sequenced single-channel helical scans were generally of poor quality, making routine sagittal imaging previously impractical. Today, producing a sagittal MPR is a trivial task; the inclu-sion of sagittal reconstructions is now a routine practice at many institutions. Sagittal images are particularly useful for evaluating the frontal sinus outflow tract and surrounding ethmoid air cells, including the agger nasi, frontal cells, and the frontal and suprabullar cells (Fig. 3); it has been re-ported that the addition of sagittal images signifi-cantly improves presurgical understanding of the

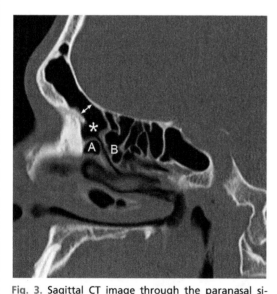

Fig. 3. Sagittal CT image through the paranasal si-nuses, which nicely demonstrates the frontal isthmus (*double-sided arrow*), frontal recess (*asterisk*), and nearby ethmoid air cells, including the agger nasi (A) and ethmoid bulla (B). Addition of reconstructed sagittal images significantly improves assessment of the size of the frontal sinus ostium and understanding of the 3D anatomy of the frontal recess.

3D anatomy of the frontal recess and that the addi-tional information provided might alter the surgical approach in more than half of ESS cases compared with having only coronal images alone.[13,14] Therefore, it is now routine at the au-thors' center to reformat all of their sinus CT exam-inations in the axial, coronal, and sagittal planes.

DOSE-REDUCTION STRATEGIES IN SINUS COMPUTED TOMOGRAPHY

Among the topics of greatest interest in CT imag-ing currently is that of radiation dose reduction, as we have all become increasingly attuned to the risks associated with exposure to ionizing radi-ation. In first world countries, CT scanning ac-counts for 7.9% of the total number of diagnostic medical examinations, yet contributes approxi-mately 47% of the total collective effective dose caused by diagnostic medical imaging.[15] Not sur-prisingly, the popularization of ESS over the last few decades has led to a significant increase in the number of sinus CTs performed today.

Therefore, significant efforts have gone into developing protocols and technologies designed to reduce to as low as reasonably achievable the radiation dose associated with a sinus CT while maintaining diagnostic image quality. However, given institutional differences in scanner hardware and practice patterns, there is likely significant variation in the protocols and radiation doses from sinus CT between centers. Guidelines regarding dose limits for sinus CT have been pub-lished in the European Union recommending a reference CT dose index (CTDI) of 35 milligray (mGy) and dose length product (DLP) of 360 mGy-cm, which in an adult patient translates to an effective dose of 0.76 milligray (mSv).[16] Although these guidelines provide a reasonable ceiling below which doses should fall, the recom-mended values serve more as a starting point than as an end goal; many centers, including the authors' use protocols requiring much lower radi-ation doses.

Among the simplest strategies to decrease the CT radiation dose is to change the acquisition pa-rameters, such as tube voltage, tube current, and pitch; but this strategy comes at the price of reducing image quality. Lowering the peak tube voltage reduces the effective dose in an exponen-tial fashion and also has the added benefit of increasing contrast for bony structures; however, substantially decreasing the peak tube voltage, while keeping other factors constant, also increases image noise in a nonlinear fashion because of the decreased tissue penetrating po-wer of the lower-energy photons.[17,18] Lowering the tube current alone reduces the dose in a linear fashion but also increases image noise because of greater quantum mottle (**Fig. 4**). Finally, although increasing the pitch also lowers the radiation dose proportionally, this degrades the section sensitivity profile and increases volume averaging. Furthermore, the effect of pitch on radiation dose is negated by scanners using an effective milliampere-second setting, which holds the effective milliampere-second value constant irrespective of pitch value.[19]

The challenge of optimizing CT in any part of the body lies in striking the right balance between dose and image quality. Studies have evaluated various low-dose sinus CT protocols in an attempt to determine how far one can reduce dose while maintaining diagnostic quality images. Most of the protocols that have been investigated to date have focused primarily on lowering the tube current,[12,20,21] but some have also looked at the effects of altering both the tube current and tube voltage.[22]

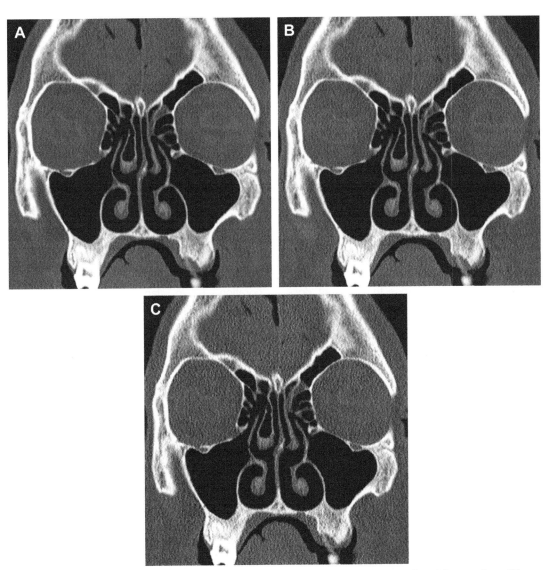

Fig. 4. Effect of lowering tube current on radiation dose and image quality. Coronal MPR images from CT scans through the paranasal sinuses of a cadaver head acquired at a fixed tube voltage of 120 kVp but different effective tube currents: 120 mAs (*A*), 60 mAs (*B*), and 30 mAs (*C*). Dose length products for the 3 settings were 251 mGy-cm for (*A*); 127 mGy-cm for (*B*); and 63 mGy-cm for (*C*). Note the increase in image noise with decreasing tube current, which results in more graininess and the osseous structures appearing less sharp on the lower dose settings.

Brem and colleagues[21] estimated that the effective tube current could be lowered to 67 mAs at a tube voltage of 120 kVp while maintaining diagnostic quality for sinus CT by using a computer simulation that artificially added image noise to emulate the effect of lowering the radiation dose. In various human studies, tube current settings as low as 10 mAs to 40 mAs have been evaluated with reported dose reductions of 59.7% to 93.0% compared with standard dose protocols and achieved average doses as low as 0.047 mSv[12,20]; these studies suggest that these low-dose settings do not seem to significantly affect ability to assess individual anatomic structures or result in discrepancies in interpretation.

Studies examining a wide variety of applications, including in the head and neck, have also shown that images acquired lower tube potentials (80–100 kVp) with an appropriately adjusted milliampere-second can substantially lower the radiation dose while still maintaining high diagnostic quality.[23–27] Abul-Kasim and colleagues[22] compared 2 low-dose protocols incorporating both reduced tube voltage and current (80 kV, 33 effective mAs and 80 kVp, 17 effective mAs) to a standard protocol (120 kVp and 59 effective mAs) and reported that the low-dose settings provided mean effective dose reductions of 74.6% and 87.9%, respectively. Although lowering dose was noted to produce lower image quality scores in the study, there was still high interobserver and intraobserver agreement for assessment of pathologic conditions across the different dose settings.

Several additional strategies for CT dose reduction that have been introduced recently by scanner manufacturers include automatic exposure control (AEC) systems, automated tube voltage selection, and noise-reducing iterative reconstruction (IR) algorithms.[17,18] AEC systems are now available on MDCT systems from all of the major scanner manufacturers and are among the most widely used automated dose-reduction techniques. These systems, which include CAREDose 4D (Siemens Medical Solutions, Erlangen, Germany); AutomA and SmartmA (GE Healthcare, Milwaukee, WI); DoseRight (Phillips Medical Systems, Andover, MA); and SureExposure 3D (Toshiba Corporation, Tokyo, Japan), vary to some degree in their basic mode of operation; but all function to modulate the radiation dose according to the patient size and attenuation while maintaining image quality.[18,28] The amount of dose savings provided by use of AEC depends on the specific system, the body part to be scanned, patient habitus, and user-specified settings; however, various studies have reported dose reductions for different body parts in the range of 15% to 60%.[18,29] More recently, an automated tube voltage selection system has been introduced for commercial use. This technology automatically calculates the optimal tube current and tube potential for each patient depending on the study type, body part, and patient habitus to maintain user-defined quality and noise preferences. To date this technology is only available on scanners manufactured by Siemens, which limits its widespread applicability.[18]

There has also been renewed interest in the use of IR techniques in CT imaging for noise reduction. IR is an alternative to filtered back projection (FBP), which had for many years been the method on which all CT reconstruction methods were based. Although IR is not a new idea, the significant computational demands and time required to perform IR precluded it from being commercially viable in the past. Faster and more powerful computers coupled with newer IR techniques have substantially reduced processing times to the point that all the major CT vendors now offer some version of IR. These versions include Image Reconstruction Iterative Reconstruction (IRIS) and Sinogram Affirmed Iterative Reconstruction (SAFIRE) (Siemens Medical Solutions, Erlangen, Germany); Adaptive Statistical Iterative Reconstruction (ASiR) and model-based IR (Veo) (GE Healthcare, Milwaukee, WI); iDose (Phillips Medical Systems, Andover, MA); and Adaptive Iterative Dose Reduction (ADIR) and ADIR 3D (Toshiba Corporation, Tokyo, Japan). Although they differ slightly, these IR techniques all basically function to reduce reconstructed CT image noise compared with traditional FBP techniques, with the user being able to determine the iteration strength and overall amount of noise reduction. Thus, theoretically, one can use lower dose settings to achieve the same contrast-to-noise ratio (CNR).[18,30] A potential disadvantage to IR is that increasing iteration strength, although it can markedly reduce image noise, also produces artificial oversmoothing of images that may impair evaluation of thin bony structures[31,32] (Fig. 5).

To date 3 studies have examined the feasibility of IR techniques in paranasal sinus imaging.[32–34] Bulla and colleagues[33] reported that application of IRIS allowed for a dose reduction of up to 60% compared with a standard low-dose (60 mAs) CT, without impairing the diagnostic quality of images. In a phantom head study, Schulz and colleagues[34] performed CT scans at different tube voltages (120 kV and 100 kV) and tube currents (100 mAs, 50 mAs, and 25 mAs) and reconstructed each scan using FBP and 5 different SAFIRE settings. Although SAFIRE reduced the

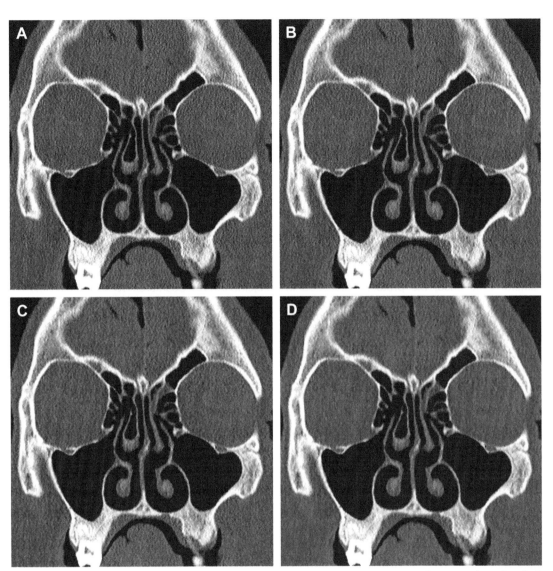

Fig. 5. Effect of increasing iterative reconstruction strength on CT images. CT image from a cadaver head obtained with 120 kVp and 30 mAs and reconstructed with FBP (A) and sinogram affirmed iterative reconstruction (SAFIRE) at progressively increasing strengths of 1 (B), 3 (C), and 5 (D). Application of SAFIRE decreases image noise, evident by decreasing graininess on the images with increasing SAFIRE strength; however, at the highest iteration strengths, the images take on an artificially smoothed and waxy appearance (in particular compare A and D).

image noise by 15% to 85% depending on the iterative strength, rendering kernel, and dose parameters, in a subjective assessment of image quality, readers invariably preferred the full tube current examinations reconstructed with FBP over the lower milliampere-second scans, regardless of SAFIRE setting; the investigators did not specifically comment on the diagnostic quality of the scans. Finally, Hoxworth and colleagues,[32] comparing standard-dose (210 mA) and low-dose (20 mA) sinus CT reconstructed with both FBP and Veo model-based iterative

reconstruction, found that although images reconstructed with Veo had the lowest image noise, none of the low-dose sinus CT scans, irrespective of the use of IR, were adequate for preoperative planning.

Ultimately, what constitutes acceptable dose and image quality in sinus CT depends, in large part, on the specific indication for the examination. A scan performed at a very low milliampere-second setting may be fine for simply confirming the presence or absence of fluid or mucosal thickening but might not provide the fine bony detail required for presurgical planning. The authors' own routine sinus CT protocol varies slightly depending on the scanner being used, but a sample protocol for a 128-slice MDCT equipped with both automated tube voltage and current systems and IR is described in Table 1. Irrespective of the specific scanner, the authors' sinus CT protocol consists of a single axial volumetric acquisition extending from the top of the frontal sinus through the hard palate using a submillimeter collimator (~0.6 mm on 64-slice scanners). Overlapping, submillimeter thick (0.6–0.75 mm) axial images that are compatible with the authors' center's intraoperative navigation systems are reconstructed using a soft tissue reconstruction kernel, whereas additional 2-mm axial, coronal, and sagittal images are reconstructed using an ultrasharp bone reconstruction kernel for general viewing. In the authors' experience, the protocol described in Table 1 produces reasonably low effective doses while being of high enough quality for routine surgical planning.

Cone Beam Computed Tomography

CBCT is a technology that has become popular for point-of-care (POC) imaging in the office setting and for intraoperative imaging, both because of its compact size and attractively low cost (compared with conventional CT) (Fig. 6). Although the reconstruction algorithm on which CBCT is based (in essence a 3D modification of traditional filtered back projection[35–37]) was first introduced

more than 30 years ago, the technology only became widely available over the last 10 to 15 years, with the first commercial dental CBCT scanner introduced in 2001 (NewTom QR DVT 9000; Quantitative Radiology, Verona, Italy). Similar systems designed primarily for imaging in the head and neck were introduced shortly thereafter (MiniCAT, Xoran Technologies, Ann Arbor, MI; Accuitomo, J Morita Technologies, Irvine, CA; ILUMA Cone Beam CT, IMTEC, Ardmore, OK; GE Healthcare, Chalfont St Giles, UK).[38,39] CBCT is now being used routinely for clinic-based dentomaxillofacial imaging, for patient positioning verification in radiotherapy,[40,41] and for imaging during operative and interventional procedures.[42]

Unlike conventional MDCT scanners, which use a multiple parallel linear detector arrays to detect incident x-ray beams as 1D projections that are then stacked to produce an imaging volume, CBCT systems use a flat panel detector which detects incident photons from the entire conical shaped x-ray beam as multiple 2D projections. As a result, CBCT systems can acquire the entire volumetric data set with a single rotation of the gantry, whereas data acquisition for conventional spiral CT data acquisition generally requires both multiple rotations and z-direction movement of the gantry to cover the volume of interest.[43]

Because of the 3D nature of data acquisition in CBCT, high-resolution isotropic images can be created in any plane without the loss of image quality that normally occurs with out-of-plane reconstruction in MDCT because of the partial-volume averaging effects. For example, the CBCT system used at the authors' center, is capable of producing a volumetric data set with isotropic voxels as small as $150 \times 150 \times 150 \ \mu m^3$, which is roughly 2 to 3 fold smaller than that of MDCT.[43–45]

Furthermore, CBCT is able to obtain comparable resolution images at a substantially lower radiation dose than MDCT. Commercial cone beam systems use tube voltages similar to MDCT (roughly 90–120 kVp) but operate at much lower tube current settings (around 10 mA vs around 80 mA).[44] Unfortunately, determining exactly how much of a dose reduction CBCT affords can be problematic because there has been a lack of agreement regarding how an effective dose in CBCT should be measured. CTDI, which is the measure widely used for MDCT, is not suitable for CBCT because the width of the cone beam in CBCT systems exceeds the width of standard 100-mm pencil ionization chambers used for measurement in MDCT systems, making it difficult to directly compare doses between MDCT and CBCT.[44] In 2011, the International Atomic Energy

Table 1 Sample sinus CT protocol (Siemens Definition AS)		
	Adult Protocol	**Pediatric Protocol**
Detector configuration	128 × 0.6 mm	128 × 0.6 mm
Automated exposure control (CAREDose)	On	On
Automated tube voltage selection (CAREkV)	On	On
Reference mAs	84 mAs	60 mAs
Reference kV	120 kV	120 kV
Rotation time	1 s	1 s
Pitch	0.8:1	0.8:1
Reconstructions	0.75 mm axial, J40s, SAFIRE 3 2-mm axial/coronal/sagittal, H70 h, SAFIRE off	

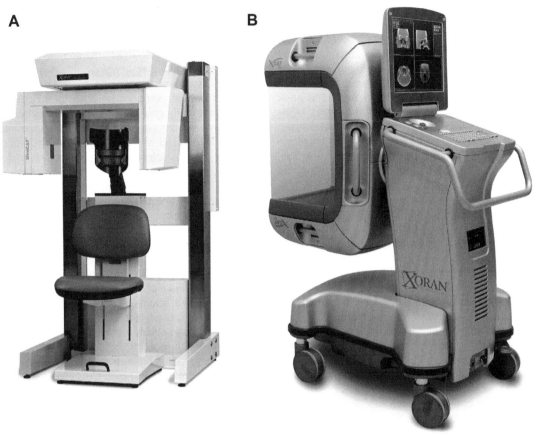

Fig. 6. Examples of CBCT scanners used for extracranial head and neck imaging (*A*) and mobile imaging (*B*). The small size of the units and the relatively low radiation emitted by these types of scanners make them attractive options for office-based POC imaging and intraoperative imaging. (*Courtesy of* Xoran Technologies, Ann Arbor, MI; with permission)

Agency published a report, proposing a standardized dosimetry method for CBCT[46]; but this method has yet to be widely adopted by scanner manufacturers.

Because of differences in scanner hardware, imaging protocols, and dosimetry techniques, studies that have attempted to quantify the potential reduction in the radiation dose of CBCT compared with MDCT have produced a broad range of numbers, making it difficult to generalize these findings across different commercial CBCT platforms. Alspaugh and colleagues[47] reported that for sinus imaging, CBCT with a spatial resolution of 12 line pairs per centimeter resulted in an effective dose of 0.17 mSv compared with 0.87 mSv for a 64-slice MDCT with a comparable spatial resolution (11 line pairs per centimeter). Dierckx and colleagues[48] reported a slightly smaller dose difference in a phantom model, with the effective dose of a standard CBCT acquisition of the sinuses being roughly 3 times lower than MDCT (0.10 mSv vs 0.33 mSv).

More recently, Leiva-Salinas and colleagues[49] compared standard CBCT and MDCT of the sinuses in 40 patients with suspected sinonasal inflammatory disease and found a much larger difference in effective dose, with CBCT demonstrating a more than 22-fold reduction in dose relative to MDCT (0.023 mSv vs 0.511 mSv, respectively). CBCT was judged to be of diagnostic quality in all patients; however, image quality was significantly lower for CBCT, with image noise for CBCT being 37.3% higher and CNR between various tissues being roughly 70% lower compared with MDCT. These findings highlight the major drawbacks of CBCT that have prevented it from overtaking conventional CT for general imaging in the head and neck (ie, noisier images and poorer contrast resolution). These shortcomings are explained in part by the higher degree of x-ray scatter in CBCT (caused in part by the lack of detector collimation) and by the reduced dynamic range and temporal resolution of current flat panel detectors.[42] Commercially available

CBCT systems have a soft tissue contrast resolution of only 5 to 10 Hounsfield units (HU) (compared with a contrast resolution of approximately 1 HU for modern MDCT scanners), meaning that these systems are not generally adequate for imaging of soft tissues. As a result, CBCT systems currently used for head and neck imaging are largely limited to evaluating high-contrast structures, such as the paranasal sinuses and temporal bones. For this reason, the American Academy of Otolaryngology-Head and Neck Surgery (AAO-HNS) recommends using conventional CT over CBCT imaging for assessing soft tissue pathology and for evaluating possible orbital and intracranial complications of sinusitis.[50]

Given that CBCT is a technology that is still, relatively speaking, in its infancy, its role in sinonasal imaging remains largely undefined. Several studies have demonstrated the utility of CBCT systems for intraoperative imaging in endoscopic sinonasal and skull base surgeries, specifically for assessing the completeness of surgical dissection, adequacy of mucocele drainage, extent of tumor resection, and for frontal stent placement, with reports suggesting that use of intraoperative CBCT results in additional intervention in 18% to 24% of cases.[51–53]

The utility of POC in office CBCT has been less well studied. Critics of POC imaging point to the lower image quality, lack of low-contrast soft tissue discrimination, potential for overuse from self-referral, inconsistency of regulation of the technology from state to state, and questions of interpretation, in some instances, by nonradiologists who lack formal training and accreditation in radiology.[38] On the other hand, a handful of studies have suggested that POC imaging, although it does result in higher imaging utilization, might reduce unnecessary antibiotic prescriptions and improve patient compliance with otolaryngologic care, particularly given the fact that patients with symptoms of chronic rhinosinusitis are currently empirically treated with antibiotics and/or corticosteroids before demonstrating objective endoscopic or imaging evidence of inflammatory disease.[54,55] Given the limited amount of data on in-office CBCT and the continued evolution of the technology, clinical guidelines outlining the indications for POC imaging with CBCT remain to be defined. Although the authors' surgeons do use CBCT as a problem-solving tool in the office setting, their own experience has been that, compared with MDCT, the amount of noise present on CBCT scans often precludes adequate visualization of the fine bone detail necessary for optimal preoperative planning (Fig. 7), particularly in the setting of revision sinus surgery, tumor, or other complex disease related to the skull base or the orbit. As a result, the authors prefer MDCT over CBCT for imaging of these operative candidates.

MR Imaging

MR imaging remains a complementary imaging tool for most sinonasal diseases, as its resolution and ability to demonstrate fine bone detail lag

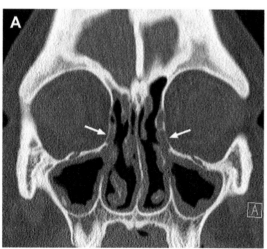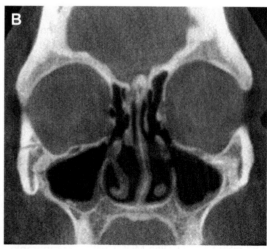

Fig. 7. Comparison of images from MDCT (*A*) and CBCT (*B*) of the paranasal sinuses using standard clinical scanner settings, obtained in the same patient on different dates. The MDCT was obtained at 120 kVp and 92 effective mAs, and the CBCT was obtained at 120 kVp and a tube current of 7 mA (exposure 48.3 mAs). Although the CBCT is associated with a lower patient dose (97.0 mGy-cm compared with 170 mGy-cm in this case) and affords superior spatial resolution compared with MDCT, it suffers from lower image contrast and greater image noise, the latter of which can limit assessment of fine bone detail. Note the difference in ability to visualize the bone of the orbital laminae, inferiorly (*arrows* in *A*). On the CBCT (*B*), this bone is not well seen.

behind that of CT. Where MR imaging outshines CT is in its ability to characterize soft tissue pathology, making it particularly useful when imaging patients with sinonasal or skull base masses or suspected intracranial and/or orbital complications of rhinosinusitis, situations in which it is crucial to assess for spread of disease beyond the paranasal sinuses and to determine the true extent of the process. The superior soft tissue resolution of MR imaging allows one to distinguish tumor in the sinonasal cavities and skull base from normal or inflamed mucosa (**Fig. 8**), trapped secretions, and, in cases of intracranial involvement, brain tissue. In addition, in patients with sinonasal malignancies, MR imaging is a must for evaluating possible perineural tumor spread (**Fig. 9**), and

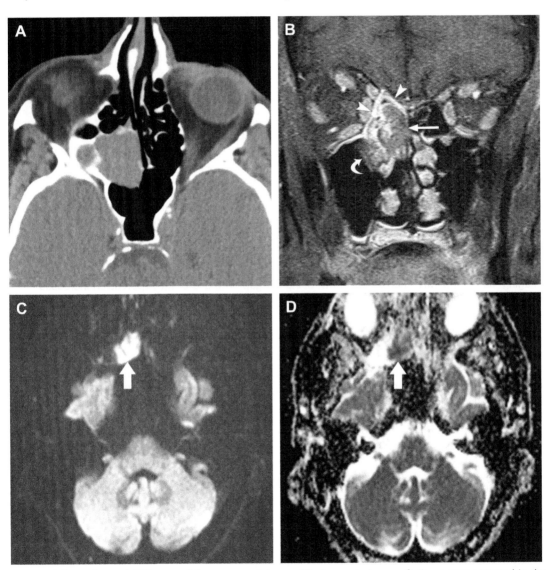

Fig. 8. Axial unenhanced CT image of the paranasal sinuses (*A*) demonstrates a soft tissue mass centered in the right posterior ethmoids and nasal cavity, with extension into the right sphenoid and maxillary sinuses. On the coronal fat-suppressed contrast-enhanced T1-weighted MR image (*B*), the lesion (*arrow*) demonstrates mild contrast enhancement compared with the adjacent inflamed and thickened sinonasal mucosa along the right ethmoid roof and lamina papyracea (*arrowheads*). Tumor extension into the right maxillary sinus (*curved arrow*) is again noted, but the mass does not seem to invade the orbit or anterior cranial fossa. Corresponding axial diffusion-weighted imaging (DWI) (*C*) and apparent diffusion coefficient (ADC) map (*D*) images demonstrate reduced diffusion within the lesion (large arrows) which is apparent as high signal intensity on DWI and markedly reduced signal on the ADC map, and which is worrisome for a malignant process. The patient had a history of a Merkel cell carcinoma of the right thigh treated 4 years earlier, and this lesion was a Merkel cell carcinoma metastasis.

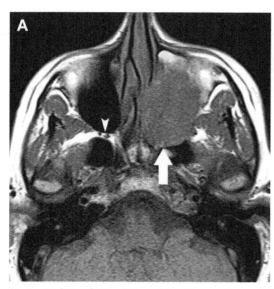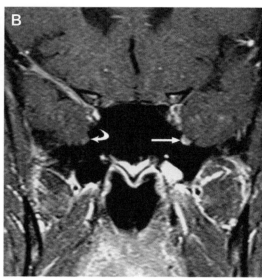

Fig. 9. Axial unenhanced T1-weighted image through the maxillary sinuses (*A*) in a patient with left-sided nasal congestion and nose bleeds demonstrates a homogeneous, intermediate signal intensity mass centered in the left maxillary sinus, with extension into the left nasal cavity and into the left pterygopalatine fossa (PPF) (*large arrow*). Compare with the normal fat-containing PPF on the right side (*arrowhead*). (*B*) Coronal contrast-enhanced, fat-suppressed T1-weighted image demonstrates perineural tumor spread, as evidenced by abnormal enlargement and enhancement of the maxillary division of cranial nerve V (CNV2) on the left (*small arrow*). Compare with the normal appearance of CNV2 on the right (*curved arrow*). This tumor was an adenoid cystic carcinoma.

imaging data from MR imaging are now being used routinely along with CT data for the purposes of presurgical planning and intraoperative navigation in the region of the skull base (see section, Image-Guided Endoscopic Sinus Surgery, later).

As most MR imaging studies ordered to evaluate the paranasal sinuses are obtained for suspected neoplastic or inflammatory conditions, protocols should include sequences obtained before and following the administration of intravenous gadolinium-containing contrast media. The exception to this rule are patients with severe renal dysfunction in whom the risk of nephrogenic systemic fibrosis becomes a concern and in whom it is appropriate to forego contrast administration in favor of an unenhanced MR imaging. For pre-contrast T1-weighted imaging, the authors prefer to use a non–fat-suppressed spin-echo T1-weighted sequences. On these images, it is useful to key in on fat-containing areas surrounding the sinonasal cavities, such as the orbits, premaxillary soft tissues, and pterygopalatine fossa, and to look for evidence of soft tissue infiltration of these normally high-signal regions, as this can be an early sign of disease extension beyond the confines of the sinuses (see Fig. 9). For postcontrast imaging, the authors acquire thin-section (≤4 mm) fat-suppressed T1-weighted images through the sinuses and skull base in the axial and coronal planes with a minimal (10%) interslice

gap. The use of fat suppression increases sensitivity for lesion enhancement and improves detection of perineural tumor spread (see Fig. 9), skull base involvement, and intracranial extension of disease. In addition, the authors' protocol also includes a contrast-enhanced 3D gradient echo T1-weighted sequence through the entire brain and skull base, which is reconstructed at 1-mm slice thickness for use in any of the authors' intraoperative guidance systems. The authors' routine protocol for imaging the skull base and paranasal sinuses is presented in Table 2.

Other sequences that can be useful in select instances include heavily contrasted 3D T2-weighted sequences, such as constructive interference in steady state (CISS; Siemens Medical Solutions, Erlangen, Germany) balanced fast field echo (balanced FFE; Philips Medical Systems, Best, the Netherlands) or fast imaging employing steady state (FIESTA and FIESTA-C; GE Healthcare, Milwaukee, WI) sequences, which can be useful for evaluating suspected cerebrospinal fistulas,[56] and diffusion-weighted imaging (DWI). DWI has been demonstrated to be useful for differentiating benign and malignant lesions in the sinonasal region, with malignant lesions having significantly lower average apparent diffusion coefficients (ADCs) compared with benign neoplasms and inflammatory lesions (see Fig. 8). However, there is a significant overlap in

Table 2
Paranasal sinus and skull base (cranial nerve 5) MR protocol at UNC

Sequence	Plane	Slice Thickness	Coverage
Precontrast			
EPI DWI	Axial	5 mm	Entire brain
Spin-echo T1W	Sagittal	4 mm	Entire brain
Fat-suppressed TSE T2	Axial	5 mm	Entire brain
FLAIR	Axial	5 mm	Entire brain
Fat-suppressed TSE T2W	Axial	4 mm	Paranasal sinuses and skull base
TSE T1W	Axial	4 mm	Paranasal sinuses and skull base
3D T1 MPRAGE	Axial	1 mm	Entire brain and skull base
Postcontrast			
Fat-suppressed SE T1W	Axial	4 mm	Paranasal sinuses and skull base
Fat-suppressed SE T1W	Coronal	3 mm	Tip of nose through brain stem
3D T1 MPRAGE	Axial Sagittal Coronal	1 mm	Entire brain and skull base
3D CISS	Axial	0.7 mm	Paranasal sinuses and skull base

Abbreviations: CISS, constructive interference in steady state; DWI, diffusion-weighted imaging; EPI, echo planar imaging; FLAIR, fluid-attenuated inversion recovery; MR, magnetic resonance; SE, spin echo; T1W, T1 weighted; T2W, T2 weighted; TSE, turbo spin echo; UNC, University of North Carolina.

the ADCs of benign and malignant processes; the overall diagnostic accuracy provided by ADC measurement (79% according to one study) is still not adequate for reliably differentiating between the two preoperatively.[57] That said, a sinonasal lesion demonstrating obviously low ADC should be viewed with a high degree of suspicion for malignancy. It has been suggested that combined imaging with both dynamic contrast-enhanced (DCE) and DWI could improve the ability to diagnose malignant sinonasal tumors, with one group reporting that they were able to discriminate malignant from benign disease with 100% accuracy by using DCE and DWI together in a small number of cases.[58] Whether these results hold up in subsequent larger-scale studies remains to be seen.

INDICATIONS FOR IMAGING OF THE PARANASAL SINUSES AND SKULL BASE

Although imaging, particularly with CT, is now a routine part of the diagnostic paradigm for most patients with chronic sinusitis or other sinonasal diseases, the benefits of imaging, as with any medical procedure, must be weighed against the costs both monetarily and in terms of potential risk to the patients. In addition to the concerns over the dangers associated with ionizing radiation exposure from CT, questions about overuse of medical imaging have also become widespread given the steadily rising cost and utilization of health care in the United States. In response to concerns over the overuse of sinus imaging, the American College of Radiology (ACR) published updated appropriateness criteria in 2013 for imaging sinonasal disease.[59] These criteria, summarized in **Table 3**, assign procedure ratings ranging from 1 to 9, with ratings of 1 to 3 indicating the test is usually not indicated; ratings of 4 to 6 indicating that the test may be appropriate for select cases; and ratings between 7 and 9 indicating the test is usually appropriate.

In addition, the AAO-HNS published a clinical consensus statement in 2012 in an effort to provide guidance to otolaryngologists on the appropriate indications for ordering CT imaging in patients with paranasal sinus disease.[50] In summary, the panel stated that CT imaging is usually appropriate for the following scenarios: chronic sinusitis refractory to appropriate medical therapy, recurrent acute or chronic sinusitis, complications of surgery or sinusitis, suspected or confirmed CSF rhinorrhea, suspicion of invasive fungal sinusitis in immunocompromised patients, tumor surveillance, or surgical planning for new or revision sinus surgery. Of note, the panel emphasized that CT is not indicated (1) in cases of clinically diagnosed uncomplicated sinusitis, (2) in patients who have had a full response to medical therapy, (3) in patients who have had uncomplicated upper respiratory infections for a duration of less than 10 days, or (4) in patients younger than 3 years with uncomplicated acute sinusitis who have not received appropriate prior medical management.

Table 3
Summary of ACR appropriate criteria for sinonasal disease

Indication	Radiologic Procedure	Rating	Comments
Acute (<4 wk) or subacute (4–12 wk) uncomplicated sinusitis	CT sinuses w/o contrast	5	Imaging may be indicated if acute frontal or sphenoid sinusitis suspected, if there are atypical symptoms, or if the diagnosis is uncertain.
	MR imaging head and sinuses w/o contrast	4	It may be useful as part of a general workup for headache.
Recurrent acute or chronic sinusitis (possible surgical candidate)	CT sinuses w/o contrast	9	Consider using it as a surgical planning protocol.
	CT sinuses w/ contrast	4	—
Acute or subacute sinusitis with associated orbital or intracranial complications with ocular or neurologic deficit	CT sinuses and orbits w/o contrast	9	MR imaging and CT are complementary. Brain imaging is essential if CNS invasion is a concern.
	MR imaging head and sinuses w/o and w/ contrast	9	—
	CT sinuses and orbits w/ contrast	8	If this is the only study that can be obtained (eg, if MR imaging is contraindicated), it would be appropriate.
	MR imaging head and sinuses w/o contrast	7	Use it if patients are unable to tolerate gadolinium (eg, severe renal dysfunction).
Acute or subacute sinusitis in immunodeficient patients	CT sinuses w/o contrast	7	These patients are at high risk for invasive fungal sinusitis, thus lowering threshold for imaging.
	MR imaging head and sinuses w/o contrast	6	—
	MR imaging head and sinuses w/o and w/ contrast	6	—
	CT sinuses w/ contrast	5	Contrast and brain imaging are essential if CNS invasion is a concern.
Sinonasal polyposis (see next indication if unilateral)	CT sinuses w/o contrast	9	—
	MR imaging head and sinuses w/o and w/ contrast	4	If it is unilateral disease, see the next indication (Sinonasal obstruction, suspected mass lesion).
	MR imaging head and sinuses w/o contrast	4	—
	CT sinuses w/ contrast	4	—
Sinonasal obstruction, suspected mass lesion	MR imaging head and sinuses w/o and w/ contrast	9	MR imaging and CT are complementary. Both are frequently needed.
	CT sinuses w/o contrast	8	—
	CT sinuses w/ contrast	6	—
	CT sinuses w/o and w/ contrast	6	—
	MR imaging head and sinuses w/o contrast	5	Use if patients are unable to tolerate gadolinium.
	Craniofacial arteriography	4	It is appropriate in selected cases (eg, vascular involvement, vascular lesion).

Rating scale: 4, 5, 6 = may be appropriate; 7, 8, 9 = usually appropriate. Note that procedures rated 1, 2, 3 (usually not appropriate) are not included in this table.
Abbreviations: CNS, central nervous system; w/, with; w/o, without.
Data from Cornelius RS, Martin J, Wippold FJ 2nd, et al. ACR appropriateness criteria sinonasal disease. J Am Coll Radiol 2013;10(4):241–6.

Furthermore, the panel also stated that plain radiographs and ultrasonography are not recommended for the evaluation of sinusitis.[50]

IMAGE-GUIDED ENDOSCOPIC SINUS SURGERY

In addition to their traditional roles in diagnosis and preoperative planning, it is now common for CT and MR imaging to be imported into computer navigation systems for image-based guidance during ESS. The concepts of modern day image-guided surgery (IGS) are rooted in techniques that were initially developed for neurosurgery; however, otolaryngologists were quick to recognize its potential in the head and neck and, in particular, in the paranasal sinuses.[60] The main goal of intraoperative navigation in ESS is to reduce surgical risk and to enable more complete exploration and dissection by providing real-time information on the position of surgical instruments relative to vital structures around the paranasal sinuses (eg, the orbits, optic nerves, skull base, and internal carotid arteries).[61–63] Although early systems primarily relied on CT data, most current IGS systems allow data from CT and magnetic resonance (MR) to be fused for preoperative viewing and navigation, providing the surgeons with both the superior bone detail of CT and the improved soft tissue and vascular visualization of MR, a feature that is particularly useful for tumor surgeries and surgeries involving the skull base (Fig. 10).

Currently, there are 2 types of systems that are widely used for IGS: electromagnetic (EM) and optical guidance systems. For the most part, the two types of navigation perform comparably; the choice of guidance system generally boils down to surgeon preference.[64] Regardless of the specific system, critical to the success of IGS is the registration process, which establishes a one-to-one relationship between corresponding points in the operative field volume and in the imaging data set volume. Assuming a satisfactory imaging data set and proper registration and calibration, both EM and optical tracking systems provide navigation accuracy to within 2 mm, which is a standard accepted by most otolaryngologists.[63] Although the various methods used for image registration are beyond the scope of this review, it is still necessary for the protocoling radiologist to be aware of the specific requirements that a guidance system may have for imaging data set acquisition, which may differ from system to system. For instance, the navigation software used at the authors' institution specifies a maximum slice thickness of 3 mm (2 mm if surface matching registration is used), a maximum pitch of 2, and a square matrix size. In addition, some older systems may require patients to wear a fiducial-containing headset during the preoperative scan. Therefore, it is important to be familiar with the types of systems being used by referring surgeons; it is often helpful to tailor protocols such that patients are not forced to undergo additional scans simply because initial diagnostic scans

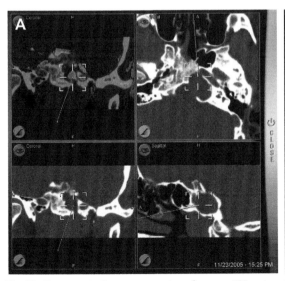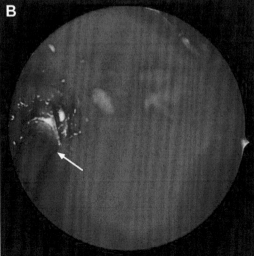

Fig. 10. Representative screen capture from an IGS system (A) obtained during endoscopic transnasal drainage of a petrous apex cholesterol granuloma. The top left image shows a coronal image fusing of the preoperative CT and MR imaging. (B) Corresponding endoscopic image demonstrating the curette (arrow on left side of the image), which is being actively tracked by the image guidance system, entering the cyst.

were not adequate for surgical planning or navigation purposes. At the authors' institution, the routine CT and MR imaging protocols used for sinonasal imaging are compatible with the authors' surgeons' IGS systems.

Although there is still some controversy as to whether the addition of intraoperative guidance actually reduces the number or severity of surgical complications, improves surgical outcomes, or justifies the added cost of its use,[65–73] the general consensus among otolaryngologists favors the view that IGS is helpful in select instances for the management of chronic rhinosinusitis, namely, when there is significant mucosal disease, altered anatomy, or obscuration of the surgical field caused by hemorrhage; the AAO-HNS has published reimbursement recommendations regarding appropriate indications for IGS (listed in **Box 1**).[74]

At the University of North Carolina, the authors use IGS for virtually all endoscopic sinus surgeries, as most cases performed at the authors' center are done for the indications outlined in the AAO-HNS position statement. In the occasional case done for an alternative indication, the authors' surgeons still find IGS to be helpful and will, therefore, still use surgical navigation; however, in those instances, the addition of IGS is not billed.

FUTURE DIRECTIONS

In the future, there will likely be further advancements in technologies aimed at dose and noise reduction in sinus CT, including application of techniques, such as organ-based current

modulation,[75] new IR methods, and various image-based filtering techniques.[76,77] It is also likely that we will see an increasing trend in the number of in-office CBCT systems as well as a narrowing of the gap in image quality and contrast resolution between MDCT and CBCT, as improvements in FPD technology and application of noise-reducing strategies, such as x-ray filtration, compensating filtration, antiscatter grids, and scatter subtraction algorithms, become incorporated into newer scanners.[43,78] Whether CBCT can eventually catch MDCT in these areas remains to be seen. Furthermore, as the authors' collective experience with CBCT both for POC and intraoperative imaging increases, guidelines defining the indications, appropriate use, and regulation of the technology are bound to be on the horizon.

Current research is also ongoing on the application of imaging for fly-through viewing techniques (virtual endoscopy), which may enhance presurgical planning and intraoperative navigation and also be useful for resident education and training.[10,79–81] Furthermore, there has also been interest in the use of computerized 3D volumetric CT scoring to assess disease severity in chronic sinusitis, as recent data suggest that use of such a scoring system may correlate better with symptoms than the widely used Lund-Mackay scoring system.[82,83]

On the MR front, it is likely that we will see continued research into the utility of functional (eg, DWI and DCE) and multiparametric imaging techniques for evaluating sinonasal malignancies; with the recent advent of combined PET/MR imaging systems, we will likely see this technology used for oncologic applications in the sinuses and skull base, particularly for posttreatment surveillance. Furthermore, with intraoperative MR imaging now being investigated for neurosurgical applications,[84,85] it is only a matter of time before we see the technology applied for guidance in resecting of complex sinonasal and skull base tumors.

Box 1
Appropriate indications for use of computer-aided image guidance for sinus and skull base surgery based on the AAO-HNS position statement

1. Revision sinus surgery

2. Distorted sinus anatomy of development, postoperative, or traumatic origin

3. Extensive sinonasal polyposis

4. Pathology involving the frontal, posterior ethmoid, and sphenoid sinuses

5. Disease abutting the skull base, orbit, optic nerve, or carotid artery

6. CSF rhinorrhea or conditions when there is a skull base defect

7. Benign and malignant sinonasal neoplasms

Data from AAO-HNS. Policy on intra-operative use of computer aided surgery. 2014. Accessed December 5, 2014.

REFERENCES

1. Ramakrishnan VR, Orlandi RR, Citardi MJ, et al. The use of image-guided surgery in endoscopic sinus surgery: an evidence-based review with recommendations. Int Forum Allergy Rhinol 2013;3(3):236–41.

2. Govindaraj S, Adappa ND, Kennedy DW. Endoscopic sinus surgery: evolution and technical innovations. J Laryngol Otol 2010;124(3):242–50.

3. Eggesbo HB. Radiological imaging of inflammatory lesions in the nasal cavity and paranasal sinuses. Eur Radiol 2006;16(4):872–88.

4. Lusk RP, Lazar RH, Muntz HR. The diagnosis and treatment of recurrent and chronic sinusitis in children. Pediatr Clin North Am 1989;36(6):1411–21.

5. Zinreich SJ. Progress in sinonasal imaging. Ann Otol Rhinol Laryngol Suppl 2006;196:61–5.

6. Zinreich J. Imaging of inflammatory sinus disease. Otolaryngol Clin North Am 1993;26(4):535–47.

7. Kennedy DW, Zinreich SJ, Rosenbaum AE, et al. Functional endoscopic sinus surgery. Theory and diagnostic evaluation. Arch Otolaryngol 1985; 111(9):576–82.

8. Hudgins PA, Mukundan S. Screening sinus CT: a good idea gone bad? AJNR Am J Neuroradiol 1997;18(10):1850–4.

9. Mafee MF, Chow JM, Meyers R. Functional endoscopic sinus surgery: anatomy, CT screening, indications, and complications. AJR Am J Roentgenol 1993;160(4):735–44.

10. Ling FT, Kountakis SE. Advances in imaging of the paranasal sinuses. Curr Allergy Asthma Rep 2006; 6(6):502–7.

11. Flohr TG, Schaller S, Stierstorfer K, et al. Multi-detector row CT systems and image-reconstruction techniques. Radiology 2005;235(3):756–73.

12. Tack D, Widelec J, De Maertelaer V, et al. Comparison between low-dose and standard-dose multidetector CT in patients with suspected chronic sinusitis. AJR Am J Roentgenol 2003;181(4):939–44.

13. Kanowitz SJ, Shatzkes DR, Pramanik BK, et al. Utility of sagittal reformatted computerized tomographic images in the evaluation of the frontal sinus outflow tract. Am J Rhinol 2005;19(2):159–65.

14. Kew J, Rees GL, Close D, et al. Multiplanar reconstructed computed tomography images improves depiction and understanding of the anatomy of the frontal sinus and recess. Am J Rhinol 2002;16(2): 119–23.

15. UNSCEAR. Sources of ionizing radiation. UNSCEAR 2008 report to the General Assembly with scientific annexes, vol. 1. New York: United Nations; 2010. Available at: www.unscear.org/docs/reports/2008/ 09-86753_Report_2008_GA_Report_corr2.pdf.

16. European Commission. EUR 16262: European guidelines for quality criteria for computed tomography. Luxembourg (Luxembourg): European Commission; 2000.

17. Parmar HA, Ibrahim M, Mukherji SK. Optimizing craniofacial CT technique. Neuroimaging Clin N Am 2014;24(3):395–405, vii.

18. Raman SP, Johnson PT, Deshmukh S, et al. CT dose reduction applications: available tools on the latest generation of CT scanners. J Am Coll Radiol 2013; 10(1):37–41.

19. Ibrahim M, Parmar H, Christodoulou E, et al. Raise the bar and lower the dose: current and future strategies for radiation dose reduction in head and neck imaging. AJNR Am J Neuroradiol 2014;35(4): 619–24.

20. Lam S, Bux S, Kumar G, et al. A comparison between low-dose and standard-dose non-contrasted multidetector CT scanning of the paranasal sinuses. Biomed Imaging Interv J 2009;5(3):e13.

21. Brem MH, Zamani AA, Riva R, et al. Multidetector CT of the paranasal sinus: potential for radiation dose reduction. Radiology 2007;243(3):847–52.

22. Abul-Kasim K, Strombeck A, Sahlstrand-Johnson P. Low-dose computed tomography of the paranasal sinuses: radiation doses and reliability analysis. Am J Otolaryngol 2011;32(1):47–51.

23. Feuchtner GM, Jodocy D, Klauser A, et al. Radiation dose reduction by using 100-kV tube voltage in cardiac 64-slice computed tomography: a comparative study. Eur J Radiol 2010;75(1):e51–6.

24. Kayan M, Koroglu M, Yesildag A, et al. Carotid CT-angiography: low versus standard volume contrast media and low kV protocol for 128-slice MDCT. Eur J Radiol 2012;81(9):2144–7.

25. LaBounty TM, Leipsic J, Poulter R, et al. Coronary CT angiography of patients with a normal body mass index using 80 kVp versus 100 kVp: a prospective, multicenter, multivendor randomized trial. AJR Am J Roentgenol 2011;197(5):W860–7.

26. Paul JF. Individually adapted coronary 64-slice CT angiography based on precontrast attenuation values, using different kVp and tube current settings: evaluation of image quality. Int J Cardiovasc Imaging 2011;27(Suppl 1):53–9.

27. Wang D, Hu XH, Zhang SZ, et al. Image quality and dose performance of 80 kV low dose scan protocol in high-pitch spiral coronary CT angiography: feasibility study. Int J Cardiovasc Imaging 2012;28(2):415–23.

28. Lee CH, Goo JM, Ye HJ, et al. Radiation dose modulation techniques in the multidetector CT era: from basics to practice. Radiographics 2008;28(5): 1451–9.

29. Kalra MK, Maher MM, Toth TL, et al. Techniques and applications of automatic tube current modulation for CT. Radiology 2004;233(3):649–57.

30. Silva AC, Lawder HJ, Hara A, et al. Innovations in CT dose reduction strategy: application of the adaptive statistical iterative reconstruction algorithm. AJR Am J Roentgenol 2010;194(1):191–9.

31. Mitsumori LM, Shuman WP, Busey JM, et al. Adaptive statistical iterative reconstruction versus filtered back projection in the same patient: 64 channel liver CT image quality and patient radiation dose. Eur Radiol 2012;22(1):138–43.

32. Hoxworth JM, Lal D, Fletcher GP, et al. Radiation dose reduction in paranasal sinus CT using model-based iterative reconstruction. AJNR Am J Neuroradiol 2014;35(4):644–9.

33. Bulla S, Blanke P, Hassepass F, et al. Reducing the radiation dose for low-dose CT of the paranasal sinuses using iterative reconstruction: feasibility and image quality. Eur J Radiol 2012;81(9):2246–50.

34. Schulz B, Beeres M, Bodelle B, et al. Performance of iterative image reconstruction in CT of the paranasal

sinuses: a phantom study. AJNR Am J Neuroradiol 2013;34(5):1072–6.

35. Feldkamp LA, Davis LC, Kress JW. Practical cone-beam algorithm. J Opt Soc Am A 1984;1(6): 612–9.

36. Gupta R, Grasruck M, Suess C, et al. Ultra-high resolution flat-panel volume CT: fundamental principles, design architecture, and system characterization. Eur Radiol 2006;16(6):1191–205.

37. Yan XH, Leahy RM. Derivation and analysis of a filtered backprojection algorithm for cone beam projection data. IEEE Trans Med Imaging 1991;10(3): 462–72.

38. Miracle AC, Mukherji SK. Cone beam CT of the head and neck, part 2: clinical applications. AJNR Am J Neuroradiol 2009;30(7):1285–92.

39. Scarfe WC, Farman AG, Sukovic P. Clinical applications of cone-beam computed tomography in dental practice. J Can Dent Assoc 2006;72(1):75–80.

40. Moore CJ, Amer A, Marchant T, et al. Developments in and experience of kilovoltage X-ray cone beam image-guided radiotherapy. Br J Radiol 2006; 79(Spec No 1):S66–78.

41. Spezi E, Downes P, Jarvis R, et al. Patient-specific three-dimensional concomitant dose from cone beam computed tomography exposure in image-guided radiotherapy. Int J Radiat Oncol Biol Phys 2012;83(1):419–26.

42. Orth RC, Wallace MJ, Kuo MD, Technology Assessment Committee of the Society of Interventional Radiology. C-arm cone-beam CT: general principles and technical considerations for use in interventional radiology. J Vasc Interv Radiol 2008;19(6): 814–20.

43. Miracle AC, Mukherji SK. Cone beam CT of the head and neck, part 1: physical principles. AJNR Am J Neuroradiol 2009;30(6):1088–95.

44. Berris T, Gupta R, Rehani MM. Radiation dose from cone-beam CT in neuroradiology applications. AJR Am J Roentgenol 2013;200(4):755–61.

45. Gupta R, Bartling SH, Basu SK, et al. Experimental flat-panel high-spatial-resolution volume CT of the temporal bone. AJNR Am J Neuroradiol 2004; 25(8):1417–24.

46. IAEA. Status of computed tomography dosimetry for wide cone beam CT scanners: IAEA human health reports No. 5. Vienna (Austria): IAEA; 2011. Available at: www-pub.iaea.org/MTCD/Publications/PDF/Pub1528_web.pdf.

47. Alspaugh J, Christogoulou E, Goodsitt M, et al. Dose and image quality of flat panel detector volume computed tomography for sinus imaging. Paper presented at: 49th Annual Meeting of the American Association of Physicists in Medicine (AAPM). Minneapolis (MN), July 22–26, 2007.

48. Dierckx D, Saldarriaga Vargas C, Rogge F, et al. Dosimetric analysis of the use of CBCT in diagnostic radiology: sinus and middle ear. Radiat Prot Dosimetry 2014;163(1):125–32.

49. Leiva-Salinas C, Flors L, Gras P, et al. Dental flat panel cone beam CT in the evaluation of patients with inflammatory sinonasal disease: diagnostic efficacy and radiation dose savings. AJNR Am J Neuroradiol 2014;35(11):2052–7.

50. Setzen G, Ferguson BJ, Han JK, et al. Clinical consensus statement: appropriate use of computed tomography for paranasal sinus disease. Otolaryngol Head Neck Surg 2012;147(5):808–16.

51. Batra PS, Kanowitz SJ, Citardi MJ. Clinical utility of intraoperative volume computed tomography scanner for endoscopic sinonasal and skull base procedures. Am J Rhinol 2008;22(5):511–5.

52. Batra PS, Manes RP, Ryan MW, et al. Prospective evaluation of intraoperative computed tomography imaging for endoscopic sinonasal and skull-base surgery. Int Forum Allergy Rhinol 2011; 1(6):481–7.

53. Chennupati SK, Woodworth BA, Palmer JN, et al. Intraoperative IGS/CT updates for complex endoscopic frontal sinus surgery. ORL J Otorhinolaryngol Relat Spec 2008;70(4):268–70.

54. Abrass LJ, Chandra RK, Conley DB, et al. Factors associated with computed tomography status in patients presenting with a history of chronic rhinosinusitis. Int Forum Allergy Rhinol 2011;1(3): 178–82.

55. Tan BK, Chandra RK, Conley DB, et al. A randomized trial examining the effect of pretreatment point-of-care computed tomography imaging on the management of patients with chronic rhinosinusitis symptoms. Int Forum Allergy Rhinol 2011; 1(3):229–34.

56. Algin O, Turkbey B. Intrathecal gadolinium-enhanced MR cisternography: a comprehensive review. AJNR Am J Neuroradiol 2013;34(1):14–22.

57. Sasaki M, Eida S, Sumi M, et al. Apparent diffusion coefficient mapping for sinonasal diseases: differentiation of benign and malignant lesions. AJNR Am J Neuroradiol 2011;32(6):1100–6.

58. Sasaki M, Sumi M, Eida S, et al. Multiparametric MR imaging of sinonasal diseases: time-signal intensity curve- and apparent diffusion coefficient-based differentiation between benign and malignant lesions. AJNR Am J Neuroradiol 2011;32(11):2154–9.

59. Cornelius RS, Martin J, Wippold FJ 2nd, et al. ACR appropriateness criteria sinonasal disease. J Am Coll Radiol 2013;10(4):241–6.

60. Klimek L, Mosges R, Schlondorff G, et al. Development of computer-aided surgery for otorhinolaryngology. Comput Aided Surg 1998;3(4):194–201.

61. Reardon EJ. Navigational risks associated with sinus surgery and the clinical effects of implementing a navigational system for sinus surgery. Laryngoscope 2002;112(7 Pt 2 Suppl 99):1–19.

62. Fried MP, Parikh SR, Sadoughi B. Image-guidance for endoscopic sinus surgery. Laryngoscope 2008; 118(7):1287–92.

63. Wise SK, DelGaudio JM. Computer-aided surgery of the paranasal sinuses and skull base. Expert Rev Med Devices 2005;2(4):395–408.

64. Citardi MJ. Surgical navigation and intraoperative imaging. In: Kennedy DW, Hwang PH, editors. Rhinology: diseases of the nose, sinuses, and skull base. New York: Thieme; 2012. p. 282–96.

65. Anon JB, Lipman SP, Oppenheim D, et al. Computer-assisted endoscopic sinus surgery. Laryngoscope 1994;104(7):901–5.

66. Mosges R, Klimek L. Computer-assisted surgery of the paranasal sinuses. J Otolaryngol 1993;22(2): 69–71.

67. Fried MP, Moharir VM, Shin J, et al. Comparison of endoscopic sinus surgery with and without image guidance. Am J Rhinol 2002;16(4):193–7.

68. Javer AR, Genoway KA. Patient quality of life improvements with and without computer assistance in sinus surgery: outcomes study. J Otolaryngol 2006;35(6):373–9.

69. Gibbons MD, Gunn CG, Niwas S, et al. Cost analysis of computer-aided endoscopic sinus surgery. Am J Rhinol 2001;15(2):71–5.

70. Metson R, Cosenza M, Gliklich RE, et al. The role of image-guidance systems for head and neck surgery. Arch Otolaryngol Head Neck Surg 1999; 125(10):1100–4.

71. Ramakrishnan VR, Kingdom TT, Nayak JV, et al. Nationwide incidence of major complications in endoscopic sinus surgery. Int Forum Allergy Rhinol 2012;2(1):34–9.

72. Tschopp KP, Thomaser EG. Outcome of functional endonasal sinus surgery with and without CT-navigation. Rhinology 2008;46(2):116–20.

73. Dalgorf DM, Sacks R, Wormald PJ, et al. Image-guided surgery influences perioperative morbidity from endoscopic sinus surgery: a systematic review and meta-analysis. Otolaryngol Head Neck Surg 2013;149(1):17–29.

74. AAO-HNS. Policy on intra-operative use of computer aided surgery. 2014. Available at: http://www.entnet.org/content/intra-operative-use-computer-aided-surgery. Accessed December 5, 2014.

75. Hoang JK, Yoshizumi TT, Choudhury KR, et al. Organ-based dose current modulation and thyroid shields: techniques of radiation dose reduction for neck CT. AJR Am J Roentgenol 2012;198(5):1132–8.

76. Szucs-Farkas Z, Bensler S, Torrente JC, et al. Nonlinear three-dimensional noise filter with low-dose CT angiography: effect on the detection of small high-contrast objects in a phantom model. Radiology 2011;258(1):261–9.

77. Yu L, Liu X, Leng S, et al. Radiation dose reduction in computed tomography: techniques and future perspective. Imaging Med 2009;1(1):65–84.

78. Roos PG, Colbeth RE, Mollov I, et al. Multiple gain ranging readout method to extend the dynamic range of amorphous silicon flat panel imagers. Proc SPIE Int Soc Opt Eng 2004;5368:139–49.

79. Dearking AC, Pallanch JF. Mapping the frontal sinus ostia using virtual endoscopy. Laryngoscope 2012; 122(10):2143–7.

80. Thomas L, Pallanch JF. Three-dimensional CT reconstruction and virtual endoscopic study of the ostial orientations of the frontal recess. Am J Rhinol Allergy 2010;24(5):378–84.

81. Haerle SK, Daly MJ, Chan H, et al. Localized Intraoperative Virtual Endoscopy (LIVE) for surgical guidance in 16 skull base patients. Otolaryngol Head Neck Surg 2015;152(1):165–71.

82. Likness MM, Pallanch JF, Sherris DA, et al. Computed tomography scans as an objective measure of disease severity in chronic rhinosinusitis. Otolaryngol Head Neck Surg 2014;150(2):305–11.

83. Pallanch JF, Yu L, Delone D, et al. Three-dimensional volumetric computed tomographic scoring as an objective outcome measure for chronic rhinosinusitis: clinical correlations and comparison to Lund-Mackay scoring. Int Forum Allergy Rhinol 2013;3(12):963–72.

84. Sommer B, Wimmer C, Coras R, et al. Resection of cerebral gangliogliomas causing drug-resistant epilepsy: short- and long-term outcomes using intraoperative MRI and neuronavigation. Neurosurg Focus 2015;38(1):E5.

85. Zhang J, Chen X, Zhao Y, et al. Impact of intraoperative magnetic resonance imaging and functional neuronavigation on surgical outcome in patients with gliomas involving language areas. Neurosurg Rev 2015;38(2):319–30.

Normal Anatomy and Anatomic Variants of the Paranasal Sinuses on Computed Tomography

CrossMark

Sanjay Vaid, MD (Radiology)[a],*, Neelam Vaid, MS, DNB (ENT)[b]

KEYWORDS

- Computed tomography (CT) • Paranasal sinuses • Anatomy • Anatomic variants
- Clinical implications

KEY POINTS

- The radiologist needs to be familiar with the complex sinonasal CT anatomy as visualized by an endoscopic sinus surgeon.
- Multiplanar region-specific reporting and preoperative identification of anatomic variants provide the endoscopic surgeon with a useful intraoperative roadmap and avoid intraoperative complications.
- This article reviews the CT anatomy of the paranasal sinuses and discusses the clinical relevance of the anatomic variants encountered in the sinonasal region.

 A video showing a coronal CT depicting multiplanar attachments of the middle turbinate accompanies this article at http://www.neuroimaging.theclinics.com/

But chiefly the anatomy
You ought to understand
If you will cure well anything
That you do take in hand!
    —John Halle, British Surgeon, 1529–1568

INTRODUCTION

Anatomic concepts of the paranasal sinuses have been known since the late nineteenth and early twentieth centuries.[1] These have assumed greater significance in recent times due to advances in functional endoscopic sinus surgery (FESS) and imaging technology. Multiplanar high-resolution CT (HRCT) of the paranasal sinuses provides a precise and reliable preoperative roadmap for the endoscopic sinus surgeon. All radiologists should be familiar with the 3-D anatomy of the paranasal sinuses and the anatomic variants that surgeons are likely to encounter. This article reviews the embryology of the paranasal sinuses and outlines the CT technique/protocols for imaging this region. CT anatomy of the nasal cavity and paranasal sinuses is described in detail together with the anatomic variants encountered in each region.

Disclosures: The authors have nothing to disclose.
[a] Head Neck Imaging Division, Star Imaging and Research Center, Connaught Place, Bund Garden Road, Pune 411001, Maharashtra, India; [b] Department of Otorhinolaryngology, K.E.M. Hospital, 489 Rastapeth, Pune 411011, Maharashtra, India
* Corresponding author.
E-mail address: svaidhn@gmail.com

neuroimaging.theclinics.com

IMAGING TECHNIQUES AND PROTOCOL

Preoperative CT imaging of the paranasal sinuses is performed after completion of the medical treatment because up to 80% of patients suffering from acute upper respiratory tract infection show evidence of mucosal disease in the sinonasal region.[2] Intranasal decongestant drops are administered 15 to 20 minutes before commencing the examination and the patient is directed to clear the nasal cavities prior to the scan to clear mucus discharge, which may interfere with the radiologic interpretation. Postoperative CT examinations are performed after a period of 8 weeks once the inflammatory changes have subsided and mucociliary clearance has returned to normal.[3] Table 1 outlines the CT protocols used at the first author's center for pre-FESS examinations of the paranasal sinuses. All examinations are carried out on a 64-channel CT scanner and viewed on a workstation to facilitate multiplanar reconstructions in standard orthogonal and nonorthogonal planes. Customized low-dose CT protocols are used while scanning pediatric population.[4] Images are reconstructed in soft tissue windows to evaluate structures surrounding the paranasal sinuses (orbits, brain, and nasopharynx) and to document any extra sinus extension of the pathology. Use of cone-beam CT or digital volume CT is advised, if available, to minimize radiation doses in children and young adults.[5,6]

All routine pre-FESS CT examinations are performed without the use of intravenous contrast medium. Contrast-enhanced CT or MR imaging examinations are indicated in unilateral pathology, suspicion of neoplastic or vascular pathology, and fungal disease for identifying associated intracranial, intraorbital, and soft tissue extension.[7]

Box 1
Learning points - 1

Multiplanar CT evaluation of paranasal sinuses in orthogonal and nonorthogonal planes is important to outline the anatomy and identify surgically important anatomic variants.

Pre-FESS CT examinations of the paranasal sinuses are usually non–contrast-enhanced studies. Contrast examinations are reserved for evaluating specific pathologies (aggressive infections, neoplasm, and vascular lesions) and for assessing extension into orbit, intracranial compartment, and surrounding soft tissues.

Knowledge of relevant embryologic events in paranasal sinus development can avoid pitfalls in diagnosis. Sinus pathologies in children younger than 4 years are uncommon except in the ethmoid sinuses because these are the only sinuses that are pneumatized at birth.

Table 1
CT imaging protocol for paranasal sinuses

Patient Position	Supine
Collimation	64 × 0.625
Reconstruction slice thickness	0.67 mm
Increment	0.33 mm
Reconstruction capability	0.20 mm
Resolution	High
Field of view	180 mm
Pitch	0.641
mA/slice	200
kV	120
Rotation time	0.5 s
Filter	Y-sharp
Image display matrix	512

EMBRYOLOGY

The embryo gets its first identifiable head and face between the fourth and fifth weeks of gestational age with a central orifice, called the stomodeum, which is surrounded by the mandibular, maxillary, and frontonasal prominences. The nasal placodes differentiate from the frontonasal prominence and later develop into the nasal cavity and choana.[8] At approximately 25 to 28 weeks of gestation, the ethmoid bone begins to develop from the folding of the cartilaginous olfactory capsule, a central structure in the forming skull base. The ethmoid sinuses that develop within are present at birth whereas the other sinuses (frontal, maxillary, and sphenoid) develop due to pneumatization beyond the confines of the olfactory capsule. Hence, the ethmoid sinus is phylogenetically, anatomically, embryologically, and functionally different from the other air-containing paranasal sinuses.[9] The further ossification pattern is complex and readers are referred to numerous excellent texts in the literature for a more detailed discussion.[10–12] The pneumatization pattern is unique to each group of sinuses and the continuous change in the size and aeration of the sinus as a child grows has a significant impact on the treatment/surgery of sinus pathology in the pediatric age group.[13] Table 2 outlines the growth pattern of each sinus group and the ostiometal complex with the resultant clinical implications.[10,14] Fig. 1 depicts the childhood development of the paranasal sinuses and related structures.

ANATOMY OVERVIEW OF THE SINONASAL REGION

The sinonasal region consists of the nose, nasal cavities, and the paranasal sinuses (frontal,

Table 2
Pneumatization/ossification pattern of paranasal sinuses and related structures

Sr.no	Sinus/Structure	Childhood Development	Clinical Implications
1.	Frontal sinus	Not seen on imaging at birth Present as a small pit or furrow at birth Slow pneumatization between 1 and 4 y, rapid growth between 4 and 8 y, reaching the orbital roof by 5–7 y of age and attaining adult appearance by 12 y of age Narrower anteroposterior diameter compared with adult	Children cannot develop frontal sinusitis before 4 y of age. Frontal trephination procedures are contraindicated in an immature frontal sinus (until it reaches the orbital plate) due to risk of inadvertent intracranial penetration, meningeal trauma and likely iatrogenic infection.
2.	Ethmoid sinus	Present and seen on imaging at birth Rapid pneumatization between 1 and 4 y Slow growth between 4 and 8 y Adult appearance by 12 y of age	Source of sinus/contiguous orbital infection in young children Accessible to both internal and external drainage procedures if required
3.	Maxillary sinus	Not seen on imaging at birth Present as a shallow rounded sac at birth Rapid pneumatization between 1 and 4 y: floor of the sinus reaches level of the inferior meatus by 7 y of age Adult appearance is attained by 12 and 14 y when the floor of the sinus reaches level of the nasal cavity floor. Slow pneumatization continues until 20 y of age.	Height discrepancy between the inferior margins of the sinus and the nasal cavity precludes the use of certain surgical techniques in children. These procedures may damage developing teeth, cause inadvertent injury to lateral sinus wall, or be ineffective in treating the pathology completely.
4.	Sphenoid sinus	Not seen on imaging at birth. Tiny mucosal sac posterior to the nasal capsule at birth. Pneumatizes between 1 and 3 y of age. Grows progressively between 7 and 14 y and may continue to pneumatize further into adulthood.	Limited clinical significance before the age of 10 y Because the posterior ethmoid sinus pneumatizes earlier, it can grow above the developing sphenoid sinus to form the Onodi cell. Location of critical neurovascular structures around the sphenoid sinus depends on the degree of pneumatization of the sinus.
5.	The ostiomeatal complex	All components are developed and present in the newborn.	All the components of the ostiomeatal complex are packed tightly together leading to a narrow caliber of the infundibulum, which must be appreciated preoperatively. Proximity of the uncinate osseous to the lamina papyracea predisposes to inadvertent intraorbital penetration.
6.	Anterior cranial fossa	The midline structures (crista galli, cribriform plates, and perpendicular ethmoid plate) are cartilaginous at birth and ossify by 2 y of age. They represent the lucent stripe on CT scans of infants as the surrounding ethmoid bone, vomer, and palate are ossified.	The lucent stripe should not be misinterpreted as a bony defect, sinus tract, cephalocoele, or bony destruction.

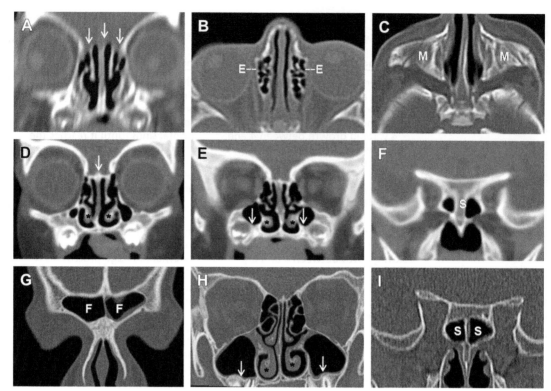

Fig. 1. Paranasal sinus development at birth (*A–C*): (*A*) unossified central anterior skull base structures resulting in lucent stripes (*arrows*); (*B*) ethmoidal labyrinth (E) are the only pneumatized cells at birth (*C*) M, non-pneumatized maxillary sinuses. Paranasal sinus development at birth at 1 year (*D–F*): (*D*) anterior skull base ossification (*arrow*) is complete; (*E*) partially pneumatized maxillary sinus floor (*arrows*) extending to level of inferior turbinates (*asterisks*); and (*F*) early sphenoid sinus (S) pneumatization. Paranasal sinus development at 5 years (*G–I*): (*G*) frontal sinus (F) pneumatized to the orbital roof; (*H*) maxillary sinus floor (*arrows*) extends to the level of inferior meatus; and (*I*) sphenoid sinus pneumatization progressively increases.

ethmoid, maxillary, and sphenoid). The sinonasal anatomy is discussed in the order of visualization during endoscopic surgery.

The Nose and Nasal Cavities

Fig. 2 depicts the imaging anatomy of the surface of the nose. The nasal cavities are triangular structures separated by the nasal septum in the midline, limited superiorly by the cribriform plate and inferiorly by the hard and soft palate. Lateral walls of the nasal cavities are complex structures that support the inferior, middle, and superior nasal turbinates and, occasionally, a fourth turbinate, known as the supreme turbinate. The middle and inferior nasal turbinates usually have a similar shape exhibiting a convex margin medially and a concave margin laterally. These turbinates divide the nasal cavity into the superior, middle, and inferior meati. The superior meatus drains the posterior ethmoidal air cells and the sphenoid sinus through the sphenoethmoidal recess. The middle meatus drains the frontal sinus via the frontal sinus

drainage pathway (FSDP), the maxillary sinus via the maxillary ostium, and the anterior ethmoidal air cells. The inferior meatus drains the nasolacrimal apparatus via the nasolacrimal duct.[15]

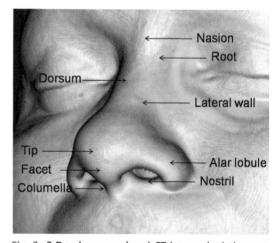

Fig. 2. 3-D volume-rendered CT image depicting surface anatomy of the nose.

The Nasal Cycle

The mucosal lining over the nasal septum and the nasal turbinates is influenced by the nasal cycle, which is responsible for alternating changes in the turbinate sizes due to mucosal engorgement.[16] This cyclic and physiologic enlargement of the turbinates alternates between both nasal cavities every 45 minutes to 1 hour and should not be mistaken for pathology.

THE NASAL SEPTUM

The nasal septum consists of an anterior cartilaginous component (the septal cartilage) and a posterior bony component (the bony septum) comprising the vomer and the perpendicular plate of the ethmoid.[17]

Anatomic variations and the implications (Fig. 3):

1. Septal deviation: Seen in 20% to 79% of the population.[18] The septum is commonly deviated in its inferior portion near the chondrovomeral junction and can also assume an S-shaped configuration with an undulating deviation onto both sides of the midline. Gross septal deviations can displace the middle turbinate and interfere with surgical access to the middle meatus. Septal deviations must be addressed to improve surgical exposure.[19]

   Septal spurs may be associated with septal

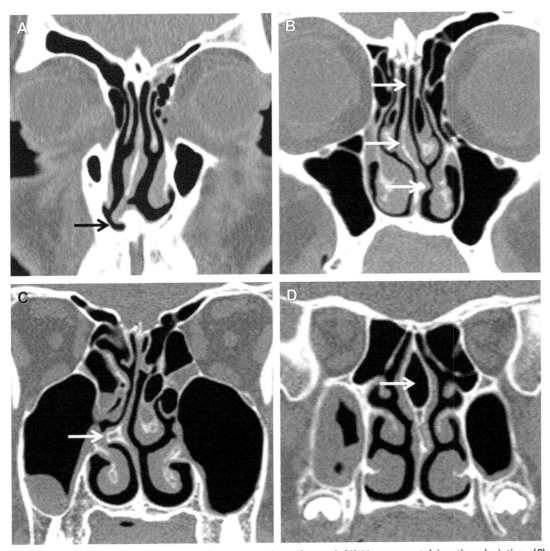

Fig. 3. Coronal CT images showing nasal septum variants (*arrows*) (*A*) Vomero-septal junction deviation, (*B*) S-shaped undulating deviation, (*C*) bony septal spur with adhesion to inferior turbinate, and (*D*) posterior septal pneumatization.

deviations and may form adhesions with the adjacent turbinates.

2. Septal pneumatization: pneumatization may occur anteriorly from the crista galli or posteriorly from the sphenoid sinus. Posterior septal pneumatization may occasionally narrow the sphenoethmoidal recess and impede access to the sphenoid ostium.

THE MIDDLE TURBINATE

The middle turbinate is a part of the ethmoid bone with attachments in all 3 planes (ie, sagittal, coronal, and axial).[20] The anterior part of the middle turbinate is oriented vertically and is attached superiorly to the anterior skull base at the lateral border of the cribriform plate. Posteriorly, the attachment becomes oblique attaching to the lamina papyracea and further posteriorly lies in a coronal plane attaching to the medial wall of the maxillary sinuses (Video 1). The obliquely directed midportion of the middle turbinate is known as the basal lamella, which is a surgical landmark marking the division between the anterior and posterior ethmoidal sinuses.[17]

Anatomic variants and the implications (Fig. 4):

1. Concha bullosa: pneumatization of the inferior bulbous portion of the middle turbinate occurs in approximately 24% to 55% of the population and is usually bilateral.[18,21] If the pneumatization is restricted to the vertical lamella of the turbinate above the level of the ostiomeatal unit, it is termed an interlamellar cell of Grunwald, lamellar bulla, or conchal neck air cell. This cell generally does not disturb sinonasal physiology. A large concha bullosa may cause septal deviation and obstruct the ethmoidal infundibulum.[17]

2. Paradoxic middle turbinate: in 26% of the population, the middle turbinate exhibits a paradoxic lateral convexity,[22] which can impede surgical access to the ostiomeatal unit and contribute to recurrent rhinosinusitis.

3. Turbinate sinus: occasionally the inferior portion of the middle turbinate curves acutely on itself producing a deep invagination called a turbinate sinus.

4. Pneumatized basal lamella: may be mistaken for an anterior ethmoidal air cell leading to incomplete exploration of the posterior ethmoid sinuses.

LAMELLAR ANATOMY

Lamellae are organizational plates, which develop within the cartilaginous olfactory capsule. They are important surgical landmarks and partition the sinonasal cavity into well-defined compartments.[14,23] The lamellae course through the ethmoidal air cells and extend superiorly up to the skull base from the lateral nasal wall. These structures are best seen in the parasagittal planes (Fig. 5) and from anterior to posterior include the uncinate process, anterior margin of the bulla ethmoidalis, lamella of the middle turbinate (basal lamella), lamella of the superior turbinate, and, if present, the lamella of the supreme turbinate. If the supreme turbinate is absent, the anterior face of the sphenoid sinus is considered the fifth lamella.

Anatomic variants and the implications:

1. The lamellae may be displaced, distorted, remodeled, or attenuated by a variety of disease processes. Visualization of intact lamellae indicates, however, a benign pathology in most cases. The lamellae are destroyed or eroded by malignant neoplastic lesions or aggressive infective pathologies like invasive fungal disease.[24]

2. The fifth lamella is not identified in case of a nonpneumatized sphenoid sinus.

3. The suprabullar and retrobullar recesses can be identified while viewing the lamellar anatomy in the sagittal plane.

THE UNCINATE PROCESS

The uncinate process is a thin crescent-shaped bone, which runs in a sagittal plane from anterosuperior to posteroinferior. It is attached anteriorly to the lacrimal bone and inferiorly to the ethmoidal process of the inferior turbinate as well as to the perpendicular process of the palatine bone.[25] Posteriorly the uncinate has a free concave margin. The superior attachment of the uncinate process may be variable. On coronal CT scan, the space between the uncinate process and the medial wall of the orbit denotes the ethmoidal infundibulum.[26]

Anatomic variants and the implications:

1. Variable attachments: the uncinate process may attach superiorly to the lamina papyracea, the anterior skull base, or the middle turbinate and may also have multiple attachments to these structures. The pattern of attachment determines the position of the FSDP (Fig. 6, Table 3).

2. The uncinate process may be pneumatized (Fig. 7A) in 4% of the population[28] or everted.[29] A pneumatized uncinate process (uncinate bulla) can narrow the infundibulum and impair normal sinus ventilation.[30] An everted uncinate process may be mistaken for a double middle turbinate on endoscopy.

3. An atelectatic uncinate process (see Fig. 7B), commonly seen in maxillary sinus hypoplasia and silent sinus syndrome, is closely related

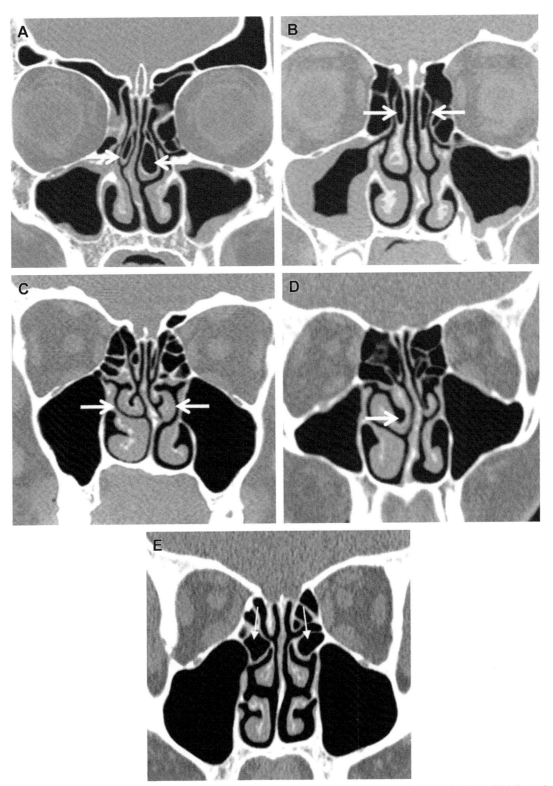

Fig. 4. Coronal CT images showing middle turbinate variants (*arrows*). (*A*) Bilateral concha bullosa, (*B*) bilateral interlamellar cells of Grunwald, (*C*) bilateral paradoxic turbinates, (*D*) right turbinate sinus, and (*E*) bilateral pneumatized basal lamella (*arrows*). (*From [A]* Vaid S, Vaid N, Rawat S, et al. An imaging checklist for pre-FESS CT: framing a surgically relevant report. Clin Radiol 2011;66(5):466; with permission.)

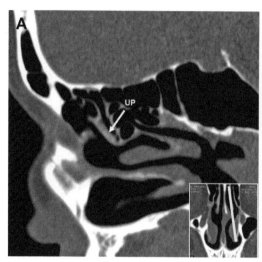
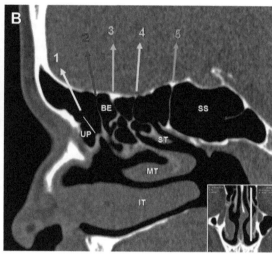

Fig. 5. Sagittal oblique (*A*) and sagittal (*B*) CT images showing lamellar anatomy. 1: Uncinate process (UP) (*white arrow* [*A*], oblique white line in [*B*]); 2: anterior margin of bulla ethmoidalis (BE); 3: basal lamella; 4: lamella of the superior turbinate (ST); and 5: anterior margin of the sphenoid sinus (SS). IT, inferior turbinate; MT, middle turbinate. Insets in figures (*A*) and (*B*) are coronal CT reference images. Yellow lines denote plane of the sagittal images (angulated obliquely in [*A*] and vertical in [*B*]).

to the inferior and medial wall of the ipsilateral orbit.[31] This increases the risk of inadvertent orbital penetration during FESS.

4. Rarely, the uncinate process may be entirely absent.[32]

THE MAXILLARY SINUS AND OSTIOMEATAL COMPLEX

The maxillary sinus occupies the body of the maxillary bone. The roof is formed by the orbital floor and the floor is formed by the alveolar process of the maxilla. The infraorbital nerve (a branch of the maxillary division of the trigeminal nerve) runs in a bony canal along the roof of the maxillary sinus. The maxillary ostium is located along the superior aspect of the medial wall of the sinus and drains into the base of the ethmoidal infundibulum.[16] The size of the ostium varies between 3 and 10 mm[33] and it can exhibit variable shapes and position. The components of the ostiomeatal complex as identified on coronal CT (**Fig. 8**)

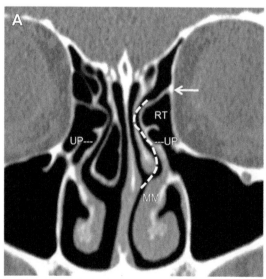
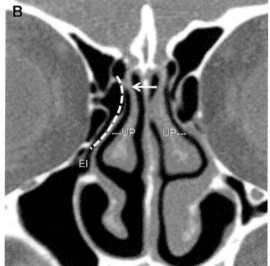

Fig. 6. Coronal CT images showing unicate process attachments. (*A*) Left uncinate process (UP) attached to lamina papyracea (*arrow*) with the FSDP (*dashed lines*) draining into the medial meatus (MM). (*B*) Right uncinate process attaching to the middle turbinate (*arrow*) with the FSDP (*dashed lines*) draining into the ethmoidal infundibulum (EI). RT, recessus terminalis.

Table 3
Pattern of superior attachment of the uncinate process

Lamina papyracea	Seen in more than 50% of individuals,[27] resulting in a medial FSDP draining into the middle meatus, creating a blind pouch laterally termed the recessus terminalis
Anterior skull base	Results in a lateral FSDP opening into the ethmoidal infundibulum, increasing chances of retrograde spread of infection into the frontal sinus from the ethmoidal sinus
Middle turbinate	FSDP is displaced posterior to the agger nasi cell, which needs to be fractured to access the FSDP.[17]

comprise the maxillary ostium, the middle meatus, the ethmoidal infundibulum, the bulla ethmoidalis, the uncinate process, and the hiatus semilunaris.[34]

Anatomic variants and the implications (Fig. 9):

1. Maxillary sinus hypoplasia is seen in up to 10% of the population. Other conditions with a reduced size of the maxillary sinus are silent sinus syndrome, posttraumatic, and postoperative sequelae. There is a higher incidence of orbital penetration during endoscopic surgery if the size of the maxillary sinus is small.[32]
2. In hyperpneumatized maxillary sinuses, there is a thin mucosal lining between the maxillary antrum and the dental roots. This can predispose to recurrent sinusitis from dental infections and to oroantral fistulas after dental extraction.[35]
3. Septae within the maxillary sinuses are common and may be fibrous or bony. They usually extend from the infraorbital nerve canal to the

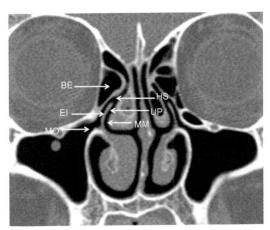

Fig. 8. Coronal CT image showing components of the ostiomeatal complex. BE, bulla ethmoidalis; EI, ethmoidal infundibulum; HS: hiatus semilunaris; MO, maxillary ostium; MM, middle meatus; UP, uncinate process.

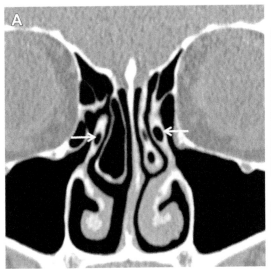

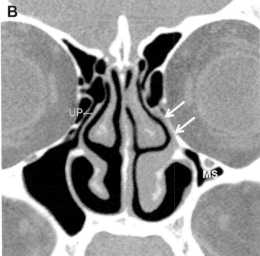

Fig. 7. Coronal CT images showing uncinate process variants (arrows). (A) Bilateral pneumatized uncinate processes (UP) and (B) left atelectatic uncinate process (arrows) due to left maxillary sinus hypoplasia (MS). (From [A] Vaid S, Vaid N, Rawat S, et al. An imaging checklist for pre-FESS CT: framing a surgically relevant report. Clin Radiol 2011;66(5):462; with permission.)

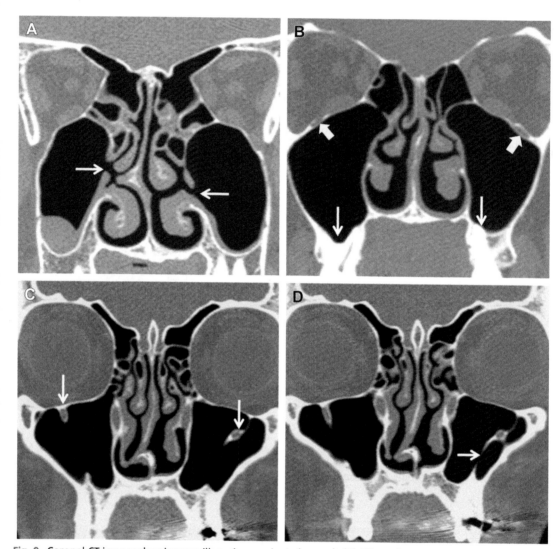

Fig. 9. Coronal CT images showing maxillary sinus variants (*arrows*). (*A*) Bilateral accessory ostia, (*B*) hyperpneumatized sinuses with exposed dental roots; normal infraorbital nerve canals (*block arrows*), (*C*) bilateral dehiscent infraorbital nerve canals, and (*D*) intrasinus septum attaching to the dehiscent canal on the left side.

lateral wall. These can affect the drainage of the maxillary sinuses.[18]

4. Accessory ostia are seen in 10% to 25% of the population, located within the region of the posterior fontanelle, behind the natural ostia.[36] It is important to surgically connect both the natural and the accessory ostia to prevent chronic recurrent sinusitis.[37]

5. Bony margins of the infraorbital nerve canal may be dehiscent in up to 14% of cases, which exposes the nerve to sinus pathology.[8]

THE FRONTAL SINUS AND FRONTAL SINUS DRAINAGE PATHWAY

The frontal sinuses develop as extensions from the anterior ethmoidal air cells. They may be absent in 5% and hypoplastic in 4% of the population.[38] Well-pneumatized frontal sinuses show typical scalloped margins with intact internal septae. Focal dehiscences within the posterior wall of the frontal sinuses can be identified on sagittal imaging.

The frontal beak (frontonasal process of the maxilla) forms an important surgical and imaging landmark in the anatomy of the FSDP.[39] It is identified on both coronal and parasagittal images (**Fig. 10**) with the frontal sinus superiorly and the FSDP inferiorly.[40] The frontal beak corresponds to the level of the frontal ostium and hence its thickness determines the size of the ostium.

The agger nasi cell is the anterior most extramural ethmoidal air cell, seen in 93% of the population,[28] and lies within the anterior portion of the

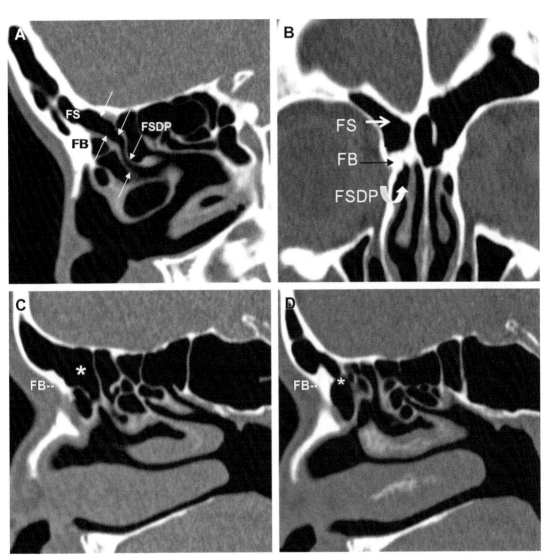

Fig. 10. Parasagittal (*A*) and coronal (*B*) CT images showing frontal beak (FB) separating the frontal sinus (FS) from the FSDP (*arrows, curved arrow*). Parasagittal CT sections (*C, D*) depict impact of the FB thickness on the size of the frontal sinus ostium (*asterisk*). (*From* Vaid S, Vaid N, Rawat S, et al. An imaging checklist for pre-FESS CT: framing a surgically relevant report. Clin Radiol 2011;66(5):463; with permission.)

FSDP. It is best viewed on parasagittal images and serves as an important surgical landmark.[41] This cell is in close proximity to the nasolacrimal duct.

The classification of frontal cells was first described by Kuhn in 1996.[42] This article discusses the modified classification of frontoethmoidal cells by Wormald[39] (**Fig. 11, Table 4**).

Anatomic variants and the implications:

1. Variability in size of the frontal sinus and prominent posterior wall dehiscences need preoperative documentation in case an external drainage procedure, like frontal sinus trephination, is considered, to prevent inadvertent intracranial penetration.[23]

2. A small agger nasi cell is associated with a thickened frontal beak with a resultant narrow frontal ostium forming an anatomic tight spot, which is a cause for recurrent frontal sinusitis.[39] Proximity of the agger nasi to the nasolacrimal duct can result in cross-infection between these 2 structures.

3. Type I and type II frontal cells do not require surgery of the frontal ostium or drilling of the frontal beak, which is unavoidable in type III and type IV frontal cells.

4. The floor of the anterior cranial fossa forms the posterior border of the frontal bullar cell (**Fig. 12A**), and caution must be exercised while

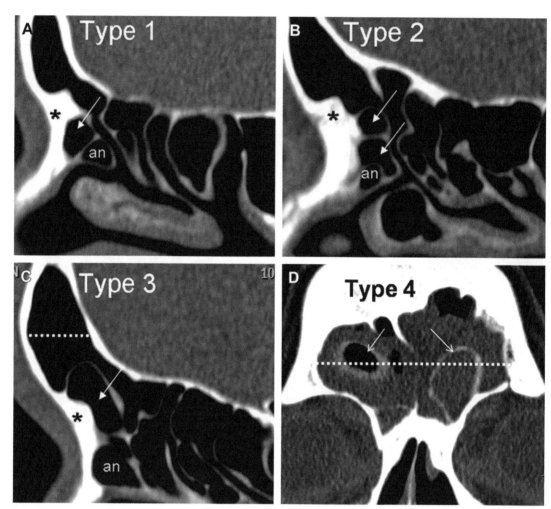

Fig. 11. Sagittal CT images (*A–C*) showing types 1 to 3 frontal cells (*arrows*). Coronal CT image (*D*) shows bilateral isolated type 4 frontal cells (*arrows*). Dotted line depicts the midpoint of the height of the frontal sinus. an, Agger nasi; FB, frontal beak (*asterisks*). (*From* Vaid S, Vaid N, Rawat S, et al. An imaging checklist for pre-FESS CT: framing a surgically relevant report. Clin Radiol 2011;66(5):465; with permission.)

Table 4 Classification of frontoethmoidal cells	
Type 1 frontal cell	Single cell above the agger nasi and below the frontal beak (below the frontal ostium)
Type 2 frontal cells	Two or more cells above the agger nasi and below the frontal beak (below the frontal ostium)
Type 3 frontal cell	Single cell above the agger nasi with extension through the frontal ostium into the frontal sinus not exceeding 50% of the vertical height of the ipsilateral frontal sinus
Type 4 frontal cell	Single cell above the agger nasi with extension through the frontal ostium into the frontal sinus exceeding 50% of the vertical height of the ipsilateral frontal sinus or an isolated cell within the frontal sinus
Frontal bullar cell	Single cell extending from the suprabullar region along the undersurface of the anterior skull base into the frontal sinus (anterior margin lies within the frontal sinus)
Interfrontal sinus septal cell	A cell associated with the frontal intersinus septum and may compromise the frontal ostium

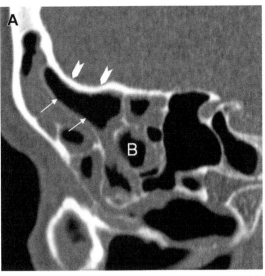
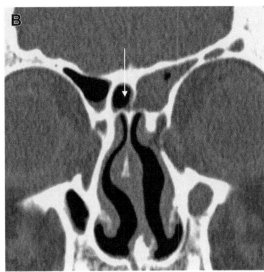

Fig. 12. Parasagittal CT image (*A*) showing a frontal bullar cell (*asterisk*), above the bulla ethmoidalis (B) with anterior margin related to the frontal sinus (*arrows*) and posterior margin formed by the anterior skull base (*arrowheads*). Coronal CT image (*B*) showing an interfrontal sinus septal cell (*arrow*). (*From* Vaid S, Vaid N, Rawat S, et al. An imaging checklist for pre-FESS CT: framing a surgically relevant report. Clin Radiol 2011;66(5):465; with permission.)

fracturing this cell to avoid inadvertent intracranial penetration.[39,40]

5. An interfrontal sinus septal cell (see **Fig. 12**B) may cause obstruction of the frontal ostium.

Anterior ethmoid sinuses:

The anterior ethmoid sinuses are located anterior to the basal lamella. The largest cell in this group is the bulla ethmoidalis, which is a key surgical landmark during endoscopic sinus surgery. It is of variable size and underdeveloped in approximately 8% of the population.[9] The cleft between the anterior margin of the bulla and the uncinate process is called the hiatus semilunaris and this further opens into a triangular cavity called the ethmoidal infundibulum.[43]

Anatomic variants and the implications:

1. An underdeveloped bulla ethmoidalis predisposes to inadvertent injury to the orbit.
2. The suprabullar recess lies between the superior wall of the bulla ethmoidalis and the roof of the ethmoid sinus. This recess can extend laterally as supraorbital cells (**Fig. 13**A). Large

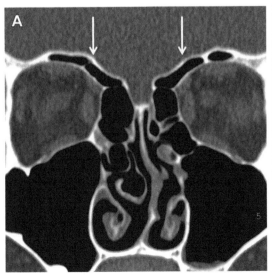
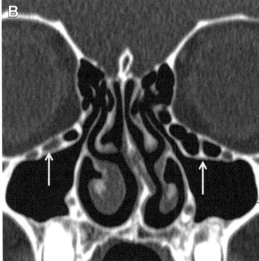

Fig. 13. Coronal CT images showing (*A*) bilateral supraorbital cells (*arrows*) and (*B*) bilateral Haller cells (*arrows*).

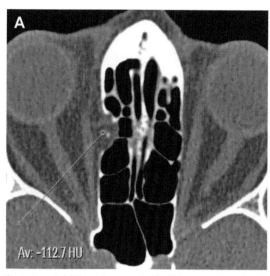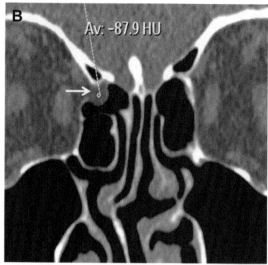

Fig. 14. Axial (*A*) and coronal (*B*) CT images showing focal dehiscence of the right lamina papyracea (*arrow*).

supraorbital cells can displace the bony canal for anterior ethmoidal artery posteriorly and may also be mistaken for frontal sinus cells.[34]

3. A retrobullar recess is formed if the posterior margin of the ethmoidal bulla does not reach the basal lamella. The bulla ethmoidalis drains into this recess.

4. Anterior ethmoidal air cells extending along the floor of the orbits, lateral to the sagittal plane of the lamina papyracea are called Haller cells (see Fig. 13B), reported in 10% to 45% of the patients.[28] These cells narrow the maxillary sinus ostium. The inferior walls of the Haller cells are at times extremely thin and seen only after adjusting the CT window settings.[38]

THE LAMINA PAPYRACEA AND ANTERIOR ETHMOIDAL ARTERY

The lamina papyracea forms the lateral walls of the ethmoid sinuses separating them from the adjacent orbits. Focal small corticated defects in the lamina papyracea are seen in up to 0.5% to 10% of the population and are not clinically significant.[34] Larger defects (congenital, post-traumatic, or postoperative) in the lamina (Fig. 14) need preoperative documentation to avoid inadvertent orbital injury. On coronal CT, the maxillary ostium and the lamina papyracea are aligned in the same sagittal plane (Fig. 15). A medially positioned lamina papyracea predisposes to orbital penetration.[44]

The anterior ethmoidal artery (branch of the ophthalmic artery) courses in a bony canal through the upper one-third of the lamina papyracea. This canal can be identified on coronal CT by a beaking

of the medial orbital wall behind the bulla ethmoidalis (Fig. 16A).[26]

Anatomic variants and the implications:

1. Defects in the posterior lamina papyracea are more significant because there is a relatively thinner fat pad between the medial rectus muscle and the lamina papyracea with increased chances of muscle laceration, orbital hematoma, and orbital fibrosis.[45]

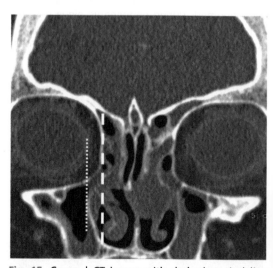

Fig. 15. Coronal CT image with dashed vertical line representing sagittal plane of the right lamina papyracea passing medial to the sagittal plane of the right maxillary ostium (*dotted line*). (*From* Vaid S, Vaid N, Rawat S, et al. An imaging checklist for pre-FESS CT: framing a surgically relevant report. Clin Radiol 2011;66(5):469; with permission.)

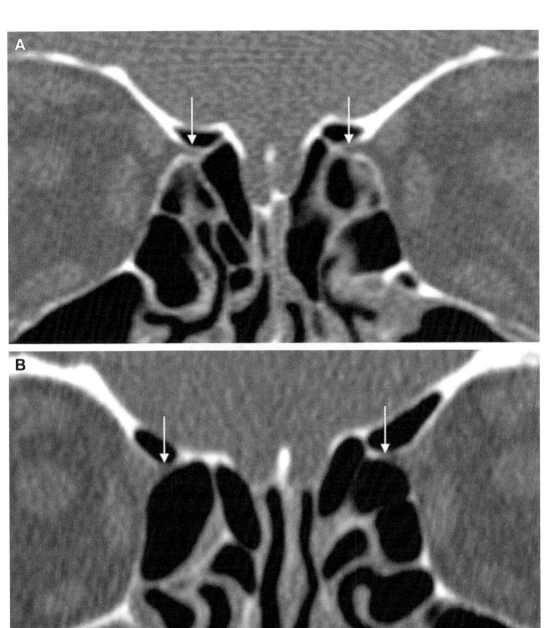

Fig. 16. Coronal CT images showing (A) normal bony canal for the anterior ethmoidal arteries (*arrows*) and (B) both arteries (*arrows*) suspended in a mesentery without bone cover. (*From* [B] Vaid S, Vaid N, Rawat S, et al. An imaging checklist for pre-FESS CT: framing a surgically relevant report. Clin Radiol 2011;66(5):468; with permission.)

2. Normal bony covering of the anterior ethmoidal artery may be absent and the canal may be dehiscent inferiorly into the anterior ethmoidal air cells in up to 40% of cases.[46] In these cases, the artery is suspended on a mucous membrane mesentery and can be injured during surgery (see **Fig. 16**B).

THE ANTERIOR SKULL BASE: OLFACTORY FOSSA AND HEIGHT OF THE ETHMOID SKULL BASE
The Olfactory Fossa

The olfactory fossa, containing the olfactory bulbs and tracts, is formed by the crista galli medially,

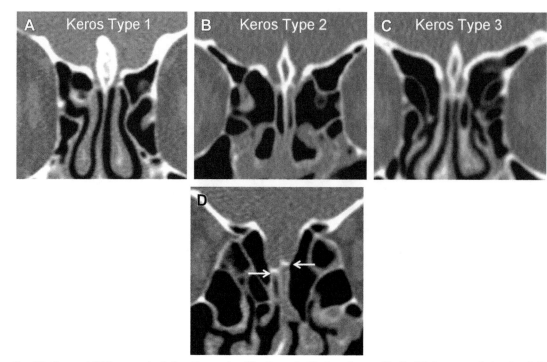

Fig. 17. Coronal CT images depicting Keros classification of olfactory fossae (A–C). (D) Asymmetric levels of the olfactory fossae (*arrows*).

medial lamella of the cribriform plate inferiorly, and lateral lamella of the cribriform plate laterally. There are 3 types of olfactory fossae described by Keros[47] based on the length of the lateral lamella of the cribriform plate (Fig. 17, Table 5). Because the lateral lamella of the cribriform plate is structurally the thinnest bone in the anterior skull base and dehiscent in up to 14% of patients,[48] there is a greater risk of intraoperative injury and iatrogenic cerebrospinal fluid (CSF) leak in this region.[49]

Anatomic variants and implications:

1. Both the type 1 and the type 3 olfactory fossae are more prone to intraoperative injury.
2. Asymmetry in the level of the olfactory fossa occurs in up to 10% to 30% of the population (see Fig. 17D). The angle between the medial and lateral lamella of the cribriform plate is also variable.[26] Inadvertent intracranial penetration is more common on the side where the olfactory fossa is lower and on the side where the angle between the medial and lateral lamella of the cribriform plate is greater.
3. An aerated crista galli is seen in 13% of patients with pneumatization occurring from the frontal sinuses.[50] When aerated, the crista galli is likely to communicate with the frontal recess and can obstruct the frontal ostium leading to chronic infections and mucocoele formation.[51]

Height of the Ethmoid Skull Base

The roof of the anterior ethmoid sinus is formed by the fovea ethmoidalis laterally and the cribriform plate medially. It is important to identify a low

---

Table 5
Keros classification of the olfactory fossa

Type 1	Length of the lateral lamella is 1–3 mm, indicating a shallow or flat olfactory fossa seen in 30% of cases.
Type 2	Length of the lateral lamella is 4–7 mm, indicating a moderately deep olfactory fossa seen in 49% of cases.
Type 3	The lateral lamella is longer, measuring 8–16 mm with a resultant deep olfactory fossa seen in 21% of cases.[26]

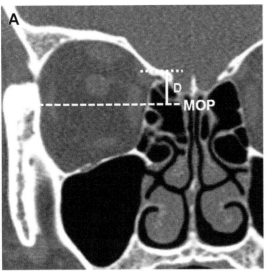 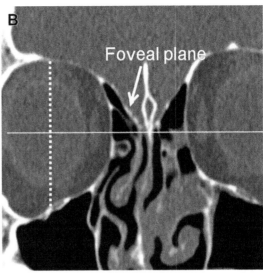

Fig. 18. ESB height. Coronal CT image (*A*) showing a normal ESB height with the vertical distance (D) between the midorbital plane (MOP) (*dashed line*) and the anterior skull base (*dotted line*) measuring more than 8.5 mm (see Table 6). Coronal CT image (*B*) showing a low-lying foveal plane (*arrow*) reaching the midorbital plane (*horizontal white line*). The dotted line depicts the vertical height of the right orbit. (*From [B]* Vaid S, Vaid N, Rawat S, et al. An imaging checklist for pre-FESS CT: framing a surgically relevant report. Clin Radiol 2011;66(5):467; with permission.)

ethmoid skull base (ESB) preoperatively to prevent potentially catastrophic intraoperative injuries.[52] The height of the ESB can be assessed by 2 methods proposed by Myers and Valvasorri[44] and more recently by Rudmik and Smith[53] (Fig. 18, Table 6).

Anatomic variants and implications:

1. A low ESB indicates a dangerously low lying and medially sloping anterior skull base with higher chances intraoperative intracranial penetration.[53]
2. A low-lying anterior skull base also indicates reduced height of the posterior ethmoid sinuses.[44]

Table 6
Estimation of the height of the ethmoidal skull base

Authors	Methodology	Interpretation
Myers & Valvasorri,[44] 1998	The vertical height of the orbit is divided into 3 equal sections. The position of the ESB is documented in reference to upper, middle, or lower third of the vertical orbital height.	If the ESB passes above the upper third of the vertical height of the ipsilateral orbit, it indicates a normal and hence a surgically safe ESB. An ESB passing through or below the midorbital plane is considered a low ESB.
Rudmik & Smith,[53] 2012	The vertical distance between the height of the ESB and the midorbital plane is measured in a coronal CT image showing the canal for the anterior ethmoidal artery.	In their study, the mean height of the ESB was found to be 8.5 mm. A vertical height of more than 8.5 mm was considered a safe and high ESB; a measurement between 4 and 7 mm was considered a moderately safe ESB; and a height less than 4 mm was deemed a low and surgically unsafe ESB with high chances of inadvertent intracranial penetration.

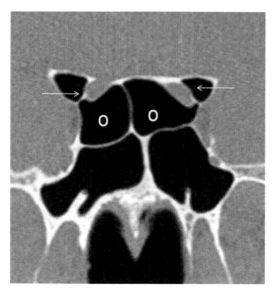

Fig. 19. Coronal CT image showing bilateral Onodi cells (O), the cruciform sign, with both optic nerves coursing through the cells (*arrows*).

Box 2
Learning points - 2

Although the middle turbinate is an exceptionally stable structure, its superior attachment to the anterior skull base is most vulnerable to intraoperative injury and resultant CSF leak.

Identification of lamellar anatomy in sinus pathologies is important to formulate a reasonably accurate differential diagnosis. An atelectatic uncinate process and a dehiscent medially located lamina papyracea are critical anatomic variants needing preoperative CT identification to avoid inadvertent orbital penetration during FESS.

Inadvertent intracranial penetration can be avoided during FESS by preoperative CT identification of a low ethmoid skull base, presence of a frontal bullar cell, Keros type 1 and type 3 olfactory fossae and asymmetric olfactory fossae.

THE POSTERIOR SINUS GROUP: POSTERIOR ETHMOID SINUS AND SPHENOID SINUS
The Posterior Ethmoid Sinus

The posterior ethmoidal air cells are located between the basal lamella and the sphenoid sinus and are fewer in number[1–4] than the anterior ethmoidal cells. The lamina papyracea lies laterally and the superior turbinate forms the medial boundary of this sinus group, which drain into the superior meatus. It is important to document the height of the posterior ethmoid sinus, which is the vertical distance between the superior margin of the maxillary sinus and roof of the posterior ethmoid sinus on coronal CT images.

Anatomic variants and implications:

1. Sphenoethmoidal cell (Onodi cell): Because the posterior ethmoidal cells pneumatize before the sphenoid sinus, they have a high propensity to grow above and lateral to the developing sphenoid sinus forming the Onodi cell. This is seen in 3.4% to 14% of the general population.[54] An Onodi cell should be suspected on coronal CT images, which show an obliquely oriented or horizontal septum within the sphenoid sinus (**Fig. 19**). Some investigators have proposed a cruciform sign to help diagnose bilateral Onodi cells, in which a coronal CT image at the level of the posterior choana demonstrates the sphenoid air cell showing cruciform septation.[17] Important critical relationships of the sphenoid sinus, namely the optic nerves and internal carotid arteries, are directly related to the posterior ethmoid sinuses and hence are at risk during surgery.

2. Reduction in the height of the posterior ethmoid sinus can lead to inadvertent intracranial penetration.

Table 7
Classification of type of sphenoid sinus

Sphenoid sinus agenesis	A nonpneumatized sphenoid sinus seen in <0.7% of individuals
Conchal sphenoid sinus	A small rudimentary air cavity within the sphenoid bone, not reaching up to the anterior wall of the sella tursica, seen in 1%–4% of the population
Presellar sphenoid sinus	The posterior sinus wall extends up to the anterior wall of the sella tursica seen in 35%–40% of the population.
Sellar sphenoid sinus	The sinus cavity extends beyond the anterior wall of the sella tursica below the pituitary fossa seen in 55%–60% of the population. Wang and colleagues[56] further classified this type of sphenoid sinus more recently based on the direction of pneumatization into sphenoid body, lateral clivus, lesser sphenoid wing, anterior rostral, and the combined variety.

545

Table 8
Critical neurovascular/congenital channels related to the sphenoid sinus

Optic nerve canals	Related to the roof of the sphenoid sinus. Bony walls can be dehiscent in up to 24% of cases.[57] Delano and colleagues classified the optic nerves into 4 categories based on the relationship of the nerve with the sphenoid and posterior ethmoid sinuses.[58]
The internal carotid artery canals	Located along the posterolateral wall of the sphenoid sinus, and the bony coverings may be dehiscent in up to 25% of cases.[43]
The pterygoid canals (vidian canals)	Along the inferior sinus walls, which transmit the combined great petrosal and deep petrosal nerve complex as well as the artery and vein of the pterygoid canal[59]
Foramen rotundum	Along the lateral sinus walls, which transmit the maxillary division of the trigeminal nerve, artery of the foramen rotundum, and an emissary vein
Lateral craniopharyngeal canal (Sternberg canal)	Represents a congenital bony defect in the lateral wall of the sphenoid sinus situated further lateral to the maxillary nerve

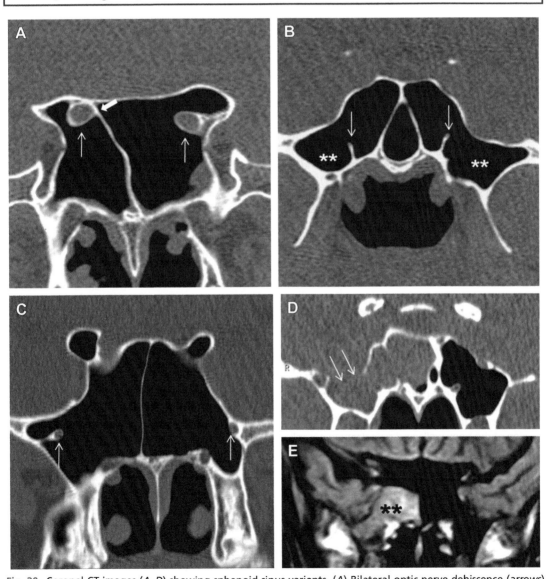

Fig. 20. Coronal CT images (A–D) showing sphenoid sinus variants. (A) Bilateral optic nerve dehiscence (arrows) with intrasinus septum attaching to right optic nerve canal (block arrow). (B) Prominent lateral recesses (asterisk) with endosinal vidian canals (arrows). (C) Endosinal right foramen rotundum. (D) Widened lateral craniopharyngeal canal on right side (arrows) with coronal T1W MR image (E) showing an associated sphenoid sinus meningoencephalocoele (asterisks). (From Vaid S, Vaid N, Rawat S, et al. An imaging checklist for pre-FESS CT: framing a surgically relevant report. Clin Radiol 2011;66(5):467; with permission.)

5. In approximately 80% of cases of anterior clinoid process pneumatization, the optic nerve is dehiscent into the superolateral aspect of the sphenoid sinus.

The Sphenoid Sinus

The sphenoid sinus develops in the body of the sphenoid bone and is generally bilateral although asymmetric in size.[8] The septae within the sphenoid sinus are usually vertical in orientation. The sphenoid sinus is classified into 4 types depending on the degree of pneumatization[55] (**Table 7**). There are several bony canals and foramina transmitting critical neurovascular structures related to the sphenoid sinus (**Table 8**).

The anterior clinoid processes may be pneumatized in up to 6% to 13% of cases[18,28] forming the opticocarotid recess between the optic nerve above and the internal carotid artery below.

Anatomic variants and the implications (**Fig. 20**):

1. A nonpneumatized sphenoid sinus and a conchal sinus are relative contraindications to transsphenoidal endoscopic skull base surgery.
2. Intrasinus septae attaching to bony walls of the internal carotid artery and optic nerve need preoperative identification because excessive traction on these septae may lead to an avulsion of the bony walls and catastrophic complications, like carotid artery injury, delayed pseudoaneurysm formation, and blindness.
3. Position of the neurovascular structures around the sphenoid sinus is determined by the degree of pneumatization. Occasionally, the structures are exposed within the sinus cavity and connected to the sinus walls by bony stalks.[60]
4. Persistence of the lateral craniopharyngeal canal in association with extensive sphenoid pneumatization and raised intracranial pressure may lead to formation of a spontaneous lateral sphenoid meningoencephalocoele and resultant CSF leak.

SUMMARY

A structured approach to reading CT scans of the paranasal sinuses using multiplanar imaging enables a better understanding of the complex anatomy of this region and its numerous anatomic variants. It is important for radiologists to be aware of the critical clinical implications of identifying these anatomic variations. A continuing interaction between the radiologist and surgeon improves the overall quality of the scan reports, resulting in better surgical outcomes.

SUPPLEMENTARY DATA

Supplementary data related to this article can be found online at http://dx.doi.org/10.1016/j.nic.2015.07.002.

REFERENCES

1. Ónodi A, Thomson SC. The anatomy of the nasal cavity and its accessory sinuses: an atlas for practitioners and students. London: H.K. Lewis; 1895.
2. Gwaltney JM Jr, Phillips CD, Miller RD, et al. Computed tomographic study of the common cold. N Engl J Med 1994;330:25–30.
3. Figueroamon R. Imaging anatomy in revision sinus surgery. In: Kountakis SE, Jacobs J, Gosepath J, editors. Revision sinus surgery. Berlin; Heidelberg (Germany): Springer; 2008. p. 1–11.
4. Aksoy EA, Özden SU, Karaarslan E, et al. Reliability of high-pitch ultra-low-dose paranasal sinus computed tomography for evaluating paranasal sinus anatomy and sinus disease. J Craniofac Surg 2014;25(5):1801–4.

5. Dahmani-Causse M, Marx M, Deguine O, et al. Morphologic examination of the temporal bone by cone beam computed tomography: comparison with multislice helical computed tomography. Eur Ann Otorhinolaryngol Head Neck Dis 2011;128: 230–5.

6. Bremke M, Leppek R, Werner JA. Digital volume tomography in ENT medicine. HNO 2010;58(8): 823–32.

7. Wormald PJ. Imaging in endoscopic sinus surgery. In: Wormald PJ, editor. Endoscopic sinus surgery: anatomy, three-dimensional reconstruction and surgical technique. 3rd edition. New York: Thieme Medical Publishers; 2013. p. 13–8.

8. Lang J. Clinical anatomy of the nose, nasal cavity and paranasal sinuses. New York: Thieme Medical Publishers; 1989.

9. Marquez S, Tessema B, Clement PA, et al. Development of the ethmoid sinus and extramural migration: the anatomical basis of this paranasal sinus. Anat Rec (Hoboken) 2008;291(11):1535–53.

10. Zeifer B. Pediatric sinonasal imaging: normal anatomy and inflammatory disease. Neuroimaging Clin N Am 2000;10(1):137–59.

11. Som PM. Sinonasal cavity. In: Som PM, Bergron RT, editors. Head and neck imaging. 2nd edition. St Louis: Mosby-Year Book; 1991. p. 51–168.

12. Sadler TW. Langman's medical embryology. 12th edition. Philadelphia: Wolters Kluwer Health/Lippincott Williams & Wilkins; 2012.

13. Wolf G, Anderhuber W, Kuhn F. Development of the paranasal sinuses in children: implications for paranasal sinus surgery. Ann Otol Rhinol Laryngol 1993; 102(9):705–11.

14. Anon JB, Rontal M, Zinreich SJ, et al. Pre-and postnatal morphogenesis of the nose and paranasal sinuses. In: Anon JB, Rontal M, Zinreich SJ, editors. Anatomy of the paranasal sinuses. New York: Thieme Medical Publishers; 1996. p. 3–10.

15. Som PM, Shugar JMA, Brandwein MS. Anatomy and physiology. In: Som PM, Curtin HD, editors. Head and neck imaging. 4th edition. St Louis: Mosby; 2003. p. 87–147.

16. Kubal WS. Sinonasal anatomy. Neuroimaging Clin N Am 1998;8(1):143–56.

17. Beale TJ, Madani G, Morley SJ. Imaging of the paranasal sinuses and nasal cavity: normal anatomy and clinically relevant anatomical variants. Semin Ultrasound CT MR 2009;30(1):2–16.

18. Sarna A, Hayman A, Laine F, et al. Coronal imaging of the ostiomeatal unit: anatomy of 24 variants. J Comput Assist Tomogr 2002;26(1):153–7.

19. Wormald PJ. Endoscopic sinus surgery: anatomy, three-dimensional reconstruction and surgical technique. 3rd edition. New York: Thieme Medical Publishers; 2013.

20. Chong V, Fan Y, Lau D, et al. Functional endoscopic sinus surgery (FESS):what radiologists need to know. Clin Radiol 1998;53:650–8.

21. Zeinrich SJ, Mattox DE, Kennedy DW, et al. Concha bullosa: CT evaluation. J Comput Assist Tomogr 1988;12:778–84.

22. Cannon CR. Endoscopic management of concha bullosa. Otolaryngol Head Neck Surg 1994;110: 449–54.

23. Stammberger H, Kopp W, Dekornfeld TJ. Special endoscopic anatomy. In: Stammberger H, Hawke M, editors. Functional endoscopic sinus surgery: the Messerklinger technique. Philadelphia: B.C. Decker; 1991. p. 61–90.

24. Aribandi M, McCoy VA, Bazan C. Imaging features of invasive and noninvasive fungal sinusitis: a review. Radiographics 2007;27(5):1283–96.

25. Stammberger HR, Kennedy DW. Paranasal sinuses: anatomic terminology and nomenclature. Ann Otol Rhinol Laryngol Suppl 1995;167:7–16.

26. Lund VJ, Stammberger H, Fokkens WJ, et al. European position paper on the anatomical terminology of the internal nose and paranasal sinuses. Rhinol Suppl 2014;24:1–34.

27. Landsberg R, Friedman M. A computer assisted anatomical study of the nasofrontal region. Laryngoscope 2001;111(12):2125–30.

28. Bolger WE, Butzin CA, Parsons DS. Paranasal sinus bony anatomic variations and mucosal abnormalities: CT analysis for endoscopic sinus surgery. Laryngoscope 1991;101:56–64.

29. El-Shazly AE, Poirrier AL, Cabay J, et al. Anatomical variations of the lateral nasal wall: The secondary and accessory middle turbinates. Clin Anat 2012; 25(3):340–6.

30. Bolger WE, Woodruff W, Parsons DS. CT demonstration of pneumatisation of the uncinate process. AJNR Am J Neuroradiol 1990;11:552.

31. Joe JK, Ho SY, Yanagisawa E. Documentation of variations in sinonasal anatomy by intra-operative nasal endoscopy. Laryngoscope 2000;110:229–35.

32. Bolger WE, Woodruff WW, Morehead J, et al. Maxillary sinus hypoplasia: classification and description of associated uncinate process hypoplasia. Otolaryngol Head Neck Surg 1990;103(5):759–65.

33. May M, Sobol SM, Korzec K. The location of the maxillary os and its importance to the endoscopic sinus surgeon. Laryngoscope 1990;100(10):1037–42.

34. Vaid S, Vaid N, Rawat S, et al. An imaging checklist for pre-FESS CT: framing a surgically relevant report. Clin Radiol 2011;66(5):459–70.

35. Sathananthar S, Nagaonkar S, Paleri V, et al. Canine fossa puncture and clearance of the maxillary sinus for the severely disease maxillary sinus. Laryngoscope 2005;115:1026–9.

36. Jog M, McGarry GW. How frequent are accessory ostia? J Laryngol Otol 2003;117:270–2.

37. Wormald PJ. Uncinectomy and middle meatal antrostomy including canine fossa puncture/trephine. In: Wormald PJ, editor. Endoscopic sinus surgery: anatomy, three-dimensional reconstruction and surgical technique. 3rd edition. New York: Thieme Medical Publishers; 2013. p. 28–44.

38. Earwacker J. Anatomic variants in sinonasal CT. Radiographics 1993;13:381–415.

39. Wormald PJ. Anatomy of the frontal recess and frontal sinus with three dimensional reconstruction. In: Wormald PJ, editor. Endoscopic sinus surgery: anatomy, three-dimensional reconstruction and surgical technique. 3rd edition. New York: Thieme Medical Publishers; 2013. p. 45–80.

40. Kew J, Rees GL, Close D, et al. Multiplanar reconstructed computed tomography images improve depiction and understanding of the anatomy of the frontal sinus and recess. Am J Rhinol 2002;16:119–23.

41. Wormald PJ. The agger nasi cell: the key to understanding the anatomy of the frontal recess. Otolaryngol Head Neck Surg 2003;129:497–507.

42. Kuhn FA. Chronic frontal sinusitis: the endoscopic frontal recess approach. Operative techniques. Otolaryngol Head Neck Surg 1996;7:222–9.

43. Stammberger H, Lund V. Anatomy of the nose and paranasal sinuses. In: Gleeson M, Browning GG, Burton MJ, et al, editors. Scott-Brown's Otorhinolaryngology, head and neck surgery, vol. 2, 7th edition. London: HodderArnold; 2008. p. 1315–43.

44. Meyers RM, Valvassori G. Interpretation of anatomic variations of computed tomography scans of the sinuses: a surgeon's perspective. Laryngoscope 1998;108:422–5.

45. Bhatti MT, Schmalfuss IM, Mancuso AA. Orbital complications of functional endoscopic sinus surgery:MR and CT findings. Clin Radiol 2005;60:894–904.

46. Moon HJ, Kim HU, Lee JG, et al. Surgical anatomy of the anterior ethmoidal canal in ethmoid roof. Laryngoscope 2001;111(5):900–4.

47. Keros P. On the practical value of differences in the level of the lamina cribrosa of the ethmoid. Z Laryngol Rhinol Otol 1962;41:809–13.

48. Ohnishi T. Bony defects and dehiscences of the roof of the ethmoid bone. Rhinology 1981;19:195–202.

49. Kainz J, Stammberger H. The roof of the anterior ethmoid: a locus minoris resistentiae in the skull base. Laryngol Rhinol Otol 1988;67:142–9.

50. Som PM, Lawson W. The frontal intersinus septal air cell: a new hypothesis of its origin. AJNR Am J Neuroradiol 2008;29(6):1215–7.

51. Reddy UM, Dev B. Pictorial essay: Anatomical variations of paranasal sinuses on multidetector computed tomography-How does it help FESS surgeons? Indian J Radiol Imaging 2012;22:317–24.

52. Stankiewicz JA, Chow JM. The low skull base: an invitation to disaster. Am J Rhinol 2004;18:35–40.

53. Rudmik L, Smith TL. Evaluation of the ethmoid skull base height prior to endoscopic sinus surgery: a preoperative CT evaluation technique. Int Forum Allergy Rhinol 2012;2(2):151–4.

54. Weinberger DG, Anand VK, Al-Rawi M, et al. Surgical anatomy and variations of the Onodi cell. Am J Rhinol 1996;10:1–6.

55. Elwany S, Elsaeid I, Thabet H. Endoscopic anatomy of the sphenoid sinus. J Laryngol Otol 1999;113(2):122–6.

56. Wang J, Bidari S, Inoue K, et al. Extensions of the sphenoid sinus: a new classification. Neurosurgery 2010;66(4):797–816.

57. Maniscalo JE, Habal MB. Microanatomy of the optic canal. J Neurosurg 1978;48:402–6.

58. DeLano MC, Fun FY, Zinreich SJ. Relationship of the optic nerve to the posterior paranasal sinuses: a CT anatomic study. Am J Neuroradiol 1996;17(4):669–75.

59. Osborn AG. The vidian artery: normal and pathologic anatomy. Radiology 1980;136(2):373–8.

60. Liu SC, Wang HW, Kao HL, et al. Three-dimensional bone CT reconstruction anatomy of the vidian canal. Rhinology 2013;51(4):306–14.

Imaging in Sinonasal Inflammatory Disease

Varsha M. Joshi, DNB, DMRD[a,b,*], Rima Sansi, DNB[a]

KEYWORDS

- Inflammatory sinonasal disease • CT • MR imaging

KEY POINTS

- Noncontrast, multiplanar, high-resolution, thin-section CT is the accepted gold standard for imaging sinonasal inflammatory disease.
- MR imaging is preferred to assess intraorbital and intracranial complications, and is not suitable as the first or sole investigation in patients with inflammatory rhinosinusitis.
- The nature of sinonasal secretions on CT and MRI and the pattern of bone changes on CT offer important information about the disease.
- Patterns of inflammatory rhinosinusitis described at CT have a bearing on the prognosis, choice of treatment options, and therapeutic outcomes for the patients.
- A pre-FESS CT report should describe the disease and address all concerns of the endoscopic surgeon, delineating pertinent anatomy, variants and critical relationships.

INTRODUCTION

Rhinosinusitis constitutes a fairly large public health problem across the globe. Chronic rhinosinusitis (CRS) affects about 12% to 16% of the US population and is one of the commonest chronic illnesses in America.[1,2] According to the statistics from the National Institute of Allergy and Infectious diseases (NIAID), about 1 in 8 Indians have this disorder.[3]

Sinusitis, in its simplest definition, means inflammation of the sinus mucosa. It is almost always accompanied by inflammation of the nasal mucosa or rhinitis. Hence, the term rhinosinusitis is used by most otolaryngologists.[4,5] Sinusitis can be viral, bacterial, allergic, vasomotor, or reactive in nature. Four basic forms are described based on the duration of symptoms:

1. Acute sinusitis: symptoms present for 4 weeks or less

2. Subacute sinusitis: continuation of the acute process and lasts anywhere between 4 and 12 weeks
3. Chronic sinusitis: persistence of the symptoms for 12 weeks or beyond
4. Recurrent acute sinusitis: occurrence of more than 4 episodes of acute sinusitis in 1 year with resolution of symptoms between the episodes

MUCOCILIARY CLEARANCE AND PATHOPHYSIOLOGY OF SINUSITIS

The paranasal sinuses are covered by mucous-secreting ciliated columnar epithelium. The cilia move continuously to propel the mucous toward the sinus ostium, the nasal cavity, and finally into the pharynx, constituting mucociliary clearance of the sinonasal cavities. This pattern of mucociliary flow is specific for each sinus and continues even if alternative openings or ostia are created

Disclosures: None.
[a] Department of CT and MRI, Vijaya Diagnostics, Hyderabad, Telangana 500034, India; [b] Visiting Consultant, Department of Imaging Tata Medical Center, Kolkata, India
* Corresponding author.
E-mail address: drjoshivarsha@gmail.com

Neuroimag Clin N Am 25 (2015) 549–568
http://dx.doi.org/10.1016/j.nic.2015.07.003
1052-5149/15/$ – see front matter © 2015 Elsevier Inc. All rights reserved.

in the sinus.[6-8] Any disturbance in this mucociliary clearance causes stagnation of secretions, secondary infection, and subsequent sinusitis. Sinus ostial obstruction causing disruption of the mucociliary flow accounts for majority of the cases of recurrent or chronic inflammatory sinusitis.[9] Commonest cause of acute sinusitis is an upper respiratory viral infection. Mucosal congestion causes apposition of the mucosal surfaces of the sinus ostia and drainage pathways, disturbing the mucociliary clearance and predisposing the sinus to secondary bacterial infection. Symptoms may resolve in about a week or may progress to subacute sinusitis. Although most cases may resolve with conservative treatment, about one-third of patients remain refractory to treatment and progress to chronic or recurrent rhinosinusitis.[9]

INDICATIONS FOR IMAGING

Sinusitis is largely a clinical diagnosis. Imaging is neither recommended nor performed for every patient who presents with sinusitis. The 1997 Task Force on Rhinosinusitis of the American Academy of Otolaryngology - Head and Neck Surgery recommended diagnosing acute rhinosinusitis (ARS) based on major and minor criteria that were further reviewed and simplified in 2007.[10,11] The American College of Radiology has also laid down appropriateness criteria for imaging in sinonasal inflammatory disease.[12] **Table 1** briefly summarizes the indications for imaging in patients with sinusitis.

IMAGING OPTIONS AND PROTOCOLS

With the developments in endoscopic sinus surgery, there has been a parallel supportive evolution in imaging technology and trends with a gradual but definite shift from the use of plain radiography toward CT for evaluating rhinosinusitis. CT has replaced plain radiography because of its greater precision in depicting sinonasal anatomy and pathology. A brief summary on the use of plain radiography, CT, and MR imaging in the evaluation of inflammatory sinonasal disease is provided in Tables 2–4.

IMAGING APPEARANCES
Acute Sinusitis

CT and MR imaging features include nonspecific mucosal thickening, submucosal edema, air-fluid levels, or sinus secretions interspersed with air bubbles (**Fig. 2**).[13-15] Acute sinonasal secretions are predominantly water and of a mucoid nature (-10 to 25 HU) on CT. They are hypointense on T1 and hyperintense on T2 sequences. An isolated air-fluid level as the only finding in the sinus is fairly characteristic for acute sinusitis, but may not be seen in all patients.[9] The distribution of disease on CT may provide a clue to the cause of the acute

Table 1
Sinusitis: Indications for imaging

Indication	Recommended Imaging Option
Acute sinusitis	Generally a clinical diagnosis; imaging adds little valuable information
Complicated acute sinusitis	Noncontrast and contrast CT or MR imaging of the paranasal sinuses including orbits and brain
Chronic sinusitis[a]	Noncontrast CT
Recurrent sinusitis[a]	Noncontrast CT

[a] Patients with symptoms of recurrent or chronic sinusitis and those who do not respond to medical treatment generally undergo intranasal endoscopy. A CT scan is requested when medical therapy fails or intranasal endoscopy suggests surgically correctable causes.[13,14]

Table 2
Imaging options for sinusitis: Plain radiography

Feature	Comment
Status	Almost obsolete
Advantages	• Low cost • Easy availability • Portability • Air-fluid levels • Low radiation dose
Concerns	• Superimposition of structures • Suboptimal delineation of the anatomy and pathology • High false-negatives
Patient preparation	None Sitting position preferred for depiction of air-fluid levels
Protocol	• Water's view • Caldwell's view • Submentomaxillary view • Lateral view

Data from Refs.[13-15]

Table 3
Imaging options for sinusitis: CT

Feature	Comments
Status	• Gold standard and primary imaging tool for recurrent and chronic rhinosinusitis • Contrast CT for complicated acute sinusitis
Advantages	• Superb delineation of sinonasal anatomy and variants • Excellent depiction of sinonasal relationships with critical regional neurovascular structures • Optimal characterization of the location, extent of disease, nature of secretions, patterns of bony changes, and intrasinus calcifications • Easy differentiation of air, dessicated secretions, and calcifications, all of which appear the same on MR imaging • Addresses all the concerns of the endoscopic surgeon • More economical than an MR imaging study
Concerns	• Differentiation from fungal infections and neoplasms can be challenging • Radiation dose to the ocular lens and thyroid gland are perhaps the major concern. However, a single-scan dose from sinonasal CT varies between 1.88 and 64 mGy and this is much lower than the threshold for damage to the lens, which ranges between 0.5 and 2 Gy. Moreover, newer multidetector CT scanners allow use of low-dose CT (20 mAs), which offers radiation doses equivalent to plain radiographs without any compromise of the image quality.[19–26] There is no clear described threshold for thyroid damage, however a single-scan dose is not considered to increase the risk of thyroid cancer[27]
Patient preparation	Considered important in eliminating reversible disease and allows better delineation of the anatomy and pathology.[16,17] These include • Resolution of symptoms of acute disease • Completion of course of antibiotics • Instillation of nasal decongestants 15 min before the scan and nasal blowing However, some studies have shown that these techniques may offer only a small reduction in mucosal thickening and hence have a limited effect on the outcome of CT[28]
Protocol	• Multidetector CT scan with multiplanar reformations preferred. Scan is performed in the axial plane with patient supine on the CT table and a neutral position of the gantry. Direct coronal acquisition is no longer performed routinely • 0.625 mm collimation, field of view of 180 mm • Multiplanar reformations are obtained from the dataset in the coronal, axial and sagittal planes. Coronal images are most preferred by the endoscopic surgeons as they simulate the appearance of sinonasal cavities at endoscopy • 0.9-mm-thick images are reconstructed in bone and soft tissue algorithms • Images are displayed at a window width of about 1500 and center of 150, that delineate the bony anatomy and inflammatory disease. Narrow windowing in the soft tissue algorithm helps with better assessment of the nature of sinonasal secretions[29] (see **Fig. 1**)

Data from Refs.[13–29]

disease. Allergic sinusitis is generally more diffuse and bacterial sinusitis is often fairly localized or asymmetric.[31]

Chronic Sinusitis

Imaging features include mucosal thickening, sinus opacification, sclerosis of the bony walls of the sinus, and intrasinus calcifications.[9,13] Air-fluid levels may be seen superimposed on chronic sinusitis (**Fig. 3**). Retention cysts, polyps, polyposis, and mucoceles may be seen as sequelae to chronic sinusitis.

Mucosal thickening
Normal mucosa is generally not seen at CT or MR imaging, and whenever sinus mucosa is seen at the interface between air and bone, that mucosa is presumed to be thickened.[9] Mucosal thickening may be smooth, irregular, or polypoid in morphology. MR is more sensitive to mucosal thickening than CT and depicts the thickened

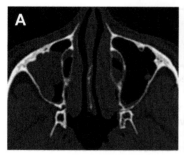 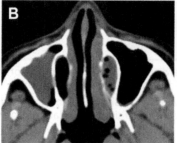 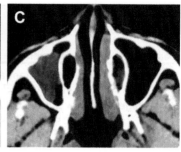

Fig. 1. Axial CT images in bone (A) and soft tissue (B) algorithms. The bone algorithm image in a wide window nicely depicts the bony anatomy and mucosal disease in the right maxillary sinus. Minimal mucosal disease is also seen in the left maxillary sinus. (B) The adjacent soft tissue anatomy is shown well but is suboptimal to assess the bones that appear thickened on such images. The narrow window in the soft tissue algorithm in (C) shows the mucoid density of the disease. The left maxillary sinus disease is not seen well in this image.

mucosa as a hyperintense signal on T2 images against the black background of sinus air and bone (Fig. 4).[13] In the maxillary sinuses, up to 3 mm mucosal thickening may be seen in healthy individuals and considered normal; any thickening in the frontal and sphenoid sinuses is always considered abnormal and is most likely to be symptomatic. In the ethmoid sinuses, mucosal thickening of up to 2 mm may be attributed to the physiologic phenomenon of the nasal cycle if there is coexistent mucosal swelling of the ipsilateral nasal cavity with prominence of the ipsilateral nasal turbinates (Fig. 5).[32,33]

Bone changes
The presence of a sclerotic thickened bone is a fairly characteristic feature of chronic sinusitis but may

not be seen in all patients.[9,34] Sclerosis of the bony walls of the sinuses reflects the chronic nature of the disease process (Fig. 6). However, with progressive obstruction and chronicity, there may eventually be gradual pressure erosion and deossification of the marginal bone that is more commonly seen with mucoceles and polyps (see Fig. 19).

Secretions and opacification
The density of the secretions at CT and their signal intensity on MR imaging is largely dependent on the proportion of proteins in the secretions.[9] With chronic obstruction, there is a gradual increase in the protein content of the secretions and the thin watery secretions become progressively more viscous and thick. This is seen as a progressive increase in the density of the secretions on CT and

Table 4	
Imaging options for sinusitis: MR imaging	
Feature	**Comment**
Status	Complementary role in assessment of complicated sinusitis when it is preferred over contrast CT.[30] Not preferred for primary evaluation or as a sole imaging tool for inflammatory sinonasal disease
Advantages	• No radiation • Superb soft tissue resolution • Assessment of intraorbital/intracranial complications is superior to CT
Concerns	• Longer scanning time • Suboptimal delineation of the intricate sinonasal anatomy compared with CT • Normal air, chronic dessicated secretions, and calcifications mimic each other appearing as signal voids, leading to diagnostic errors
Patient preparation	• None
Protocol	• Head coil • 3 or 4 mm T1-weighted and T2-weighted sequences in coronal and axial planes. Contrast T1-weighted sequences with fat suppression in coronal and axial planes. Sagittal images whenever required • Include the adjacent orbits and intracranial cavity along with the sinuses

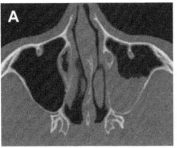
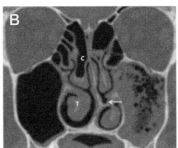
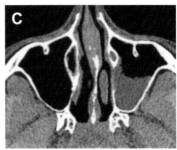

Fig. 2. Axial CT image (*A*) shows the air-fluid level in the left maxillary sinus with overlying air bubbles that are seen better in the coronal CT image (*B*). Nasal septal deviation to left side (*white arrow*), right concha bullosa (*C*), enlarged right inferior turbinate (T). The narrow window in (*C*) depicts the mucoid density of the secretions.

the chronic inspissated secretions are hyperdense on CT. A thin hypodense line is usually seen separating the dense sinus secretions from the bony wall and represents the thickened mucosa and submucosal edema (**Fig. 7**). On MR imaging, various combinations of signal intensities on T1 and T2 images have been described with increasing protein concentration of the secretions (see **Fig. 7**; **Figs. 8** and **9**).[9,13,35,36] These are tabulated in **Table 5**. On contrast administration, if the thickened mucosa does not enhance, it is probably not actively infected and is fibrotic and scarred. Active infection has a thin zone of mucosal enhancement with a zone of submucosal edema separating this mucosa from the bony wall (**Fig. 10**).

Calcifications
Calcifications are uncommon in CRS and, when seen, are more peripheral and scattered.[37] Yoon and colleagues[37] found that round or egg-shell calcifications are more common in patients with chronic inflammatory rhinosinusitis (see **Fig. 7A**).

Sequelae or Local Complications with Chronic Sinusitis

Retention cyst
Retention cyst is the most common finding in patients with chronic sinusitis and is also seen as an incidental finding in the general population. Two forms of retention cysts have been described: serous and mucous retention cysts; the mucous variety is more common. Mucous retention cysts are formed as a result of obstruction of a submucous mucinous gland and serous cysts occur as a result of accumulation of fluid in the submucosal layer of the sinus mucosa.[9] They are most commonly found in the maxillary sinuses. Both forms cannot be distinguished from one another and are seen as mucoid, low-density, well-defined, outwardly convex lesions on CT, with

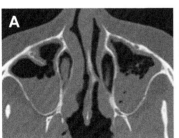
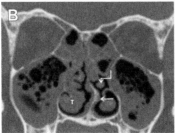
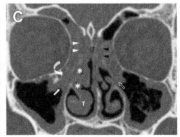

Fig. 3. Axial (*A*) coronal (*B, C*) CT images show air-fluid levels, air bubbles, and mucosal disease in the maxillary sinuses. (*B*) Opacification of anterior ethmoid air cells, nasal septal deviation (*white arrow*), paradoxic curvature of the left middle turbinate (*elbow arrow*), and mildly enlarged right inferior turbinate (T) are seen. (*C*) Opacified Haller cell (*curved white arrow*), right maxillary ostium and infundibulum (*thick white arrow*), middle meatus (*white asterisks*), and frontal recess (*white arrowheads*) indicate the OMU pattern of chronic sinusitis. Infundibular narrowing (*white outlined arrow*) and frontal recess disease (*black arrowheads*) seen on the left side with patent left middle meatus.

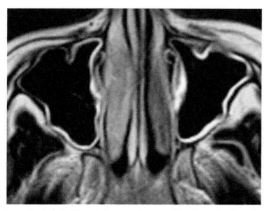

Fig. 4. Axial T2 MR image in a patient with chronic headache shows a thin rim of hyperintense mucosal thickening along the walls of the maxillary sinuses.

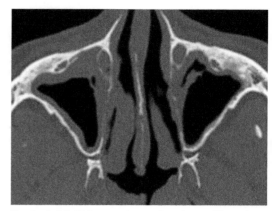

Fig. 6. Axial CT image shows chronic maxillary sinusitis with mucosal disease bordering the thickened sclerotic walls.

low signal on T1-weighted images and high signal on T2-weighted MR imaging sequences (Fig. 11).

Polyp

Polyps are the commonest expansile inflammatory masses in the sinuses and may be solitary or multiple (see Fig. 11; Fig. 12). They are generally small, but may grow and become very deforming with pressure erosion and deossification of the bony walls of the sinuses. They result from accumulation of fluid in the deeper lamina propria of the sinus mucosa. Larger polyps are seen as expansile masses with areas of high attenuation caused by chronic secretions in a background of mucoid matrix. They are generally separated from the adjacent bones by a thin zone of mucoid material and when they do extend into the orbit or

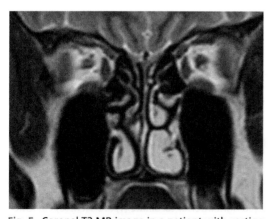

Fig. 5. Coronal T2 MR image in a patient with vertigo shows prominence of the left middle and inferior turbinates without nasal septal deviation or sinonasal disease; likely attributable to the nasal cycle.

the cranial cavity, they regain their outwardly convex polypoid shape (Fig. 13).[38] Polyposis is often associated with a superadded noninvasive fungal infection. An antrochoanal polyp is usually unilateral, solitary, and seen in young adults. It is a large polyp in the maxillary sinus that expands and fills the antrum, prolapses through and widens the primary or accessory ostium into the nasal cavity. It fills the nasal cavity and extends behind into the nasopharynx (Fig. 14).[39,40] Ethmochoanal and sphenochoanal polyps are rare (Fig. 15).[41] Polyps and cysts cannot be differentiated on CT or MR imaging, however it is of little consequence as they are both treated in the same manner.

Mucocele

Mucocele is the commonest expansile lesion of the paranasal sinuses, most commonly seen in the frontal sinus (60%), followed by ethmoid air cells (25%), and the maxillary sinuses (10%). It rarely develops in the sphenoid sinus. Mucocele forms as a result of obstruction of a sinus ostium or a compartment of a septate sinus and hence is lined by the sinus mucosa. CT shows an expanded airless sinus cavity with bony remodeling of the sinus walls filled with fairly homogeneous mucoid attenuation. The sinus cavity must be expanded to make the diagnosis of a mucocele (Figs. 16 and 17). When the sinus is not expanded, it is called obstructed sinus (Fig. 18).[9] At first, the sinus cavity expands and results in remodeled intact surrounding bone. However, with continued obstruction, the sinus cavity may balloon and the walls may show deossification (Fig. 19). The imaging appearance of the secretions is again largely dependent on the protein content as described earlier. Mucoceles can occur in an Onodi cell,

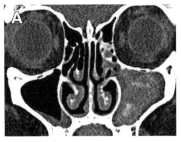
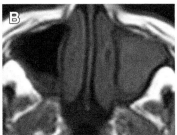
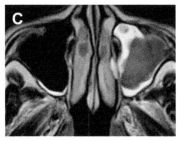

Fig. 7. Coronal CT image (A) shows hyperdense secretions and scattered calcifications in the left maxillary sinus with a peripheral hypodense rim. The secretions are hyperintense on axial T1 MR images and hypointense on T2 MR images (B, C). Minimal mucosal disease seen in right maxillary sinus.

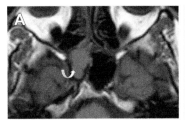
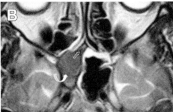
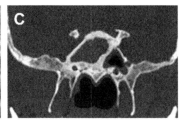

Fig. 8. Axial T1 MR image (A) shows hyperintense signal in the right sphenoid sinus that is hypointense on the T2 image in (B) (white curved arrow). The outlined white arrow points to the sphenoid sinus ostium in (B). Coronal CT image in (C) shows thickening of the walls of the right sphenoid sinus. Chronic sphenoid sinusitis with chronic inspissated secretions.

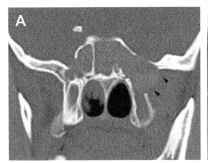
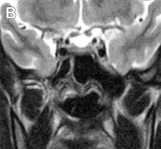
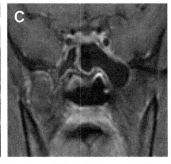

Fig. 9. Coronal CT image (A) shows opacified sphenoid sinuses with marked thinning of the left sinus wall (black arrowheads). T2 MR image (B) and contrast T1 image (C) show a signal void in the sinus with enhancing peripheral sinus mucosa in (C). Chronic sphenoid sinusitis with inspissated secretions mimicking normal sinus on MR imaging.

| Table 5 | | |
| Sinonasal secretions at MR imaging | | |
Protein Content	T1 Images	T2 Images
Up to 5%	Hypointense	Hyperintense
5%–25%	Hyperintense	Hyperintense
25%–30%	Hyperintense	Hypointense (see Figs. 7 and 8)
30%–35%[a]	Hypointense	Hypointense
>35%[a]	Signal void	Signal void (see Fig. 9)

[a] These chronically dessicated secretions can be easily misinterpreted as normal aerated sinuses on MR imaging, but CT allows easy identification because of their hyperdense attenuation (see Fig. 9).

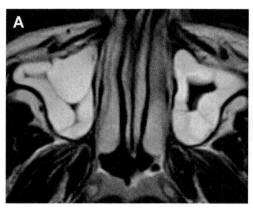
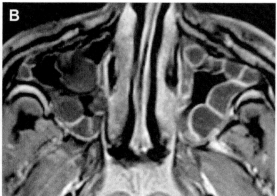

Fig. 10. Axial T2 image (*A*) shows polypoid mucosal disease with submucosal edema underlying the thin mucosa in both maxillary sinuses. Contrast T1 image (*B*) shows mucosal enhancement outlining the nonenhancing submucosal edema suggesting active infection.

pneumatized anterior clinoid process, and a concha bullosa (**Fig. 20**).

Staging of Chronic Rhinosinusitis

Box 1 provides the modified Lund-Mackay system; it is the easiest to use and well accepted compared with the other proposed staging systems.[42,43] The score calculated from this system has been found to correlate well with other markers of disease severity, the nature of surgery offered, and its outcome.[44]

Complications of Sinusitis

The common complications that arise from sinusitis are broadly grouped into intraorbital and intracranial forms and are listed in **Box 2**. MR imaging is superior to CT in assessment of such complications.[30,45] Orbital complications are commonly seen with frontal or ethmoid sinusitis. Orbital cellulitis is well seen with CT and MR imaging. Evaluation of the orbital apex, superior ophthalmic vein, and the cavernous sinus thrombosis is better achieved with contrast-enhanced fat-suppressed T1 images. Orbital abscesses are typically seen as rim-enhancing collections especially along the medial wall or the roof of the orbit. Intracranial abscesses as a complication of

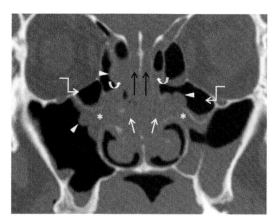

Fig. 12. Coronal CT image shows multiple polypoid masses (*white arrowheads*) filling the ethmoid sinuses, nasal vault, frontal recesses (*curved white arrows*), infundibula (*white asterisks*), middle meati (*straight white arrows*) bilaterally, with a widened gap between vertical attachment of the middle turbinate and the nasal septum (*straight black arrows*). Haller cells (*white elbow arrows*) and intrasinus septum in the left maxillary sinus with partial opacification of the sinus are noted. OMU pattern of sinusitis.

Fig. 11. Coronal CT image shows retention cysts/polyps in both maxillary sinuses. Minimal mucosal disease noted along the roof of the right maxillary sinus. Haller cells (*white arrowhead*), pneumatized uncinate (*elbow arrow*), lamellar concha (*straight white arrow*). Enlarged left inferior turbinate.

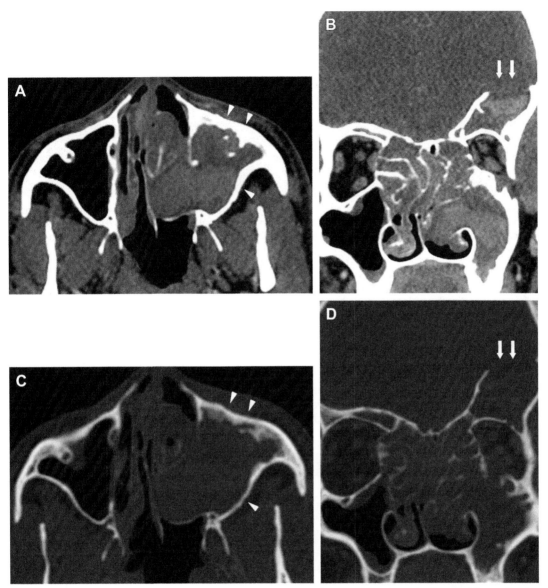

Fig. 13. Axial (*A*) and coronal (*B*) CT images show polyposis with expansile masses and central hyperdensities filling the maxillary and ethmoid sinuses and nasal cavity, extending intracranially (*thick white arrows*) with upward convex contour. (*C, D*) show sclerosis of maxillary sinus walls (*white arrowheads*) with deossification of the ethmoid trabeculae. Outward expansion and erosion of the roof of the fronto-ethmoid sinuses (*thick white arrows*) and the lamina papyracea noted.

sinusitis are infrequent and when seen, develop as a sequelae to frontal sinusitis especially in children (**Fig. 21**).

Patterns of Sinonasal Inflammatory Disease

Sinonasal inflammatory disease has been categorized into 5 patterns for better understanding, interpretation, prognostication, and grouping of patients into nonsurgical (normal CT), routine surgical (I and II), and complex surgical groups (III and IV).[46,47] Groups I–III are the obstructive

patterns and are based on the major routes of mucociliary drainage described previously. While reading sinonasal CT scans, the interpreting radiologist must try and categorize the inflammatory disease process into 1 of these patterns.

Pattern 1: infundibular pattern
The level of obstruction is at the maxillary sinus ostium and inferior infundibulum with the disease limited to the ipsilateral maxillary sinus only (**Fig. 22**). Common causes of such obstruction include mucosal swelling, polyps, anatomic

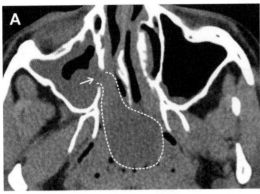

Fig. 14. Axial CT image (*A*) shows a right antrochoanal polyp (*dashed white line*) prolapsing through the accessory ostium of the right maxillary sinus (*straight white arrow*). Coronal CT image (*B*) shows the polyp widening the accessory ostium (*straight white arrow*). The curved white arrow shows the normal accessory ostium of the left maxillary sinus.

variants such as Haller cells, enlarged ethmoid bulla, pneumatized uncinate, and hypoplastic maxillary sinuses.[24] This type of disease requires the least amount of endoscopic intervention and is associated with low recurrence rates.[48]

Pattern II: osteomeatal unit pattern

The level of obstruction is at the middle meatus. Depending on the amount of obstruction in various components of the osteomeatal unit (OMU), the disease may involve some or all of the ipsilateral maxillary, frontal, and anterior ethmoid air cells (see **Fig. 12**; **Fig. 23**). The frontal recess pattern is a limited form of OMU pattern that is seen when the disease is limited to the frontal sinus, as a result of obstruction of the frontal recess draining in the anterior aspect of the middle meatus. OMU opacification correlates well with the development of sinusitis. Yousem and colleagues[49] found that the specificity of middle meatus opacification for maxillary or ethmoid sinus disease was 93%. Conversely, isolated OMU disease without maxillary, ethmoid, or frontal disease is uncommon.[50] Common causes of OMU obstruction include mucosal swelling, hypertrophied turbinates, polyps, adhesions, anatomic variants such as concha bullosa, paradoxic middle turbinates, and nasal septal deviation.[50,51] This type of disease pattern requires more extensive surgery and is associated with higher recurrence rates compared with the infundibular pattern.[48]

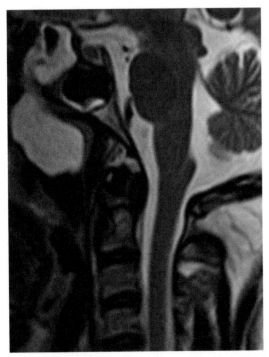

Fig. 15. Sagittal T2 MR image shows an ethmochoanal polyp reaching the nasopharynx. Mucosal disease noted in the sphenoid sinus.

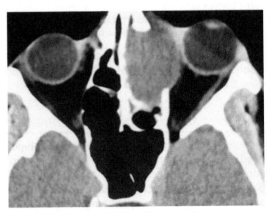

Fig. 16. Left anterior ethmoid mucocele.

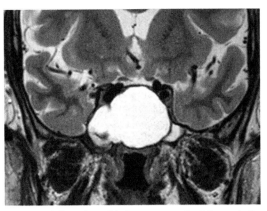

Fig. 17. Right sphenoid sinus mucocele. Mucosal disease noted in the left sphenoid sinus.

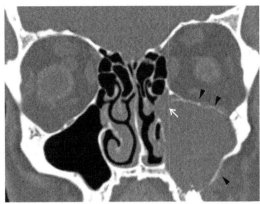

Fig. 19. Coronal CT image shows mucocele in the septate compartment of the left maxillary sinus. The opacified sinus is expanded with thinning of the walls (*black arrowheads*). Thin bony septum is seen toward the sinus ostium (*straight white arrow*).

Pattern III: spheno-ethmoid recess pattern

The obstruction is at the spheno-ethmoid recess (SER) causing inflammatory disease limited to the sphenoid sinus and the posterior ethmoid air cells. Isolated sphenoid disease, without posterior ethmoid sinus disease, can be seen in the SER pattern because the sphenoid sinus drains directly into the SER and the posterior ethmoid initially drains more anteriorly into the superior meatus (**Fig. 24**). Surgery is more difficult and treatment failures and complications are higher.[52]

Pattern IV: sinonasal polyposis

This pattern of disease is characterized by polyps diffusely present within the nasal cavity and paranasal sinuses, filling the nasal vault and sinuses, causing bilateral infundibular enlargement, convex (bulging) ethmoid sinus walls, and attenuation of the bony nasal septum and ethmoid trabeculae (**Fig. 25**). Truncation of the bulbous portion of the middle turbinates may be seen.[53] Polyposis often shows the presence of central areas of hyperdensity as a result of inspissated secretions against a background of mucoid matrix. Isolated polyps are not included in this disease pattern. The disease is generally treated medically and surgery is offered for medically refractory cases. Surgery is more extensive and difficult with higher rates of recurrence and treatment failure.[48]

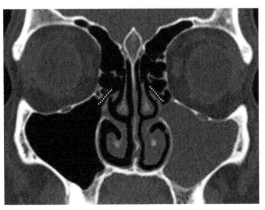

Fig. 18. Coronal CT image shows completely opacified left maxillary sinus caused by ostial obstruction without sinus expansion. The dotted lines show normal infundibulum on both sides. Obstructed sinus.

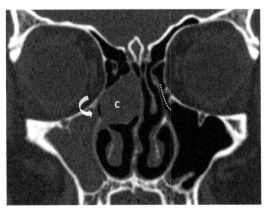

Fig. 20. Coronal CT image shows mucocele of the right concha bullosa (C) obstructing the right infundibulum (*curved white arrow*) and disease in the right maxillary sinus. Normal left infundibulum (*dotted line*).

Box 1

Staging of chronic sinusitis: modified Lund-Mackay system

Sinus

0 – normal

1 – partial opacification

2 – total opacification

OMC

0 – no obstruction

2 – obstructed

Normal variants

0 – absent

1 – present

Absent frontal sinus

Concha bullosa

Paradoxic middle turbinate

Haller cells

Everted uncinate process

Agger nasi cell pneumatization

Pattern V: sporadic pattern

The sporadic pattern is diagnosed when inflammatory sinonasal disease is not attributable to obstruction of known mucous drainage routes or polyposis and there is randomly placed disease noted anywhere within the sinuses. This group includes individual inflammatory lesions such as retention cysts and mucoceles.

Box 2

Complications of sinusitis

Orbital complications

Orbital cellulitis

Subperiosteal abscess

Superior ophthalmic vein thrombosis

Intracranial complications

Cavernous sinus thrombosis

Meningitis

Epidural abscess

Subdural abscess

Cerebritis

Cerebral abscess

Silent Sinus Syndrome

Silent sinus syndrome is a unilateral atelectasis of the maxillary sinus caused by negative pressure within the sinus consequent to chronic occlusion of the sinus ostium, seen in the adult population. There is complete resorption of the sinus air with near complete opacification of the sinus. The sinus wall eventually collapses. Although most cases are idiopathic, trauma to the lateral nasal wall may be the cause in some patients. History of previous chronic maxillary sinusitis is obtained in only about 36% of patients.[29] The primary imaging finding is reduced caliber of a fully formed maxillary sinus caused by inward retraction of the sinus walls, occlusion of the maxillary ostium and infundibulum, sinus opacification, and reactive osteitis of the sinus walls (Fig. 26).[54,55] The orbital floor is almost always retracted downward and patients present generally with enophthalmos.

Atrophic Rhinosinusitis

Atrophic rhinosinusitis is a fairly common, although often underdiagnosed form of chronic sinusitis. The normal ciliated sinonasal epithelium is replaced by nonciliated epithelium. Two forms are described: primary and secondary. The primary form is seen in young adults from developing countries; the secondary form is more common and associated with previous nasal injury, surgery, or inflammation. Nasal and paranasal mucosal thickening, small inferior and middle turbinates with atrophic mucosa, widened sinonasal passages, and partial or total bony erosion are seen.[29,56]

SINONASAL INFLAMMATION IN SYSTEMIC DISEASES

CRS is described as a part of many systemic diseases such as Wegener granulomatosis, sarcoidosis, cystic fibrosis, and various other syndromes including immotile cilia syndrome, primary ciliary dyskinesia, Young syndrome, Yellow Nail syndrome, Wiskot Aldrich syndrome, Sertoli cell only syndrome, Churg Strauss disease, and so forth.[57] The imaging findings in most cases are nonspecific and a complete clinical, laboratory, and imaging work-up may be necessary for an accurate diagnosis.

Imaging findings described in Wegener granulomatosis include nonspecific mucosal thickening, sinus opacification, granulomas that show low signal on T1-weighted sequences and intermediate to high signal on T2-weighted sequences, and bony erosions mainly involving the septum, turbinates, and medial walls of the maxillary

---

Box 3
Pearls and pitfalls

- Sinonasal CT interpretation is best done by viewing interactive multiplanar reformations on the workstation
- Disease extent should be mapped with the intermediate or wide window technique on CT; the narrow window should be used for assessing the nature of the secretions
- Persistent unilateral sinus opacification, extrasinus disease, bone erosion should alert the radiologist to noninflammatory causes of sinonasal disease
- Hyperdensity on CT is seen in chronic rhinosinusitis with inspissated secretions, chronic fungal disease, and intrasinus hemorrhage; although intrasinus hemorrhage can be reliably excluded based on the clinical history, differentiation of CRS from fungal infection is extremely difficult on CT and MR imaging in the absence of bony erosion
- Hyperdensity on CT and hypointense signal on T2 images suggest concern for fungal infection or chronic sinusitis with inspissated secretions; these features almost completely exclude a sinonasal tumor
- MR imaging should not be used as the first or the sole imaging tool for evaluation of inflammatory sinonasal disease; chronic dessicated secretions and fungal infection show low signal on T1 and T2 images and eventually appear as signal voids leading to serious diagnostic errors when they are interpreted as normal aerated sinuses
- On MR imaging, if a contrast study is performed, a noncontrast T1 sequence should be obtained; without such a sequence, apparent enhancement cannot be distinguished from T1 high-signal lesions.

---

sinuses followed by sclerosing osteitis of the sinus wall.[58,59] A characteristic finding described in cystic fibrosis is medial bulging of the lateral nasal walls and bilateral maxillary pyoceles.[60] The medial maxillary sinus wall may reach the nasal septum and obstruct the nasal cavities. The secretions show a high signal on T1 images and a low signal on T2 images.[61]

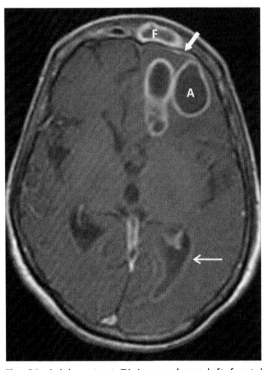

Fig. 21. Axial contrast T1 image shows left frontal sinusitis with enhancing mucosa (F), thin leptomeningeal enhancement (*thick white arrow*), lateral ventricular ependymal enhancement (*straight white arrow*), and ring-enhancing abscesses (A) in the left frontal lobe. Frontal sinusitis with meningitis and frontal lobe abscesses. (*Courtesy of* Dr V.S.V. Rammohan, Hyderabad, India.)

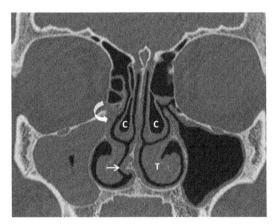

Fig. 22. Coronal CT image shows obstruction at the right infundibulum (*curved white arrow*) and opacified right maxillary sinus. Nasal septal deviation to the right side (*straight white arrow*), bilateral concha bullosa (C), mildly enlarged left inferior turbinate (T). Infundibular pattern of sinusitis.

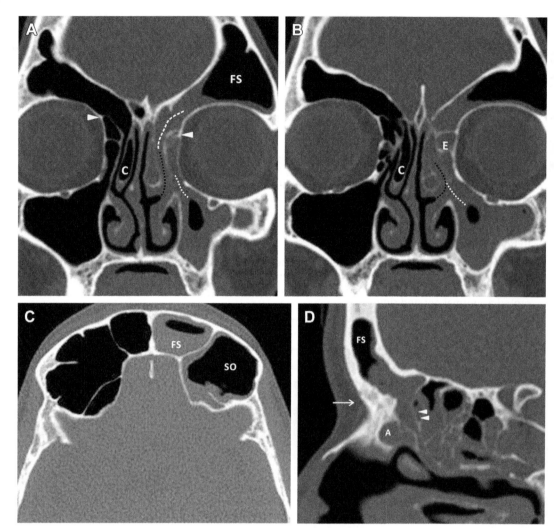

Fig. 23. Coronal CT images (*A*, *B*) show mucosal disease in the left infundibulum (*dotted white line*), frontal recess (*dashed white line*), middle meatus (*dotted black line*), opacified left frontal sinus (FS), anterior ethmoid air cells (*E*), and maxillary sinus. Opacified concha bullosa (C) is seen on the left side. Type II uncinate (*white arrowhead*) with frontal recess opening into the middle meati bilaterally. (*C*) shows disease in the left frontal sinus (FS) and left supraorbital cell (SO). Sagittal CT image (*D*) shows disease in the frontal sinus (FS), frontal sinus ostium, and frontal recess (*white arrowheads*), and agger nasi cell (A). OMU pattern of sinusitis.

DIFFERENTIAL DIAGNOSIS

The most important condition that inflammatory rhinosinusitis needs to be differentiated from is fungal infection. When evaluating sinonasal CT scans, persistent unilateral opacification is one important sign that should alert the radiologist to the possibility of an alternate diagnosis of a fungal or neoplastic nature of the disease process.

Differentiation of acute inflammatory sinusitis from an acute invasive fungal sinusitis (AIFS) is of paramount importance because of the highly aggressive and fulminant nature of the latter. It is

almost impossible to distinguish the two forms, but imaging features of early extrasinus spread into the periantral region and the orbital fat across normal-appearing sinus walls in an immunosompromised or a patient with uncontrolled diabetes serve as useful pointers for the diagnosis of AIFS.[62] Chronic fungal sinusitis and mycetoma are hyperdense on CT and show a dark signal on T2-weighted MR images, closely mimicking the imaging appearances of chronic sinusitis with dessicated secretions (**Fig. 27**).[63,64] At the present time, it is extremely difficult to differentiate the two conditions on CT or MR imaging with or

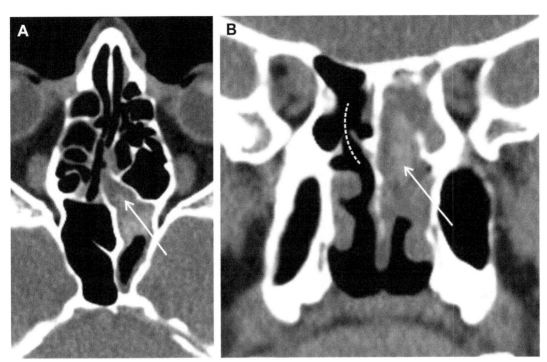

Fig. 24. Axial (A) and coronal (B) CT images with the soft tissue algorithm show polyposis in the left sphenoid sinus with widening of the sphenoid sinus ostium (*dashed line*) and the spheno-ethmoid recess (*white arrow*). SER pattern of sinusitis.

without contrast. Irregular bone erosion on CT is perhaps the only imaging sign that may help in the diagnosis of fungal infection.[65]

Diagnosis and evaluation of sinonasal neoplasms requires a contrast study, preferably a contrast MR imaging. Malignant sinonasal tumors are isodense to muscle on CT and show erosive destruction of the sinus walls unlike the hyperdensity and sclerosis seen with chronic sinusitis or smooth pressure erosion seen with mucoid masses such as polyps and mucoceles.[38] On MR imaging, tumors show a hypointense signal on T1 images and an intermediate signal on T2 images that is always slightly brighter than the T1 signal (**Fig. 28**). CRS with inspissated secretions shows hypointense signal on T2 images that may fall below the T1 signal with progressing chronicity. Moreover, on contrast studies,

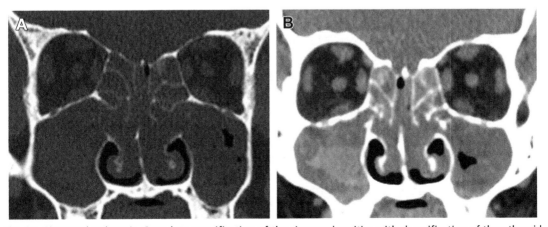

Fig. 25. Sinonasal polyposis. Complete opacification of the sinonasal cavities with deossification of the ethmoid trabeculae and widening of the ethmoid infundibuli and osteomeatal units noted on bone (A) and soft tissue (B) images.

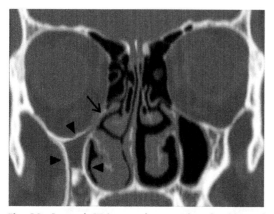

Fig. 26. Coronal CT image shows reduced caliber of the right maxillary sinus, thickened sinus walls, opacification of the sinus and the ethmoid infundibulum (*black arrow*), and inward retraction of the sinus walls (*black arrowheads*). Note the increased right orbital volume. Silent sinus syndrome.

inflammatory masses show peripheral rim enhancement of the surrounding mucosa, unlike tumors, which enhance completely as they arise from the mucosa itself.[66–68]

PEARLS AND PITFALLS

Box 3 provides a brief summary on important issues in sinonasal imaging, highlighting some pertinent pearls and pitfalls that the radiologist must be familiar with while interpreting sinonasal studies in day to day practice.

WHAT THE REFERRING CLINICIAN WANTS TO KNOW: PREPARING A CLINICALLY RELEVANT REPORT

A pre–functional endoscopic sinus surgery (FESS) CT report that is typically limited to describing the presence and extent of the disease process in the

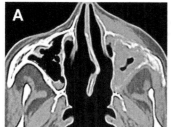
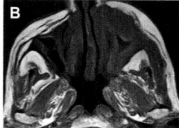
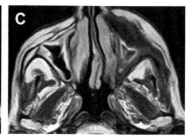

Fig. 27. Axial CT image (*A*) shows irregular thickening with intervening lysis of the left maxillary sinus walls and zygomatic arch with abnormal soft tissue thickening along the sinus walls and premaxillary and retroantral regions. The soft tissue is hypointense on the axial T1 MR image (*B*) with further lowering of the signal on the axial T2 image (*C*). Chronic invasive fungal sinusitis.

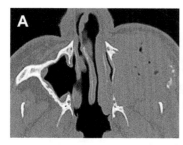
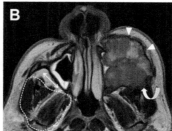
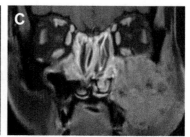

Fig. 28. Axial CT section in (*A*) shows significant destruction of the walls of the left maxillary sinus caused by a large soft tissue mass. Squamous cell carcinoma of the left maxillary sinus. Axial T2 image (*B*) shows an intermediate signal mass in the sinus extending into the periantral soft tissues (*white arrowheads*), retroantral fat, left masticator space (*curved white arrow*). Normal retroantral fat (*double-headed white arrow*) and masticator space (*dotted white line*) posterior to the right maxillary sinus. Contrast T1 image with fat suppression (*C*) shows minimal intraorbital extension and heterogeneous enhancement of the whole mass unlike the mucosal enhancement seen in inflammatory sinus disease (see **Fig. 10**B). Chronic right-sided maxillary sinusitis is seen.

Box 4
Recommended algorithm for systematic evaluation of pre-FESS noncontrast sinonasal CT

Step 1: Nasal cavity, lateral nasal wall, anterior skull base

- Nasal septal deviation
- Presence of septal spur
- Middle turbinate variations
  - ○ Concha bullosa
  - ○ Lamellar concha
  - ○ Paradoxic curvature
- Inferior turbinate
- Superior turbinate
- Uncinate process variations
  - ○ Medialized or lateralized
  - ○ Pneumatized uncinate
- Attachments of middle turbinate uncinate process (type I–III)
- Anterior skull base
  - ○ Depth of olfactory fossa (Kero's types)
  - ○ Canal for anterior ethmoid artery
  - ○ Dehiscence of cribriform plate
- Any dehiscence in lamina papyracea

Step 2: Sinuses and drainage pathways

Middle meatus and related anatomy

- Maxillary sinus
- Anterior ethmoid cells
- Maxillary sinus ostium
- Ethmoid infundibulum
- Ethmoid bulla
- Uncinate process
- Middle meatus
- Basal lamella
- Sinus lateralis
- Haller cells
- Infraorbital foramen

Frontal sinus and frontal sinus drainage pathway

- Frontal sinus
- Frontal ostium
- Frontal recess
- Frontal beak
- Agger nasi cell
- Frontal recess cells

- Frontal bullar cell
- Supraorbital cell

Spheno-ethmoid sinus-related anatomy

- Sphenoid sinus
- Posterior ethmoid cells
- Sphenoid sinus ostium
- Spheno-ethmoid recess
- Onodi cell
- Optic canal types
- Attachment of intersphenoid sinus septum to carotid canal

Step 3: Disease characterization

1. Description of the disease process: location and extent, CT attenuation of the secretions, pattern of bone changes
2. Diagnosis or diagnostic differentials, concern for possibility of a fungal or neoplastic nature
3. Status of visualized orbits and cranial cavity
4. Any further recommendations for contrast CT or MR imaging/tissue characterization if needed

sinuses almost always falls short of the endoscopic surgeon's expectations from this imaging study. It is important for the interpreting radiologist to be aware of the potential of this imaging tool; it extends beyond disease definition to provision of a precise presurgical anatomic roadmap delineating the important anatomy, anatomic variants, and relationships of the sinuses with critical neurovascular structures that have an important bearing on the surgery and surgical outcomes. Lack of attention or comment on the presence of certain important anatomic variants can influence the surgery and surgical outcomes.[69,70] A systematic approach to the interpretation of sinonasal CT is recommended; all the findings needs to be compiled to make a clinically relevant report that addresses all the concerns of the endoscopic surgeon that affect patient management (**Box 4**).

SUMMARY

CT is the accepted gold standard for evaluating inflammatory rhinosinusitis and is routinely ordered as a part of a pre-FESS work-up in patients with inflammatory rhinosinusitis. The manifestations of CRS are varied, but careful analysis of the imaging features on CT frequently enables a fairly accurate diagnosis. MR imaging is essentially a secondary tool and is used to evaluate complicated sinusitis or when there is suspicion of an alternate diagnosis. Imaging offers useful clues to differentiate inflammatory sinonasal disease from the more ominous fungal infections and sinonasal neoplasms. In addition to making a diagnosis and delineating the extent of the disease process, the interpreting radiologist must systematically evaluate the sinonasal cavities to generate a report that addresses all the issues before any intervention.

REFERENCES

1. Anon JB. Upper respiratory infections. Am J Med 2010;123:S16–25.
2. Hamilos DL. Chronic rhinosinusitis: epidemiology and medical management. J Allergy Clin Immunol 2011;128(4):693–707.
3. Khanna S, Gharpure AS. Correlation of increased sinusitis and urban air pollution. Ind J Sci Res Tech 2012;1:14–7.
4. Lanza DC, Kennedy DW. Adult rhinosinusitis defined. Otolaryngol Head Neck Surg 1997;117: S1–7.
5. Benninger MS, Ferguson BJ, Hadley JA, et al. Adult chronic rhinosinusitis: definitions, diagnosis, epidemiology, and pathophysiology. Otolaryngol Head Neck Surg 2003;129:S1–32.
6. Proctor DF. The mucociliary system. In: Proctor DF, Andersen IH, editors. The nose: upper airway physiology and the atmospheric environment. New York: Elsevier; 1982.
7. Stammberger H. Functional sinus surgery. Philadelphia: B.C. Decker; 1991. p. 273–82.
8. Nouraei SA, Elisay AR, Dimarco A, et al. Variations in paranasal sinus anatomy: implications for the pathophysiology of chronic rhinosinusitis and safety of endoscopic sinus surgery. J Otolaryngol Head Neck Surg 2009;38(1):32–7.
9. Som PM, Brandwein MS. Inflammatory diseases. In: Som PM, Curtin DC, editors. Head and neck imaging. 4th edition. St Louis (MO): Mosby; 2003. p. 193–259.
10. Rosenfeld RM, Andes D, Bhattacharyya N, et al. Clinical practice guidelines: adult sinusitis. Otolaryngol Head Neck Surg 2007;137(3 Suppl): S1–31.
11. Bhattacharyya N. Clinical and symptom criteria for the accurate diagnosis of chronic rhinosinusitis. Laryngoscope 2006;116(7 Pt 2 Suppl 110):1–22.
12. Cornelius RS, Martin J, Wippold FJ 2nd, et al. ACR appropriateness criteria sinonasal disease. J Am Coll Radiol 2013;10:241–6.
13. Zeifer B. Update on sinonasal imaging: anatomy and inflammatory disease. Neuroimaging Clin N Am 1998;8:607–30.
14. Yousem DM. Imaging of sinonasal inflammatory disease. Radiology 1993;188:303–14.
15. Dodd G, Jing B. Radiology of the nose, paransal sinuses and nasopharynx. Baltimore (MD): Williams and Wilkins; 1977. p. 59–65.
16. Harnsberger R. Imaging of the sinus and the nose. In: Harnsberger R, editor. Head and neck imaging handbook. St Louis (MO): Mosby-Year Book; 1990. p. 377–419d.
17. Babbel R, Harnsberger HR, Nelson B, et al. Optimisation of techniques in screening CT of the sinuses. AJNR Am J Neuroradiol 1991;12:849–54.
18. Som PM. Sinonasal cavities. In: Som PM, Curtin HD, editors. Head and neck imaging. 4th edition. St. Louis, Missouri: Mosby; 2003. p. 1–438.
19. Momeni AK, Roberts CC, Chew FS. Imaging of chronic and exotic sinonasal disease: a review. AJR 2007;189:S35–45.
20. Fatterpekar GM, Delman BN, Som PM. Imaging the paranasal sinuses: where we are and where we are going. Anat Rec (Hoboken) 2008;291:1564–72.
21. Bassim MK, Ebert CS, Sit RC, et al. Radiation dose to the eyes and parotids during CT of the sinuses. Otolaryngol Head Neck Surg 2005;133:531–3.
22. Czechowski J, Janeczek J, Kelly G, et al. Radiation dose to the lens in sequential and spiral CT of the facial bones and sinuses. Eur Radiol 2001; 11:711–3.
23. Sohaib SA, Peppercorn PD, Horrocks JA, et al. The effect of decreasing mAs on image quality and patient dose in sinus CT. Br J Radiol 2001;74: 157–61.
24. Aalokken TM, Hagtvedt T, Dalen I, et al. Conventional sinus radiography compared with CT in the diagnosis of acute sinusitis. Dentomaxillofac Radiol 2003;32(1):60–2.
25. Hagtvedt T, Aaløkken TM, Nøtthellen J, et al. A new low-dose CT examination compared with standard-dose CT in the diagnosis of acute sinusitis. Eur Radiol 2003;13(5):976–80.
26. Hein E, Rogalla P, Klingebiel R, et al. Low-dose CT of the paranasal sinuses with eye lens protection: effect on image quality and radiation dose. Eur Radiol 2002;12:1693–6.
27. Zammit-Maempel I, Chadwick CL, Willis SP. Radiation dose to the lens of eye and thyroid gland in paranasal sinus multislice CT. Br J Radiol 2003;76: 418–20.
28. Mahmutyazicioglu K, Ozer T, Gundogdu S. How does nose blowing effect the computed tomography of paranasal sinuses in chronic sinusitis? Eur J Radiol 2005;53:182–8.
29. Eggesbo HB. Radiological imaging of inflammatory lesions in the nasal cavity and paranasal sinuses. Eur Radiol 2006;16:872–88.
30. Younis RT, Anand VK, Davidson B. The role of computed tomography and magnetic resonance

imaging in patients with sinusitis with complications. Laryngoscope 2002;112(2):224–9.

31. Madani G, Beale TJ. Sinonasal inflammatory disease. Semin Ultrasound CT MR 2009;30:17–24.

32. Zinreich SJ, Kennedy DW, Kumar AJ, et al. MR imaging of normal nasal cycle: comparison with sinus pathology. J Comput Assist Tomogr 1988;12: 1014–9.

33. Rak KM, Newell JD 2nd, Yakes WF, et al. Paranasal sinuses on MR images of the brain: significance of mucosal thickening. AJR Am J Roentgenol 1991; 156:381–4.

34. Som PM, Curtin HD. Inflammatory lesions and tumors of the nasal cavities and paranasal sinuses with skull base involvement. Neuroimaging Clin N Am 1994;4:499–513.

35. Som PM, Dillon WP, Fullerton GD, et al. Chronically obstructed sinonasal secretions: observations on T1 and T2 shortening. Radiology 1989; 172:515–20.

36. Zinreich SJ, Abayram S, Benson ML, et al. The osteomeatal complex and functional endoscopic surgery. In: Som PM, Curtin HD, editors. Head and neck imaging. 4th edition. St Louis (MO): Mosby; 2003. p. 149–74.

37. Yoon JH, Na DG, Byun HS, et al. Calcification in chronic maxillary sinusitis: comparison of CT findings with histopathologic results. AJNR Am J Neuroradiol 1999;20:571–4.

38. Chow JM, Leonetti JP, Mafee MF. Epithelial tumors of the paranasal sinuses and nasal cavity. Radiol Clin North Am 1993;31:61–73.

39. Pruna X, Ibanez JM, Serres X, et al. Antrochoanal polyps in children: CT findings and differential diagnosis. Eur Radiol 2000;10:849–51.

40. Chung SK, Chang BC, Dhong HJ. Surgical, radiologic, and histologic findings of the antrochoanal polyp. Am J Rhinol 2002;16:71–6.

41. Ozcan M, Ozlugedik S, Ikinciogullari A. Simultaneous antrochoanal and sphenochoanal polyps: a rare clinical entity. J Laryngol Otol 2005;119: 152–4.

42. Zinreich SJ. Imaging for staging of rhinosinusitis. Ann Otol Rhinol Laryngol Suppl 2004;193:19–23.

43. Lund VJ, Mackay IS. Staging in rhinosinusitis. Rhinology 1993;31:183–4.

44. Hopkins C, Browne JP, Slack R, et al. The Lund-Mackay staging system for chronic rhinosinusitis: how is it used and what does it predict. Otolaryngol Head Neck Surg 2007;137(4):555–61.

45. Koopmann CF Jr. Intracranial complications of paranasal sinusitis: a combined institutional review. Laryngoscope 1991;101:234–9.

46. Babbel RW, Harnsberger HR, Sonkens J, et al. Recurring patterns of inflammatory sinonasal disease demonstrated on screening sinus CT. AJNR Am J Neuroradiol 1992;13:903–12.

47. Sonkens JW, Harnsberger HR, Blanch GM, et al. The impact of screening sinus CT on the planning of functional endoscopic sinus surgery. Otolaryngol Head Neck Surg 1991;105(6):802–13.

48. Stankiewicz JA. Complications of endoscopic sinus surgery. Otolaryngol Clin North Am 1989;22:749–58.

49. Yousem DM, Kennedy DW, Rosenberg S. Osteomeatal complex risk factors for sinusitis: CT evaluation. J Otolaryngol 1991;20:419–24.

50. Zinreich SJ, Kennedy DW, Rosenbaum AE, et al. Paranasal sinuses: CT imaging requirements for endoscopic surgery. Radiology 1987;163:769–75.

51. Pollei SR, Harnsberger HR. The radiologic evaluation of the sinonasal region. Postgrad Radiol 1989; 9:242–64.

52. Schaefer SD. Endoscopic total sphenoethmoidectomy. Otolaryngol Clin North Am 1989;22: 727–32.

53. Liang EY, Lam WW, Woo JK, et al. Another CT sign of sinonasal polyposis: truncation of the bony middle turbinate. Eur Radiol 1996;6(4):553–6.

54. Hourany R, Aygun N, Santina CC, et al. Silent sinus syndrome: an acquired condition. AJNR Am J Neuroradiol 2005;26:2390–2.

55. Illner A, Davidson HC, Harnsberger HR, et al. The silent sinus syndrome: clinical and radiographic findings. AJR Am J Roentgenol 2002;178:503–6.

56. deShazo RD, Stringer SP. Atrophic rhinosinusitis: progress toward explanation of an unsolved medical mystery. Curr Opin Allergy Clin Immunol 2011;11(1):1–7.

57. Alobid I, Guilemany JM, Mullol J. Nasal manifestations of systemic illnesses. Curr Allergy Asthma Rep 2004;4:208–16.

58. Muhle C, Reinhold-Keller E, Richter C, et al. MRI of the nasal cavity, the paranasal sinuses and orbits in Wegener's granulomatosis. Eur Radiol 1997;7(4): 566–70.

59. Yang C, Talbot JM, Hwang PH. Bony abnormalities of the paranasal sinuses in Wegener's granulomatosis. Am J Rhinol 2001;15(2):121–5.

60. Eggesbo HB, Dølvik S, Stiris M, et al. Complementary role of MR imaging of ethmomaxillary sinus disease depicted at CT in cystic fibrosis. Acta Radiol 2001;42(2):144–50.

61. Eggesbo HB, Dølvik S, Stiris M, et al. CT characterisation of developmental variations of the paranasal sinuses in cystic fibrosis. Acta Radiol 2001;42(5): 482–93.

62. Aribandi M, McCoy VA, Bazan C III. Imaging features of invasive and noninvasive fungal sinusitis: a review. Radiographics 2007;27:1283–96.

63. Khattar VS, Hathiram BT. Radiologic appearances of fungal sinusitis. Otorhinolaryngol Clin Int J 2009; 1(1):15–23.

64. Dillon WP, Som PM, Fullerton GD. Hypointense MR signal in chronically inspissated sinonasal secretions. Radiology 1990;174:73–8.

65. Fatterpekar G, Mukherji S, Arbealez A, et al. Fungal diseases of the paranasal sinuses. Semin Ultrasound CT MR 1999;20:391–401.

66. Som PM, Shapiro MD, Biller HF, et al. Sinonasal tumors and inflammatory tissues: differentiation with MR imaging. Radiology 1988;167:803–8.

67. Som PM, Shugar JM. The significance of bone expansion associated with the diagnosis of malignant tumors of the paranasal sinuses. Radiology 1980;136:97–100.

68. Som P. Tumors and tumor-like conditions of sinonasal cavity. In: Som P, Bergeron RT, editors. Head and neck imaging. 4th edition. St Louis (MO): Mosby; p. 261–373.

69. Vaid S, Vaid N, Rawat S, et al. An imaging checklist for pre-FESS CT: framing a surgically relevant report. Clin Radiol 2011;66:459–70.

70. Caughey RJ, Jameson MJ, Gross CW, et al. Anatomic risk factors for sinus disease: fact or fiction? Am J Rhinol 2005;19(4):334–9.

Fungal Sinusitis

Eytan Raz, MD, William Win, MD, Mari Hagiwara, MD, Yvonne W. Lui, MD,
Benjamin Cohen, MD, Girish M. Fatterpekar, MD*

KEYWORDS

- Invasive fungal sinusitis • Noninvasive fungal sinusitis • Granulomatous fungal sinusitis
- Allergic fungal sinusitis

KEY POINTS

- Fungal sinusitis is classified into invasive and noninvasive forms based on histopathologic evidence of tissue invasion by fungi.
- The invasive category includes acute invasive, chronic invasive, and granulomatous forms.
- The noninvasive category includes allergic fungal sinusitis and mycetoma.
- Each of the subtypes of fungal sinusitis has a different clinical presentation, distinct from the other forms, is associated with unique radiologic features, and a specific treatment plan.

INTRODUCTION

Among causes of sinonasal inflammatory disease, fungal sinusitis is a relatively uncommon but well-established clinical entity. Fungi are ubiquitous in the environment, and can colonize the upper respiratory tract mucosa when fungal spores are inhaled. In people with normal immune function, the fungal growth is kept in check. With impaired host immunity, fungi can invade host mucosa and cause invasive disease. Clinicians should therefore maintain a high index of suspicion of fungal sinusitis in immunocompromised patients with sinusitis, and those with chronic sinusitis. Fungal sinusitis consists of a heterogeneous group of disorders, with diversity in the affected patient population, offending agents, mechanism of disease, clinical presentation, histopathology, imaging appearances, treatment, and overall prognosis.[1]

Fungal sinusitis is broadly classified into two major groups: invasive and noninvasive forms. Although fungal sinusitis can be caused by any fungus, most result from *Aspergillus* infection. The invasive form is distinguished from the noninvasive variety depending on the presence of fungal elements outside the paranasal sinuses. It should be noted that although the distinction between invasive and noninvasive forms is suggested based on the clinical presentation, imaging evidence and/or histopathologic confirmation is required. Patients with noninvasive form typically present with chronic sinusitis that fails to respond to repeated courses of antibiotics and surgeries.[2] Invasive fungal sinusitis usually occurs with an acute onset characterized by fever, cough, and occasionally nasal mucosal ulceration. Usually this invasive form is seen in immunocompromised patients. There are chronic forms of invasive disease that can have an innocuous presentation, but usually demonstrate progressive worsening of symptoms suggestive of involvement of adjacent structures, such as associated visual disturbance suggesting orbital invasion.

This article first explains the classification of fungal sinusitis, and then evaluates separately the different entities with a particular focus on the radiologic appearance, and the information that the clinician needs to know to institute an appropriate therapy.

CLASSIFICATION OF FUNGAL SINUSITIS

The first attempt to classify fungal sinusitis was made in 1965, when two subtypes were recognized: a noninvasive form, clinically similar to chronic bacterial sinusitis; and an invasive form,

Department of Radiology, NYU School of Medicine, 660 First Avenue, 2nd Floor, New York, NY 10016, USA
* Corresponding author.
E-mail address: Girish.Fatterpekar@nyumc.org

Neuroimag Clin N Am 25 (2015) 569–576
http://dx.doi.org/10.1016/j.nic.2015.07.004
1052-5149/15/$ – see front matter Published by Elsevier Inc.

where the infection mimicked a disease similar to a tumor with bone erosion with invasion into adjacent tissues.[3] The most commonly accepted classification system, based on International Society for Human and Animal Mycology Group, February 2008, categorizes fungal sinusitis into invasive and noninvasive types based on histopathologic evidence of tissue invasion by fungi.[4] The noninvasive subtypes include allergic fungal sinusitis (AFS) and mycetoma; the invasive subtypes include acute invasive fungal sinusitis, chronic invasive fungal sinusitis, and granulomatous invasive fungal sinusitis.[4]

GENERAL IMAGING CONSIDERATIONS

There are certain characteristic computed tomography (CT) and MR imaging findings that are highly suggestive of fungal sinusitis.[5,6] Imaging overall therefore plays a key role in evaluating patients with suspected fungal sinusitis. Noncontrast CT remains the initial imaging study of choice in the work-up of fungal sinusitis.[7,8] In cases of complicated especially invasive fungal sinusitis, MR imaging can be performed for a more definitive evaluation.[7] CT in general is better in assessing for hyperattenuation within the opacified sinus, which in an appropriate clinical setting can suggest fungal infection. MR imaging is better at evaluating disease extension into adjacent soft tissues, including soft tissues of the neck, such as pterygomaxillary fissure, orbit, intracranial compartment, and vasculature.[6]

On CT, inflammatory watery secretions are seen as low-attenuation. As the inflammatory sinus disease persists, the secretions become inspissated and demonstrate a higher attenuation than muscle. In cases of fungal sinusitis, calcium and magnesium salts become deposited in areas of fungus growth and fungus-infected mucin.[6] These fungal concretions appear hyperdense on noncontrast CT.

MR imaging appearance of secretions depends on their protein content, viscosity, and presence of calcifications. Watery secretions usually contain less than 5% protein content; they appear as low signal intensity on T1-weighted images and high signal intensity on T2-weighted images. As they become inspissated, the secretions contain higher percentage of protein content (between 5% and 25%). Increasing T1 signal intensity is noted on T1-weighted images and a variable signal is seen on T2-weighted images. Within sludge or mycetoma where protein content can be between 25% and 40%, low signal intensity on T1-weighted images, and low signal or signal void on T2-weighted images are seen. This last pattern has been described to be highly suggestive of fungal sinusitis.[6]

NONINVASIVE FUNGAL SINUSITIS
Allergic Fungal Sinusitis

AFS is the most common form of fungal sinusitis, and is common in humid climates.[9] The overall incidence of AFS is estimated at 5% to 10% of all hypertrophic sinus disease cases going to surgery.[10] It was first reported as allergic aspergillosis by Millar and colleagues in 1981[11] who noted the similarity of the fungal-containing sinus exudate characteristic of this condition to the one found in the bronchi of patients affected by allergic bronchopulmonary aspergillosis.

AFS refers to noninvasive collection of impacted mucus and cellular debris, resulting from an allergic response to fungal colonization within the sinus cavity.[4] It should be noted that the amount of fungal elements within the opacified sinus is variable, often times scanty. The secondary inflammatory process that results does not depend on the quantity of fungus present. Hence, the role of fungi in initiating or promoting this disease is controversial and by some, thought to be circumstantial.[4]

The typical patient with AFS is young, atopic, immunocompetent, and presents clinically with hypertrophic sinus disease experiencing chronic headaches, nasal congestion, and chronic sinusitis for several years.[9] Fungal-specific IgE as detected by type I hypersensitivity skin testing is a constant feature. Total serum IgE is elevated, up to 5000 IU/mL, with a mean of 600 IU/mL commonly seen.[12] Originally considered to be caused solely by *Aspergillus* species, other causative fungi commonly reported include dematiaceous fungi, such as *Bipolaris*, *Curvularia*, *Alternaria*, and *Fusarium*.

Within affected sinuses, "allergic mucin" is found, characterized by a purulent, yellow-green and sometimes black mucus, which at histopathologic analysis reveals the presence of eosinophil granulocytes and Charcot-Leyden crystals, which are eosinophil degradation products.[13–15] Fungal hyphae are sparse and noninvasive, and may be identifiable by special stains, such as Gomori methenamine silver stain. Given the specific histopathologic findings, the presence of allergic mucin is virtually diagnostic for AFS, sometimes even in the absence of fungal identification.

Imaging features
On imaging, there is unilateral or asymmetric involvement of the sinuses. Characteristically, multiple sinuses are involved. Maxillary and ethmoid sinuses are most commonly involved. Noncontrast CT shows hyperdense areas within the sinus cavities outlined by hypodense-appearing thickened

and inflamed mucosa (**Fig. 1**).[16,17] Depending on the contents of the material, the MR imaging signal is variable, ranging from isointense to hypointense signal to signal void on T1- and T2-weighted images. This signal heterogeneity is related to the presence of deposited heavy metals, such as iron and manganese. On contrast-enhanced studies, the intrasinus contents usually demonstrate no masslike enhancement. Because of the expansive nature of allergic mucin, and its propensity to incite local inflammatory response, sinus expansion along with osseous remodeling and erosive changes of the sinus walls are seen.[18]

Treatment
Endoscopic removal of polyps and inflammatory material, including mucin, to re-establish aeration and drainage of involved sinuses is essential for successful treatment.[19] Following surgery, additional measures including the use of topical steroids for immune response suppression is important to prevent recurrences; this concept was actually derived from experience with allergic bronchopulmonary aspergillosis. Other therapies, such as immunotherapy, antihistamines, oral anti-leukotrienes, oral steroids, and nasal irrigation, are helpful in certain clinical situations.[12,20]

Fungus Ball

Fungus ball, also referred to as a fungal mycetoma or aspergilloma, is reported as a distinct clinical entity and a discrete form of noninvasive fungal sinus disease.[6] It refers to an indolent growth of fungal hyphae in a sinus cavity until a masslike lesion is formed. Affected patients are immuno-competent, nonatopic, and otherwise healthy. Some studies have reported the disease to be more common in older women. However, patients of all ages are affected. The maxillary sinus by far is the most common site of occurrence. It has been postulated that the host's deficient mucociliary clearance mechanism is accountable for the disease. This allows the uncleared fungal elements to colonize and proliferate in the retained secretions within the sinonasal cavity, inciting an inflammatory response. Previous endodontic treatment and radiotherapy are sometimes implicated in the development of a mycetoma. *Aspergillus fumigatus* is the most commonly implicated pathogen.[21]

Clinical diagnosis
Typically, medical attention is sought for mild sinus pressure. In some cases, patients are asymptomatic and the diagnosis is made incidentally on imaging. A surgical specimen of a fungal mycetoma has been described as a thick, semisolid mass with "claylike" consistency. Histopathologic examination reveals tightly packed fungal hyphae without allergic mucin, a feature distinct from AFS.[2] Calcium oxalate deposition often accompanies the growth of *Aspergillus*, and appears as radiating clusters of birefringent crystals on histochemistry.

Imaging features
Characteristic imaging findings are critical to the diagnosis. Typically, a single sinus cavity is affected, a distinct feature from other forms of

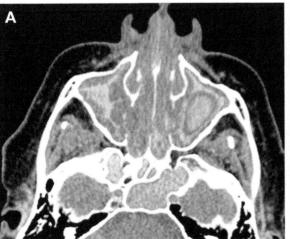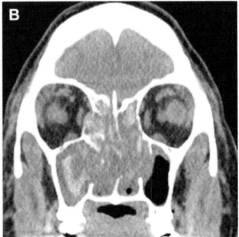

Fig. 1. Allergic fungal sinusitis in a 72-year-old woman with history of nasal polyposis. Noncontrast (*A*) axial and (*B*) coronal CT scans demonstrate opacified paranasal sinuses and nasal cavity relatively sparing the left maxillary sinus. Hyperdensity seen within opacified sinuses suggests a mixture of inspissated secretions and fungal concretions.

fungal sinusitis.[5,8] Maxillary sinuses are most commonly affected, followed by sphenoid, frontal, and ethmoid sinuses. Another unique feature is the lack of sinus expansion. Because of its chronic nature, osseous remodeling of the sinus wall can be seen, noted as thickening and sclerosis. There is opacification of the involved sinus with central areas of high density and fine, round-to-linear matrix calcifications (**Fig. 2**). T1-weighted images demonstrate low signal intensity of the thick, solid, mycetomatous mass, although the signal can be heterogeneous depending on the content.[5,8] Because of the presence of calcifications and paramagnetic metals, such as magnesium, iron, and manganese, low T2 signal intensity is also observed. Contrast-enhanced studies demonstrate thickening and enhancement of the surrounding inflamed mucosa. There is no involvement of the soft tissues surrounding the involved sinus cavity.[5]

Treatment and prognosis

Good prognosis is noted following surgical excision and reestablishing adequate sinus aeration.[2]

INVASIVE FUNGAL SINUSITIS
Acute Invasive Fungal Sinusitis

Acute invasive fungal sinusitis is a fungal infection of nasal cavity and paranasal sinuses with a rapid progressive time course (<4 weeks).[22,23] There is associated invasion of fungal elements into vessels and adjacent soft tissues. Affected patients tend to be critically ill, and demonstrate some degree of compromised immune function. Such

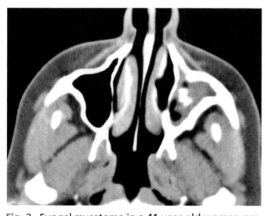

Fig. 2. Fungal mycetoma in a 41-year-old woman presenting with sinus pressure. Noncontrast axial CT scan demonstrates an opacified left maxillary sinus. Central hyperdensity seen within is suggestive of fungal concretions. Note the circumferential thickening of the osseous walls of the left maxillary sinus, a finding consistent with a chronic inflammatory process.

patients typically include those with decreased host cell-mediated immunity, specifically with impaired neutrophil function, hematologic malignancies, aplastic anemia, hemochromatosis, poorly controlled diabetes, acquired immunodeficiency syndrome, or organ transplantation; or are undergoing immunosuppressive treatments, such as systemic steroids or chemotherapeutic agents. Infrequently, acute invasive disease has been reported in patients with normal immune function.[24]

Aspergillus sp and members of the family *Mucoraceae* (*Mucor*, *Rhizopus*, and *Absidia*) are implicated in most cases of acute invasive fungal sinusitis. In poorly controlled diabetics, *Mucor*, *Rhizopus*, and *Absidia* predominate, and in neutropenic patients, *Aspergillus* sp account for most cases.[22]

As expected in this patient population, the disease course is rapidly progressive and can prove to be fatal within days to weeks. Therefore, it is important for clinicians to maintain a high level of awareness, and for radiologists to proactively look for subtle changes that can be identified in the early stages of the disease.

Clinical features

The presenting symptoms are nonspecific and include fever, headache, rhinorrhea, facial pain, and diplopia, which can also be seen with acute bacterial sinusitis. Therefore, when sinusitis is considered in patients with impaired immune function, appropriate diagnostic work-up, including imaging studies and nasal endoscopy with possible biopsy, must be initiated in a timely manner.

Involvement of the nasal cavity is common, with the middle turbinate being the most commonly affected site, thus a high-yield target for nasal biopsy. On nasal endoscopy, the infected mucosa appears pale, progressing to ulceration and tissue necrosis with worsening disease. The affected area is commonly painless. Definitive diagnosis is made with microscopic identification of invasive fungi in the biopsy samples of mucosa, submucosa, vessels (angioinvasion), and bone. Infarcted tissue and inflammatory cellular infiltrates are also seen.

Imaging features

Maxillary and ethmoid sinuses are most commonly affected. On CT, mucosal thickening with partial or complete opacification of the affected sinus is a typical imaging feature[8,23] Hyperattenuation areas within the opacified sinuses are commonly seen, and in an immunocompromised state should raise a red flag for an underlying fungal cause. This is especially concerning when associated soft tissue/vascular invasion, as suggested of effacement of fat, beyond intact sinus walls is seen (**Fig. 3**). In such cases, disease spread is thought to occur through microvascular channels present within the bone. The areas to be particularly mindful of to evaluate for such soft tissue infiltration are spaces adjacent to maxillary sinuses, such as pre-maxillary and retroantral fat, and pterygopalatine fossa. Occasionally, focal areas of bone erosion can be seen.[23] On MR imaging, opacified sinuses are seen. Within these opacified sinuses are areas of signal drop-out suggestive of fungal concretion. It should therefore be noted that appreciation of such fungal concretion is therefore best made on noncontrast CT, and can be a limitation of MR imaging. However, invasion of adjacent soft tissues is best assessed on MR imaging. With involvement of the spaces around the sinuses, there is T1 signal intensity similar to soft tissue replacing normal fat signal intensity. Edematous change on T2-weighted images, and enhancement within these soft tissues is commonly seen. A unique feature on imaging suggestive of invasive fungal sinusitis is the lack of enhancement in areas that should typically enhance following contrast administration, such as the nasal mucosa and the turbinates. Lack of enhancement of the affected mucosa of the turbinates, described as the black-turbinate sign on imaging, is highly suggestive of tissue necrosis, and is consistent with the angioinvasive nature of fungal sinusitis (**Fig. 4**).[23] For radiologists, it is also crucial to identify and alert clinicians of the extension of the disease, especially to the orbits and intracranial compartment. In addition, the angioinvasive nature of some of the fungi makes it important to assess adjacent intracranial vessels,

such as the cavernous segment of internal carotid arteries for thrombosis, dissection, and pseudoaneurysm formation (**Fig. 5**).

Treatment

Treatment consists of emergency surgical debridement and systemic antifungal agents. Aggressive management of any inciting factor, such as diabetic ketoacidosis, is crucial in the management. The mortality associated with acute invasive fungal sinusitis has been traditionally cited up to 50% to 80%.[25] Despite a recent downward trend, likely caused by better understanding of the disease and timely diagnosis and initiation of treatment, the mortality remains high, with some studies reporting up to 18%.[26] Studies have shown that overall mortality is higher in patients infected with *Mucor* compared with those infected with *Aspergillus* sp.

Chronic Invasive Fungal Sinusitis

Chronic invasive fungal sinusitis is characterized by an indolent course of the disease (>4–12 weeks), in contrast to the rapidly progressive course of its acute counterpart.[2,21] As with acute invasive disease, patients in immunocompromised states, such as poorly controlled diabetes mellitus or undergoing immunosuppressive treatments, show predisposition to the disease. Patients with normal immune function are uncommonly affected.

Clinical diagnosis

Patients usually seek medical attention for symptoms of chronic sinusitis, for which findings of

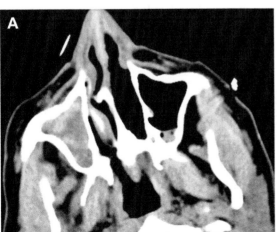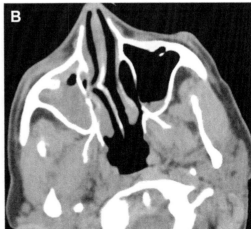

Fig. 3. Acute invasive fungal sinusitis in a 58-year-old man with neutropenia and right maxillary pain. (*A*) Non-contrast axial CT scan demonstrates complete opacification of the right maxillary sinus with mixed attenuation material. (*B*) At a level slightly cranial, CT scan demonstrates ill-defined soft tissue infiltration in the region of the right pterygomaxillary fissure and soft tissues of the cheek. Also, note edematous change involving the right masseter, temporalis, and pterygoid muscles suggestive of masticator space invasion.

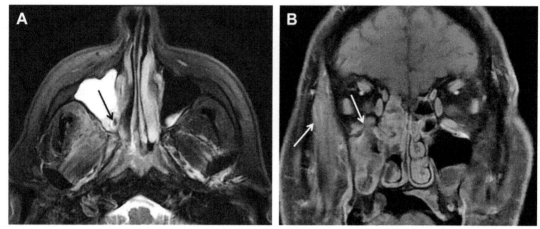

Fig. 4. Acute invasive fungal sinusitis in a 33-year-old man with immunosuppression and acute right facial pain and swelling. (A) Axial T2-weighted image demonstrates an opacified right maxillary sinus. Focus of hypoattenuation (arrow) is likely suggestive of fungal concretion. There is a suggestion of soft tissue infiltration within the right pterygomaxillary fissure and edematous change within the right pterygoid muscles. (B) Contrast-enhanced fat-suppressed coronal MR imaging demonstrates lack of "normal" enhancement of the right middle and inferior turbinates suggestive of black turbinate sign. There is a suggestion of right orbital invasion and masticator space invasion (arrows).

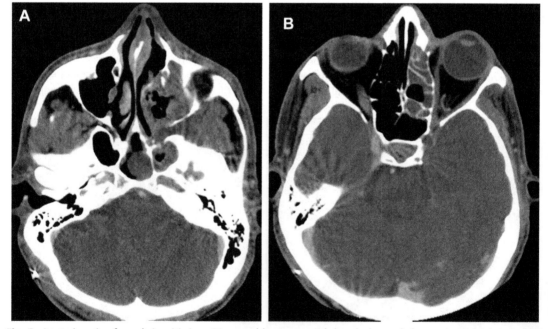

Fig. 5. Acute invasive fungal sinusitis in a 61-year-old woman with headache and change in mental status. (A) Contrast-enhanced axial CT scan demonstrates nonvisualization of the medial wall of the left maxillary sinus suggestive of recent surgical intervention. Opacified left sphenoid sinus is also seen. There is a suggestion of effacement of the fat in the left pterygomaxillary fissure and edema within the left infratemporal fossa suggestive of tissue invasion. (B) At a slightly more cranial level, there is no enhancement of the cavernous segment of the left internal carotid artery suggestive of thrombosis and reflecting vascular invasion secondary to the angioinvasive nature of fungal infection.

protracted disease course, slow progression, and refractoriness to standard antibiotic treatment are common. In some cases, patients report decreased vision and ocular immobility, known as orbital apex syndrome. This has been reported to be associated with disease extension to the orbital apex in patients with chronic invasive fungal sinusitis. The causative agent is known to be of *Aspergillus* genus with *A fumigatus* being the most common species. Except for the difference in time course compared with the acute disease, the clinical and imaging work-up should be identical. Clinical examination reveals evidence of nasal congestion and nasal polyposis. On histology, the specimen includes material containing densely packed hyphae, mixed with scattered, chronic, inflammatory infiltrates. Evidence of fungal invasion into the paranasal mucosa and adjacent tissues is often seen.

Imaging features

Intrasinus and extrasinus imaging features are mostly similar to the acute counterpart. However, there is a difference in the pattern of calcifications between acute and more chronic diseases. On CT, intrasinus calcifications in an acute stage show fine punctate appearance. With a protracted course of the disease, more calcium metabolites are deposited in the fungal mass, taking on a more dense and coarse appearance.[27] Otherwise, in keeping with its invasive nature, localized erosive changes in the sinus walls are seen with extension into adjacent tissues (**Fig. 6**). Extension to the orbits and intracranial compartments is seen.

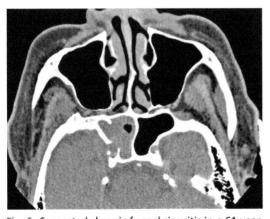

Fig. 6. Suspected chronic fungal sinusitis in a 61-year-old man with symptoms of chronic sinusitis. Axial non-contrast CT scan demonstrates mixed-attenuation material filling the right sphenoid sinus. Note the focal dehiscence of the right carotid canal.

Treatment and prognosis

Treatment typically includes surgical debridement, followed by systemic antifungal agents, a strategy similar to acute invasive fungal sinusitis. Although the overall mortality is lower than the acute disease, when there is invasion into adjacent structures, such as cavernous sinus or intracranial compartment, a high mortality rate is reported.[2]

Granulomatous Invasive Fungal Sinusitis

Similar to chronic invasive fungal sinusitis, the disease course is slowly progressive. The affected patients are usually immunocompetent and report a history of chronic sinusitis.[2] This disease is prevalent in Africa and Southeast Asia, with rare reported cases in the United States. The causative agents are of *Aspergillus* genus, with *Aspergillus flavus* being most commonly implicated.

Clinical diagnosis

Microscopic features include evidence of fungal invasion, noncaseating granulomas with giant cells, plasma cells, central small granulomas containing eosinophils, fibrinoid necrosis, fibrosis, and vasculitic changes.

Imaging features

The imaging features are nonspecific and similar to other invasive fungal sinusitis. There is soft tissue opacification of the involved sinus, and evidence of surrounding tissue invasion. Extension to soft tissues around the sinuses and the orbits and intracranial compartment is also seen. Typically, only one or two sinuses are involved. Sinus expansion is uncommon. Bone erosion is localized to the area of extrasinus extension and extrasinus component of the disease tends to be more extensive than intrasinus component.[28]

Treatment and prognosis

Surgical resection is the mainstay of treatment. If surgical intervention is not initiated in a timely manner, the disease can invade adjacent structures, resulting in worse prognosis. Concurrent antifungal agents are usually used to lower relapse rate.[2]

SUMMARY

Fungal sinusitis is classified into the noninvasive (AFS, fungal ball) and invasive (acute invasive, chronic invasive, and chronic granulomatous) forms. These different types and subtypes of fungal sinusitis present with clinical features similar to the viral and bacterial forms of sinusitis. However, the associated morbidity and mortality of fungal sinusitis is worse when compared with the other pathogens. The radiologist based on imaging features can help suggest the diagnosis of fungal sinusitis in an appropriate clinical setting. Such accurate assessment by the radiologist, especially when assessing invasive forms, is crucial with regards to further management, and therefore the overall prognosis of the patient.

REFERENCES

1. Wise SK, Ghegan MD, Gorham E, et al. Socioeconomic factors in the diagnosis of allergic fungal rhinosinusitis. Otolaryngol Head Neck Surg 2008; 138(1):38–42.

2. deShazo RD, Chapin K, Swain RE. Fungal sinusitis. N Engl J Med 1997;337(4):254–9.

3. Hora JF. Primary aspergillosis of the paranasal sinuses and associated areas. Laryngoscope 1965; 75:768–73.

4. Chakrabarti A, Denning DW, Ferguson BJ, et al. Fungal rhinosinusitis: a categorization and definitional schema addressing current controversies. Laryngoscope 2009;119(9):1809–18.

5. Zinreich SJ, Kennedy DW, Malat J, et al. Fungal sinusitis: diagnosis with CT and MR imaging. Radiology 1988;169(2):439–44.

6. Aribandi M, McCoy VA, Bazan C III. Imaging features of invasive and noninvasive fungal sinusitis: a review. Radiographics 2007;27(5):1283–96.

7. Cornelius RS, Martin J, Wippold FJ II, et al. ACR appropriateness criteria sinonasal disease. J Am Coll Radiol 2013;10(4):241–6.

8. Fatterpekar G, Mukherji S, Arbealez A, et al. Fungal diseases of the paranasal sinuses. Semin Ultrasound CT MR 1999;20(6):391–401.

9. Glass D, Amedee RG. Allergic fungal rhinosinusitis: a review. Ochsner J 2011;11(3):271–5.

10. Katzenstein AL, Sale SR, Greenberger PA. Allergic Aspergillus sinusitis: a newly recognized form of sinusitis. J Allergy Clin Immunol 1983;72(1):89–93.

11. Millar JW, Johnston A, Lamb D. Allergic aspergillosis of the maxillary sinuses. Thorax 1981;36:710.

12. Schubert MS, Goetz DW. Evaluation and treatment of allergic fungal sinusitis. II. Treatment and follow-up. J Allergy Clin Immunol 1998;102(3):395–402.

13. Bent JP III, Kuhn FA. Allergic fungal sinusitis/polyposis. Allergy Asthma Proc 1996;17(5):259–68.

14. Bent JP III, Kuhn FA. Diagnosis of allergic fungal sinusitis. Otolaryngol Head Neck Surg 1994;111(5): 580–8.

15. Marple BF. Allergic fungal rhinosinusitis: current theories and management strategies. Laryngoscope 2001;111(6):1006–19.

16. Braun J, Riehm S, Veillon F. Value of CT in allergic fungal sinusitis (AFS). J Radiol 2008;89(4):480–6 [in French].

17. Mukherji SK, Figueroa RE, Ginsberg LE, et al. Allergic fungal sinusitis: CT findings. Radiology 1998;207(2):417–22.

18. Wise SK, Rogers GA, Ghegan MD, et al. Radiologic staging system for allergic fungal rhinosinusitis (AFRS). Otolaryngol Head Neck Surg 2009;140(5): 735–40.

19. Manning SC, Vuitch F, Weinberg AG, et al. Allergic aspergillosis: a newly recognized form of sinusitis in the pediatric population. Laryngoscope 1989; 99(7 Pt 1):681–5.

20. Bent JP III, Kuhn FA. Antifungal activity against allergic fungal sinusitis organisms. Laryngoscope 1996;106(11):1331–4.

21. deShazo RD, O'Brien M, Chapin K, et al. Criteria for the diagnosis of sinus mycetoma. J Allergy Clin Immunol 1997;99(4):475–85.

22. Gillespie MB, O'Malley BW Jr, Francis HW. An approach to fulminant invasive fungal rhinosinusitis in the immunocompromised host. Arch Otolaryngol Head Neck Surg 1998;124(5):520–6.

23. Groppo ER, El-Sayed IH, Aiken AH, et al. Computed tomography and magnetic resonance imaging characteristics of acute invasive fungal sinusitis. Arch Otolaryngol Head Neck Surg 2011;137(10): 1005–10.

24. Del Valle Zapico A, Rubio Suarez A, Mellado Encinas P, et al. Mucormycosis of the sphenoid sinus in an otherwise healthy patient. Case report and literature review. J Laryngol Otol 1996;110(5): 471–3.

25. Waitzman AA, Birt BD. Fungal sinusitis. J Otolaryngol 1994;23(4):244–9.

26. Parikh SL, Venkatraman G, DelGaudio JM. Invasive fungal sinusitis: a 15-year review from a single institution. Am J Rhinol 2004;18(2):75–81.

27. Yoon JH, Na DG, Byun HS, et al. Calcification in chronic maxillary sinusitis: comparison of CT findings with histopathologic results. AJNR Am J Neuroradiol 1999;20(4):571–4.

28. Reddy CE, Gupta AK, Singh P, et al. Imaging of granulomatous and chronic invasive fungal sinusitis: comparison with allergic fungal sinusitis. Otolaryngol Head Neck Surg 2010;143(2):294–300.

Imaging Approach to Sinonasal Neoplasms

Saugata Sen, MD[a,b,*], Aditi Chandra, MD[a,b], Sumit Mukhopadhyay, MD[a,b],
Priya Ghosh, MD[a,b]

KEYWORDS

- CT • MR imaging • Sinonasal • Tumors • Neoplasms

KEY POINTS

- Imaging of sinonasal neoplasms is critical to map the entire extent of the lesion for management.
- A systematic approach is required to evaluate involvement of the critical areas related to the sinonasal space as well as nerves.
- Computed tomography and MR imaging complement each other in a complete evaluation of a sinonasal neoplasm.

INTRODUCTION

Sinonasal neoplasms are rare and account for 3% of all head and neck cancers.[1] A large variety of neoplasms are possible, mainly of epithelial and mesenchymal origin; malignant lesions are more common than benign ones. Squamous cell carcinoma is by far the commonest, accounting for 80% of all the neoplasms in this region, and the maxillary sinus most frequently involved.[2]

The closely apposed and communicating air-filled spaces allow for clinically silent tumor progression within the sinonasal tract. The clinical symptoms (commonly nasal congestion, epistaxis, and nasal obstruction) are so akin to the ubiquitous inflammatory and infective conditions, that the treating physician is often caught unawares. Occasionally, the neoplasm coexists with the inflammatory pathology, leading to misdiagnosis. Hence, most lesions are large at presentation and palliative options can only be offered. Many of the pathologies in this region are very aggressive, further contributing to poor prognosis. The small, restricted sinonasal space with its rich lymphatic supply as well as proximity to vital anatomic structures like orbits, skull base, palate and pterygopalatine fossa (PPF) account for early extracompartmental disease extension. There is a paucity of pain in sinonasal neoplasms until late in the disease, another important factor that leads to delayed diagnosis (**Fig. 1**). Bony destruction, which is an important imaging feature, rarely causes pain. When there is pain, it usually is a sign of nerve or skull base involvement and heralds a poor prognosis.

The optimal assessment and treatment of sinonasal neoplasms require a multidisciplinary approach. Both surgery and radiotherapy have contributed to the management of these conditions. When curative surgery is possible, there is significant cosmetic deformity and functional morbidity. Plastic surgical reconstruction procedures are often undertaken for cosmesis. An often ignored feature of these advanced lesions and potentially morbid management options is the patient's inability to eat, leading to early onset of cancer cachexia, which significantly contributes to poor outcome.

Disclosures: Authors do not have any conflict of interest or financial disclosure to declare.
[a] Department of Radiology, Tata Medical Center, 14, Main Arterial Road, Rajarhat, New Town, Kolkata 700156, India; [b] Department of Nuclear Medicine, Tata Medical Center, 14, Main Arterial Road, Rajarhat, New Town, Kolkata 700156, India
* Corresponding author. Department of Radiology, Tata Medical Center, 14, Main Arterial Road, Rajarhat, New Town, Kolkata 700156, India.
E-mail addresses: drsaugatasen@gmail.com; saugata.sen@tmckolkata.com

Neuroimag Clin N Am 25 (2015) 577–593
http://dx.doi.org/10.1016/j.nic.2015.07.005

neuroimaging.theclinics.com

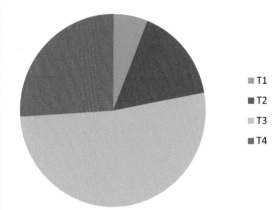

- ■ T1
- ■ T2
- ■ T3
- ■ T4

Fig. 1. Stage at presentation of sinonasal carcinomas at the authors' institution.

Both computed tomography (CT) and MR imaging have complimentary roles in the management of sinonasal tumors. The radiologist is called upon not only to detect the disease, but also to map the entire extent of surgical margins as well as radiotherapy planning.

COMPUTED TOMOGRAPHY AND MR IMAGING

Only the superficial extent of a sinonasal neoplasm is visible on clinical examination and nasal endoscopy. The complete investigation of a sinonasal neoplasm mandates cross-sectional imaging. Both CT and MR imaging have played synergistic roles in the assessment of neoplasms of the sinonasal space.

COMPUTED TOMOGRAPHY

CT is usually the first radiologic modality to investigate a sinonasal neoplasm. It provides excellent anatomic detail of the sinonasal skeleton. CT is superior to MR imaging in evaluating matrix of fibroosseous lesions, which can aid in specific histologic diagnosis. Bony destruction of sinuses and orbital walls, as well as involvement of the anterior and middle skull base are precisely depicted in the newer multidetector CT scanners, with reconstruction in different planes. Neural foraminal widening owing to perineural spread (PNS) can be observed on thin sections and reconstructions. Fat is easily depicted on CT. Hence, for lesions that are invading the orbits, coronal CT images are reliable. All these features are of paramount surgical consideration and CT is usually a mandatory requirement from the surgical stand point. CT sections are generally reconstructed at 1- to 1.25-mm sections in the axial, coronal, and sagittal planes. When contrast is administered,

the sections are taken 80 to 90 seconds after the initiation of the contrast bolus to achieve good tumor to nontumor interface as well as good visualization of the vessels of the neck. Rate of contrast injection generally is 1.5 to 2.0 mL/s. Both narrow and wide window settings need review for the soft tissue lesion as well as bone changes.

Radiation issues for CT continue to stimulate debate around the world. The new, sensitive multidetector scanners are significantly dose efficient, with resultant low mAs scans reducing the radiation dose delivered, yet maintaining spatial resolution. Because the coronal reconstructions from axial scans in multidetector CT allow the required quality, there is no need for the direct coronal scans, thereby reducing radiation dose further. Of particular concern has been the dose delivered to the lens and thyroid gland. It has been shown conclusively that, even after multiple scans, patients have a negligible risk for premature cataract formation and thyroid cancer.[3]

MR IMAGING

MR imaging has excellent soft tissue resolution and is accepted widely as the best radiologic modality to evaluate the extent of soft tissue component of tumors in the sinonasal space. The multiparametric capabilities, contrast administration, and multiplanar sequences make MR imaging a potent tool. The extension of tumors along the nerves contiguously or as skip lesions are best evaluated on contrast MR imaging. The orbital fat involvement, dural involvement, reactive changes in dura, and brain involvement are some of the areas where MR imaging plays a decisive role in formulating management options.

The protocol for MR imaging of the sinonasal space includes high resolution T1-weighted, T2-weighted, and diffusion-weighted images as well as T1-weighted, fat-suppressed, contrast-enhanced images. The sections are generally taken at 3-mm thickness with interslice gap of 0.3 mm. Axial and coronal planes are routine, but sagittal sequences are preferred when anterior skull base needs evaluation. The plane of imaging in axial sequences should be parallel to hard palate. Sagittal T1- and T2-weighted images are also indicated when evaluation of anterior skull base is required.

For evaluating PNS, high-resolution images with a small field of view of 16 to 18 cm are preferred. Thin section T1- and T2-weighted axial and coronal images with and without fat saturation are required that cover the entire course of the nerve. Contrast images are acquired in axial and coronal planes, both with and without fat suppression.[4]

MR imaging contrast (gadolinium gadopentetic acid) is administered at a dose of 0.1 to 0.2 mmol/kg body weight.

At the authors' institution, the radiologic evaluation of sinonasal tumors consist of contrast enhanced MR imaging and multidetector CT with reconstruction in bone algorithm.

RADIOLOGIC FEATURES OF A MALIGNANT SINONASAL NEOPLASM

The radiologic features of a malignant sinonasal neoplasm can be varied. Enough evidence cannot be derived from imaging to arrive at a conclusive pathologic diagnosis in most cases. A structured approach narrows down the imaging differential. The following radiologic points raise the suspicion of a malignant tumor in the sinonasal space:

1. Single site/compartment of involvement.
2. Large soft tissue mass with heterogeneous enhancement and necrosis. Intermediate signal on T2-weighted images generally.
3. Bone erosion/destruction.
4. Contiguous multicompartmental disease with destruction of intervening boundary, be it bone or cartilage. Extracompartmental invasion to adjacent structures.
5. PNS.

The sinonasal inflammatory diseases usually involve all or several sinuses on both sides. The changes are usually not confined to 1 side or 1 sinus only, suggesting generalized hypersensitivity of the mucosa of the entire sinonasal region. Malignant sinonasal diseases arise from a single compartment and grow into another in a contiguous manner with destruction of the intervening bone or boundary. A single site of involvement with no other sign of disease in the other compartments may suggest neoplastic disease (**Fig. 2**). Again, large soft tissue lesions involving contiguous sites with destruction of the intervening boundary raise the suspicion of a malignant lesion (**Fig. 3**).

The soft tissue component of a malignant disease is large at the time of diagnosis. Areas of necrosis and heterogeneous enhancement are observed both on CT and MR imaging. The differentiation between an inflammatory polyp and a neoplastic lesion can be made on the T2-weighted images where intermediate signal of the neoplastic lesion makes the diagnosis evident. The neoplastic lesions are typically of intermediate signal intensity on T2-weighted images owing to low water content and high cellularity. Polyps are hyperintense on T2-weighted images, reflecting

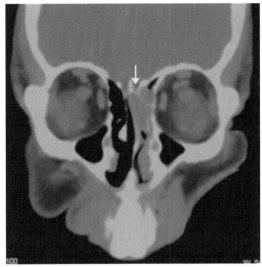

Fig. 2. Single site involvement (olfactory niche; *yellow arrow*) by olfactory neuroblastoma. Single site involvement is suggestive of neoplastic change.

their higher water content, and show uniform linear enhancement of the margins (**Fig. 4**).

Although most neoplastic lesions seem to be of intermediate signal on T2-wieghted imaging, there are certain exceptions, as in the case of low-grade adenoid cystic carcinoma, which can show high T2 signals owing to paucicellularity[5] (**Box 1**).

Inspissated secretions can lead to ambiguity in diagnosis of a neoplastic lesion or delineating the exact margins of the tumor. MR imaging is the best modality to resolve this problem, because the secretions have an increased water content and show high signal intensity on T2-weighted images (**Fig. 5**).

Chronic inspissated secretions from inflammatory conditions can produce a variety of signals on T1- and T2-weighted images.[6] Secretions with high protein content render them hyperintense in T1-weighted images. But if the protein content is more than 28%, both T1 and T2 signals are hypointense with appearance of a pseudoaerated sinus on MR imaging. CT can be helpful in such cases. Smooth, marked peripheral enhancement is observed in inflammatory conditions. Most malignant tumors, especially large ones, are pathologically heterogeneous in nature, and this is represented on imaging. Contrast administration amplifies the heterogeneous nature of the tumor, with moderate enhancement at some parts and poor enhancement at other areas, representing necrosis. Necrosis is the hallmark of tumors, because the lesions grow rapidly, outstripping their own blood supply. Necrosis of a malignant tumor is a key differentiating feature from benign and

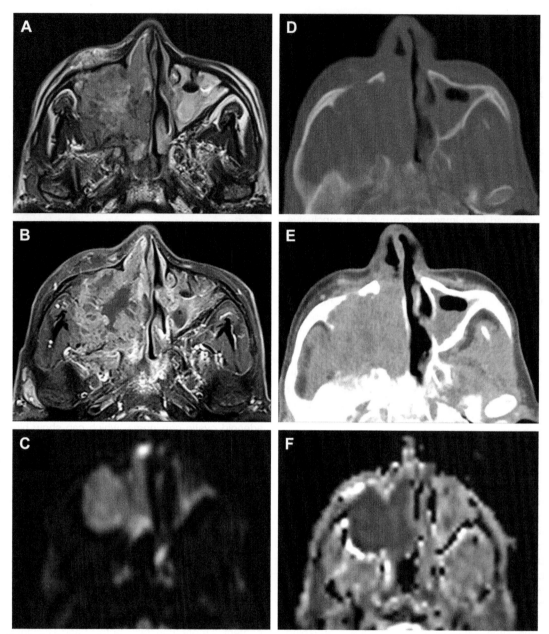

Fig. 3. Typical imaging features of sinonasal carcinoma. Large, multicompartmental, soft tissue mass is seen with intermediate signal in T2-weighted MR image (*A*), heterogeneous enhancement with necrotic areas in postgadolinium T1-weighted image (*B*), and extensive bone destruction on computed tomography (*D, E*). Diffusion restriction is demonstrated in diffusion-weighted imaging (*C*) and apparent diffusion coefficient map (*F*).

inflammatory conditions. Hemorrhage may also be encountered in malignant lesions, appearing as focal bright areas on T1-weighted imaging and further contributing to the heterogeneous nature.[7]

T2-weighted MR imaging is the most helpful sequence for delineating tumor boundaries. Even though contrast enhancement of the lesion may be prominent, the adjacent soft tissue and muscles can enhance significantly owing to

inflammatory and desmoplastic changes induced by the tumor (**Fig. 6**).

Diffusion-weighted MR imaging of neoplastic lesions (see **Fig. 3**) show restriction and low apparent diffusion coefficient values.[8] This is owing to tightly packed cells in the neoplastic lesions with resultant restricted diffusion of water molecules in the intercellular space. Perfusion MR imaging has also been studied to differentiate

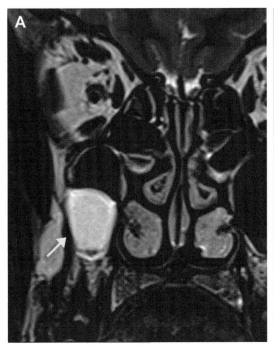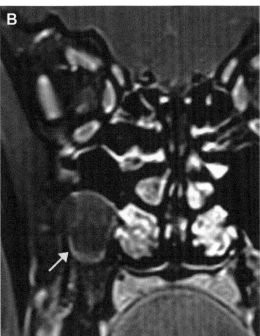

Fig. 4. Mucosal polyp (*yellow arrows*). T2-weighted coronal MR imaging (*A*) shows hyperintense mass with smooth convex superior border in right maxillary antrum, which demonstrates thin peripheral enhancement in a postgadolinium T1-weighted image (*B*). Compare with T2 signal and enhancement pattern of a carcinoma in Fig. 3.

a benign from malignant lesion. Time intensity curves plotted from dynamic contrast-enhanced MR imaging have been proven to be reliable when used together with apparent diffusion coefficient values in establishing the malignant nature of lesions.[9]

Several bone changes are possible in a malignant lesion and they are best depicted on CT. Bone erosion and destruction are encountered in most aggressive sinonasal carcinomas. Once the bony boundary is breached, the lesions are free to involve critical areas such as the PPF, infratemporal fossa, orbits, palate, and anterior cranial fossa. Such changes, however, can be seen in certain benign conditions such as Wegener's granulomatosis, rhinocerebral mucormycosis, and giant cell reparative granuloma.[10] Bone remodeling is seen in several neoplasms of the sinonasal space like minor salivary gland neoplasm, lymphoma and melanoma. Natural killer–T-cell lymphoma can, however, cause aggressive bone destruction. Melanoma, despite being very aggressive, causes only bone remodeling (Fig. 7). New bone formation is seen in osteosarcoma where there may be a typical aggressive periosteal reaction of the sunburst type. A chondroid type of matrix calcification is observed in chondrosarcoma. Both of these lesions usually have a large, heterogeneously enhancing soft tissue mass with necrosis. Chondroid calcification shows low signal on T1-weighted images and high signal on T2-weighted images.

Bone disease is evaluated optimally by CT. However, in the skull base, MR imaging is superior to CT in evaluating bone involvement and marrow edema.

Transgression of disease through the medullary spaces leading to disease on both sides of a bony wall with no intervening destruction has been described in literature.[11]

PNS is common in cases of adenoid cystic carcinoma (Fig. 8). This phenomenon is also seen in melanoma and lymphoma. A few benign lesions like sarcoidosis can also show PNS.

Box 1
Neoplastic lesions with high signals on T2-weighted imaging sequences in sinonasal spaces

1. Low-grade adenoid cystic carcinoma
2. Other low-grade minor salivary gland tumors, pleomorphic adenoma
3. Nerve sheath tumors
4. Inverted papilloma
5. Hemangioma
6. Chondrosarcoma

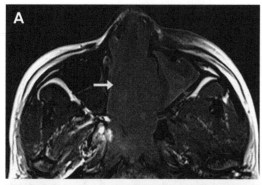

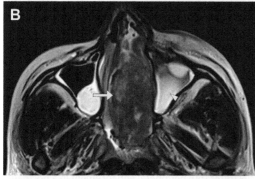

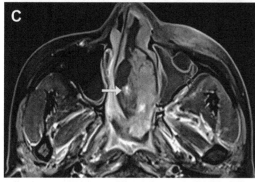

Fig. 5. Differentiating inspissated mucous from tumor. The nasal cavity contains heterogeneously enhancing tumor (*yellow arrow*) with areas of necrosis (*C*; postgadolinium T1-weighted image), having intermediate signal intensity in T2-weighted image (*B*). The adjacent left maxillary antrum contains inspissated mucous, showing marked hyperintense signals in T1-weighted image (*yellow arrowhead* in *B*) and smooth thin margin with marked enhancement (*red open arrow* in *C*). Areas of high protein content demonstrate mild hyperintense signals in T1-weighted image (*red arrowhead* in *A*).

ROUTES OF DISEASE SPREAD WITH RELEVANT ANATOMY

The sinonasal space is restricted and complex. It is close to the skull base and is rich in lymphatic supply. Several small neural foramina are in close association. Because local recurrence is the major cause of treatment failure, the regional radiologic assessment needs to be precise. The tumors disseminate by direct extension, lymphatics, and perineural route. Distant metastasis may also be encountered. Hence, detailed knowledge of anatomy and natural routes of dissemination is an essential part of mapping of sinonasal tumors. Erosion and destruction of bony boundaries of the sinonasal space leads to extracompartmental extension of disease. The vulnerable areas are the:

1. Anterior cranial fossa from lesions of frontal and ethmoidal sinuses (Fig. 9);
2. Middle cranial fossa from sphenoid sinus;
3. Orbits from lesions of ethmoidal and maxillary sinuses;
4. Palate from lesions of nasal cavity and maxillary sinuses (Fig. 10);
5. Premaxillary space and skin from disease of maxillary sinus; and
6. PPF and infratemporal fossa from disease of maxillary sinus (Fig. 11).

Anterior and Middle Cranial Fossa

The roof of the nasal cavity is formed by the cribriform plates (part of ethmoid bone), which have sievelike pores for the olfactory nerves. The anterior ethmoidal air cells are limited superiorly by the fovea ethmoidalis (part of frontal bone; Figs. 12 and 13). The superior boundary of posterior ethmoidal air cells and sphenoid sinus are the planum ethmoidale and planum sphenoidale, respectively (Fig. 14). Superior extension of aggressive lesions of the nasal cavity, and ethmoidal and sphenoid sinuses to the dura and brain are limiting factors for aggressive curative surgery. Hence, these review areas are vital for complete radiologic assessment. Coronal CT evaluates the bony integrity of the cribriform plate best.

Pterygopalatine Fossa

The PPF is a box-shaped space that lies posterior to the maxillary sinus and derives its name from its boundaries, anteriorly the perpendicular plate of palatine bone and posteriorly the pterygoid plate of sphenoid. Contents are usually fat with hyperintensity on both T1- and T2-weighted images. Early sign of involvement of PPF in MR imaging is replacement of the fat signal (Fig. 15). The aggressive maxillary sinus lesions can easily destroy the posterior wall of the sinus and the perpendicular plate of palatine bone. Once in the PPF, there are several pathways of disease extension directly and along the nerves:

1. To the infratemporal fossa through the pterygomaxillary fissure;

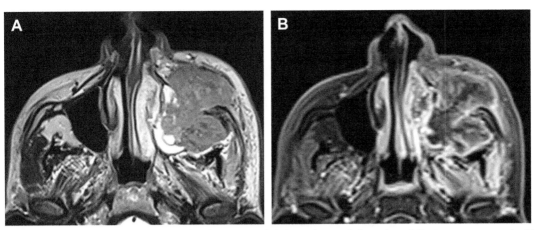

Fig. 6. T2 delineation of tumor. T2-weighted MR image (*A*) shows better delineation of the tumor compared with postgadolinium T1-weighted image (*B*), where surrounding structures without involvement may enhance.

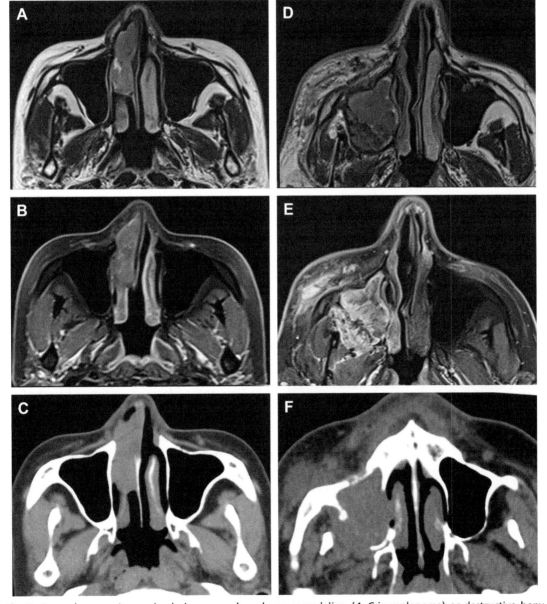

Fig. 7. Bone changes. Aggressive lesions may show bone remodeling (*A–C* in melanoma) or destructive bony changes (*D–F* in carcinoma).

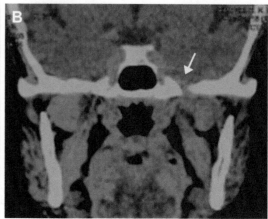
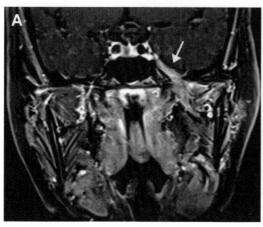

Fig. 8. Perineural spread in adenoid cystic carcinoma. (A) Coronal postgadolinium T1-weighted MR image shows enhancement of the left mandibular nerve (*yellow arrow*). (B) Coronal computed tomography image shows widened left foramen ovale (*yellow arrow*).

2. To the orbits through the inferior orbital fissure (Fig. 16);
3. To the ethmoid sinuses and nasal space through the sphenopalatine foramen;

4. To the palate and oral cavity through the ptery-gopalatine canal/greater and lesser palatine foramina; and
5. To the skull base in middle cranial fossa through the vidian canal and foramen rotundum.

The applied anatomy of PPF in relation to pathways of disease extension are enumerated in Figs. 17–26.

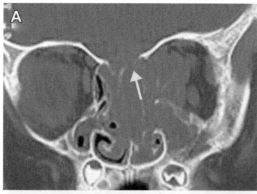
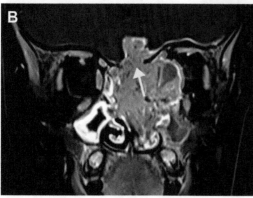

Fig. 9. Extension of olfactory neuroblastoma into anterior cranial fossa by erosion of cribriform plate and fovea ethmoidalis (*yellow arrows*). (A) Coronal computed tomography image. (B) Coronal postgadolinium T1-weighted MR image.

Orbits

Orbital involvement by sinonasal neoplasms is a poor prognostic indicator. Orbits can be involved by the following routes:

1. Direct extension of a maxillary or ethmoidal lesion, by violation of the intervening bone (Fig. 27).
2. Along the nasolacrimal duct from a nasal lesion or a maxillary antral lesion, which has invaded the nasal cavity (Fig. 28).
3. Through the inferior orbital fissure from the PPF and infratemporal fossa.
4. Along the infraorbital nerve by a maxillary sinus tumor, which has involved the premaxillary region, through the infraorbital foramen.

Because significant involvement of the orbit requires operative exenteration, radiologic assessment needs to be accurate. Several criteria have been proposed to evaluate the orbit in cases of direct extension.[12,13] They are:

1. Orbital fat stranding;
2. Relation of tumor and periorbita (periorbital displacement, abutment, tumor-periorbital nodular interface);

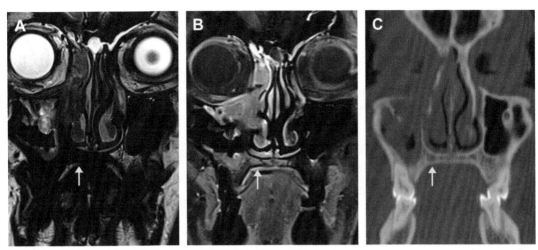

Fig. 10. Involvement of hard palate by maxillary carcinoma. Yellow arrows indicate replacement of marrow fat in T2-weighted coronal MR image (*A*), enhancement in postgadolinium T1-weighted MR image (*B*), and subtle bony erosion of hard palate in coronal computed tomography image (*C*).

3. Extraocular muscle abnormality (enhancement, signal abnormality, displacement); and
4. Integrity of the bony orbit.

The periorbita is the periosteum of the orbital bones and is a tough structure that acts as a potent barrier to neoplastic invasion. Its integrity is the key to determining involvement of the orbit. Both CT and MR imaging can assess the orbit reliably. An advantage of CT is better evaluation of bone and orbital fat. MR imaging cannot differentiate between cortical bone and periorbita, both

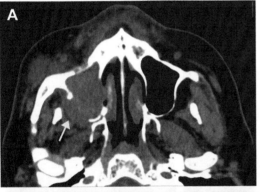

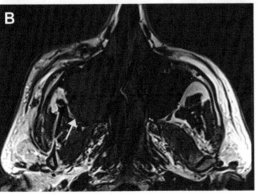

Fig. 11. Retromaxillary fat involvement (*yellow arrows*) in a patient with maxillary carcinoma. (*A*) Axial computed tomography image. (*B*) Axial T1-weighted MR image.

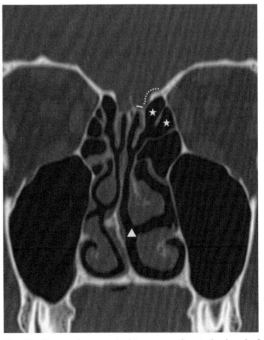

Fig. 12. Coronal computed tomography at the level of orbits. Yellow line, cribriform plate forming roof of nasal cavity (*yellow triangle*); white dotted line, Fovea ethmoidalis forming roof of ethmoidal air cells (*yellow stars*).

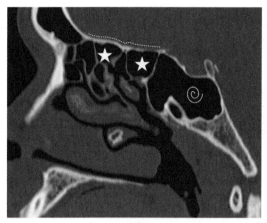 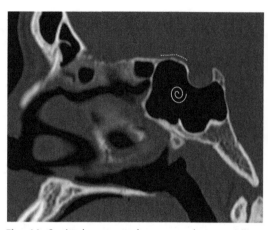

Fig. 13. Sagittal computed tomography at the level of ethmoid sinuses. White stars, ethmoidal air cells; yellow spiral, sphenoid sinus; yellow dotted line, Fovea ethmoidalis.

Fig. 14. Sagittal computed tomography at midline. Yellow spiral, sphenoid sinus; yellow dotted line, planum sphenoidale.

of which appear hypointense on all sequences.[13] Displaced periorbita appears as an elevated hypointense layer on T2-weighted images and does not indicate orbital violation. On the other hand, infiltration of the periorbita leads to loss of hypointensity and indicates orbital involvement.[14]

The accuracy of detecting orbital involvement by imaging does not exceed 79% if any individual or all criteria are taken together.[13] Because loss of sight is a major handicap for the patient and imaging accuracy remains less than perfect, frozen

sections are used in all equivocal cases. However, CT and MR imaging done together offer sufficient information to prepare and counsel the patient for such a major undertaking.

Dura

Contrast-enhanced MR imaging precisely characterizes dural disease. Focal nodular enhancement, thickness of the enhancing region of more than 5 mm and pial enhancement

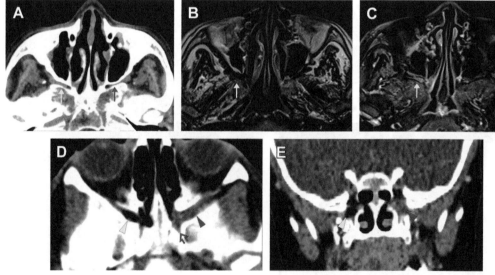

Fig. 15. Pterygopalatine fossa (PPF) involvement. Yellow arrows indicate replacement of fat in right PPF by soft tissue density in an axial computed tomography (CT) (*A*), hypointense lesion in axial T2-weighted image (*B*), which enhances in postgadolinium T1-weighted image (*C*). Normal fat in left PPF (*red arrows*) is seen as hypodense stripe in (*A*), hyperintense area in (*B*), without any contrast enhancement in C. In another patient with acute myelogenous leukemia, soft tissue (chloroma) is seen to fill the left PPF (*red arrowheads* in *D, E*; axial and coronal CT images). Extension into left vidian canal is seen in *D* (*red open arrow*). Note normal right PPF fat (*yellow arrowheads* in *D, E*).

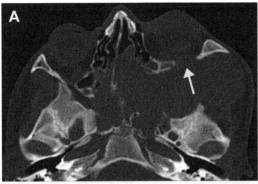

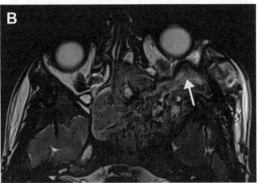

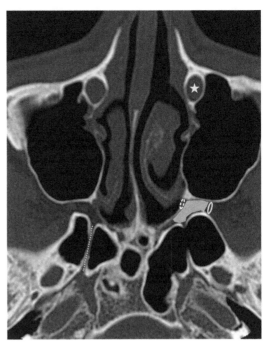

Fig. 18. Axial computed tomography at the level of maxillary sinus. Yellow star, nasolacrimal duct; yellow shaded area, pterygopalatine fossa; yellow ring, pterygomaxillary fissure; white dotted ring, sphenopalatine foramen; yellow dotted line, vidian canal.

Fig. 16. Inferior orbital fissure (IOF) involvement in a patient of juvenile nasopharyngeal angiofibroma. (A) Axial computed tomography shows widening of the IOF (*yellow arrow*). (B). Axial T2-weighted MR image shows soft tissue bulging from pterygopalatine fossa into orbits (*yellow arrow*).

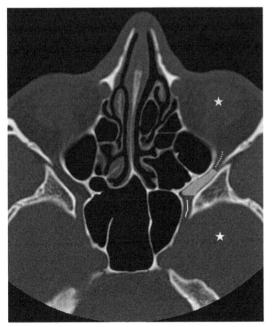

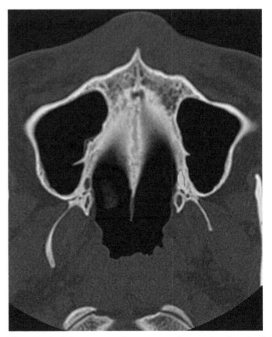

Fig. 17. Axial computed tomography at the level of orbit. Yellow star, orbit; white star, middle cranial fossa; yellow shaded area, pterygopalatine fossa; white dotted line, inferior orbital fissure; yellow solid line, foramen rotundum.

Fig. 19. Axial computed tomography at the level of pterygoid plates. Yellow shaded area, greater palatine foramen; red dots, lesser palatine foramina.

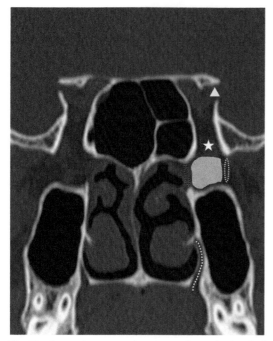

Fig. 20. Coronal computed tomography at the level of pterygopalatine fossa. Yellow shaded area, pterygopalatine fossa; yellow triangle, superior orbital fissure; white star, inferior orbital fissure; white ring, pterygomaxillary fissure; red ring, sphenopalatine foramen; yellow dotted line, greater palatine canal.

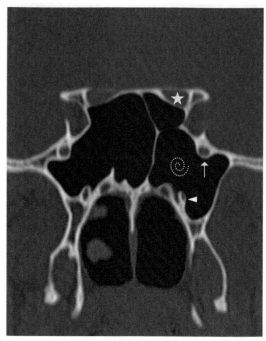

Fig. 22. Coronal computed tomography at the level of sphenoid sinus (a few millimeters posterior to **Fig. 21**). Yellow star, optic canal; spiral, sphenoid sinus; yellow arrow, foramen rotundum; white arrowhead, vidian canal.

indicates dural involvement[15] (**Fig. 29**). Reactive dural enhancement represented by a thin linear enhancement can mimic dural involvement. Large dural disease may require craniofacial resection and reconstruction. Thus, preoperative detection of dural disease has major operative and prognostic implications.

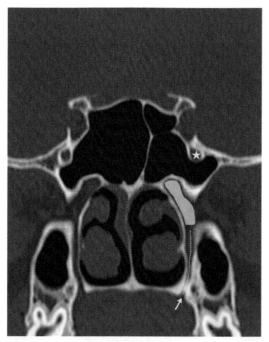

Fig. 21. Coronal computed tomography at the level of sphenoid sinus. Yellow shaded area, pterygopalatine fossa; yellow star, foramen rotundum; white dotted line, greater palatine canal; yellow arrow, greater palatine foramen.

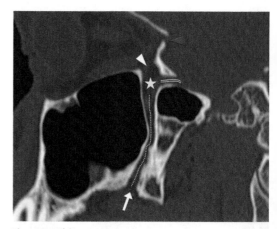

Fig. 23. Oblique sagittal computed tomography at the level of pterygopalatine fossa. Yellow star, pterygopalatine fossa; red arrowhead, superior orbital fissure; white arrowhead, inferior orbital fissure; parallel white lines, foramen rotundum; dotted yellow line, greater palatine canal; white arrow, greater palatine foramen.

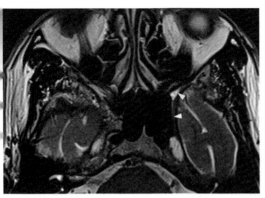

Fig. 24. Axial T2-weighted MR image demonstrating course of maxillary nerve (V2). Red arrowhead, Meckel's cave; white arrowhead, curvilinear course of V2; yellow arrowhead, pterygopalatine fossa.

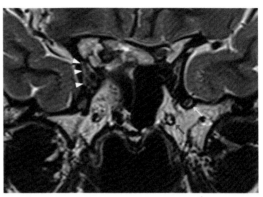

Fig. 26. Coronal T2-weighted MR image. White arrowheads, cranial nerves within cavernous sinus (seen as *black dots*); yellow arrow, foramen rotundum; red arrow, vidian canal.

Perineural Spread

PNS of malignant conditions of the sinonasal space is along the perineurium or nerve sheath. Most lesions that show PNS express neural cell adhesion molecule, a protein that enables malignant cells to bind to the perineural sheath of the nerve.[16,17] Involvement can be contiguous and in a retrograde fashion toward the skull base and brain. Skip lesions and antegrade extension have also been described. Because the lesions are silent clinically in nearly 40% of cases,[18] the radiologist needs to develop a "neutropic mind" to evaluate and detect such disease. The detection of PNS has adverse prognostic value because it denotes high incidence of local recurrence, nodal secondaries, and poor overall survival.[16] MR imaging is the preferred modality and the optimum technique has been described in an appropriate section elsewhere in this article. MR imaging

features of PNS are enlargement or thickening of the nerve with irregular margins. Excessive enhancement, more than can be explained by enhancement of the perineural venous plexus present in the perineural foramina and bony canals, is also helpful. Beyond the bony canals, obliteration of the perineural fat pad is another important feature that helps the radiologist to identify PNS.[4] Loss of cerebrospinal fluid signals in Meckel's cave, cavernous sinus involvement, as well as encasement of the carotid arteries can be encountered in advanced cases.[7] CT can demonstrate widened neural foramina at the skull base (see **Fig. 8**). The neoplastic lesions that commonly show PNS in the sinonasal space are adenoid cystic carcinoma, squamous cell carcinoma, desmoplastic melanoma, lymphoma, and leukemia. Several benign lesions can show PNS, namely sarcoidosis and rhinocerebral mucormycosis.

Nodal Disease

Nodal disease and extracapsular invasion are poor prognostic markers. Hence, the knowledge of lymphatic drainage of the sinonasal region needs to be revisited (**Box 2**). The retropharyngeal nodal chain (**Fig. 30**) can only be evaluated by cross-sectional imaging, whereas other nodes may be clinically detected if enlarged. CT and MR imaging demonstrate metastatic lymph nodes in 38% to 67% of patients with no palpable disease.[19]

The radiologic features of metastatic disease in a node are size greater than 1 cm, capsular invasion, and necrosis. Diffusion-weighted MR imaging and apparent diffusion coefficient values as well as dynamic contrast-enhanced MR imaging have been used to enhance the specificity of this diagnosis.[13]

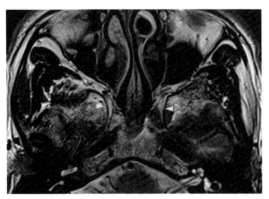

Fig. 25. Axial T2-weighted MR image a few millimeters below **Fig. 24**. Yellow arrowheads, vidian canals; red arrowhead, pterygopalatine fossa.

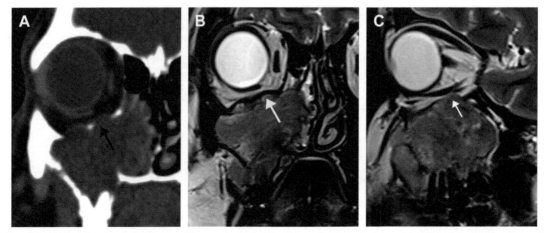

Fig. 27. Orbital involvement by maxillary sarcoma. (A). Coronal computed tomography showing erosion of orbital floor (*black arrow*). (B) Coronal T2-weighted MR image showing intact periorbita seen as elevated black line (*yellow arrow*). (C). Sagittal T2-weighted MR image showing focal breach of periorbita (*white arrow*) and involvement of orbital fat.

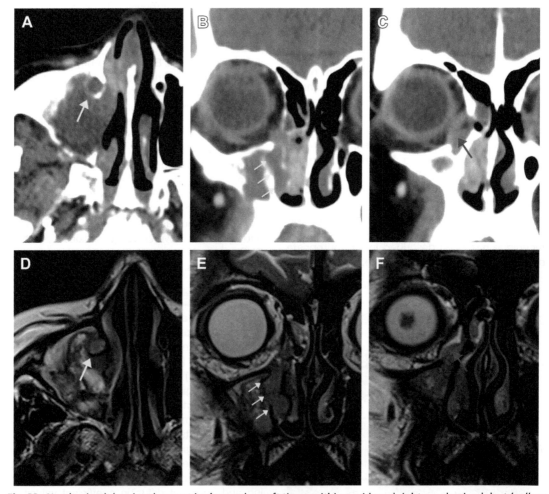

Fig. 28. Nasolacrimal duct involvement is observed as soft tissue within a widened right nasolacrimal duct (*yellow arrows*). (A) Axial and (B, C) coronal computed tomography images. (D) Axial and (E, F) coronal T2-weighted MR images. (C, F) Involvement of lacrimal sac (*red arrow*), and thus, the orbit. Note contralateral normal nasolacrimal duct.

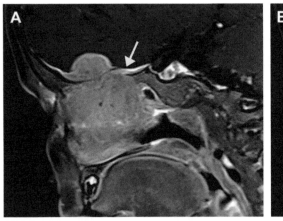
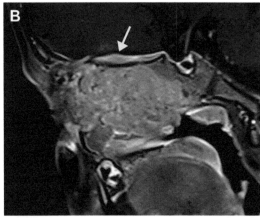

Fig. 29. Dural involvement by olfactory neuroblastoma. Nodular and plaquelike dural enhancement (*yellow arrow*) is seen in T1 postgadolinium parasagittal (*A*) and mid sagittal (*B*) MR images.

Box 2	
Lymphatic drainage of sinonasal space	
Site/Region	**Drainage Station**
Anterior half of nasal cavity	Level IB
Posterior half of nasal cavity	Retropharyngeal node, levels II, III, IV, and V
Frontal and anterior ethmoidal sinuses	Level IB
Sphenoid sinus and posterior ethmoidal sinus	Retropharyngeal node
Maxillary sinus	Levels IB, II, III, and IV

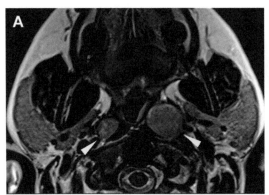
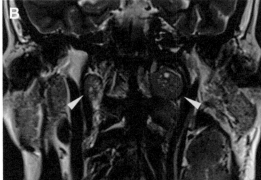

Fig. 30. Bilateral enlarged retropharyngeal lymph nodes (*arrowheads*). (*A*) Axial T2-weighted MR image. (*B*) Coronal T2-weighted MR image.

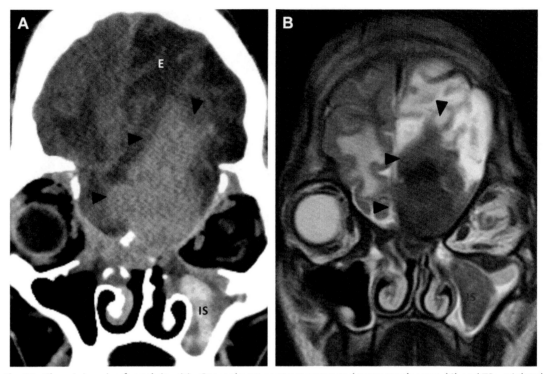

Fig. 31. Chronic invasive fungal sinusitis. Coronal post contrast computed tomography scan (*A*) and T2-weighted image (*B*) show an aggressive, enhancing mass with bone destruction arising from the superior nasal cavity and ethmoidal air cells and extending intracranially, which is hypointense in T2-weighted image (*black arrowheads*). Note left frontal lobe edema (E) and inspissated secretions (IS).

WHAT THE PHYSICIANS NEED TO KNOW (DIFFERENTIALS AND RESECTABILITY)

Aggressive fungal lesions (chronic invasive fungal sinusitis) may mimic malignancy. They present with soft tissue mass with erosive as well as sclerotic bone changes. On CT, the lesions are hyperdense and diagnosis is conclusive. MR imaging is also helpful in determining the etiology. The highly cellular neoplasms show intermediate to low signals on T2-weighted images. Chronic fungal lesions, on the other hand, may be hypointense on T2-weighted imaging owing to mineral content (Fig. 31).[20]

Palatal lesions or lesions of the orbit can extend and invade the adjacent sinonasal space. They are easily differentiated clinically as well as on imaging (Fig. 32).

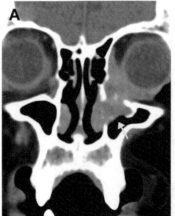
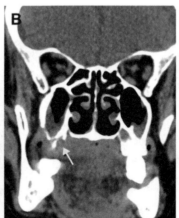
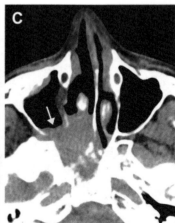

Fig. 32. Secondary involvement of paranasal sinus (*yellow arrow*) by (*A*) basal cell carcinoma of the orbit, (*B*) carcinoma of hard palate, and (*C*) nasopharyngeal carcinoma.

Contraindications for surgical extirpation of sinonasal neoplasms are controversial at best. Every case needs a multidisciplinary approach for management based on their merit. However, contraindications for surgery can include involvement of the nasopharynx, clivus, bilateral orbital cavities, or optic nerves. Involvement of the carotid artery is a relative contraindication for surgery. Brain or cavernous sinus involvement has been considered unresectable, but surgical management has also been described.[21] Spread to the brain from sinonasal neoplasms is in a contiguous manner and resection of the portion of the gyrus rectus of the frontal lobe usually results in minimal functional deficits. Surgical resection of the cavernous sinus, in view of the extensive venous network and carotid artery, is an extremely challenging task and is associated with significant morbidity and a poor outcome. Very carefully selected patients must be considered for surgical resection in cases of cavernous sinus involvement. The limitations and indications for excision also depend on the abilities and experience of the surgical team.

SUMMARY

The anatomic extent of a tumor in the sinonasal framework and involvement of critical structures such as PPF, orbits, palate, skull base, and nerves determine the type of therapy offered and impact prognosis. All such parameters are best evaluated by the synergistic information derived from CT and MR imaging done together.

REFERENCES

1. Barnes L. Diseases of the nasal cavity, paranasal sinuses, and nasopharynx. In: Leone Barnes, editor. Surgical Pathology of the Head and Neck. 3rd edition. New York: Informa Healthcare; 2009. p. 343–422.
2. Rao VM, el-Noueam KI. Sinonasal imaging. Anatomy and pathology. Radiol Clin North Am 1998;36(5): 921–39, vi.
3. Fatterpekar GM, Delman BN, Som PM. Imaging the paranasal sinuses: where we are and where we are going. Anat Rec 2008;291(11):1564–72.
4. Gandhi D, Gujar S, Mukherji SK. Magnetic resonance imaging of perineural spread of head and neck malignancies. Top Magn Reson Imaging 2004;15(2):79–85.
5. Mosesson RE, Som PM. The radiographic evaluation of sinonasal tumors: an overview. Otolaryngol Clin North Am 1995;28(6):1097–115.
6. Loevner LA, Sonners AI. Imaging of neoplasms of the paranasal sinuses. Magn Reson Imaging Clin N Am 2002;10(3):467–93.
7. Madani G, Beale TJ, Lund VJ. Imaging of sinonasal tumors. Semin Ultrasound CT MR 2009; 30(1):25–38.
8. Sasaki M, Eida S, Sumi M, et al. Apparent diffusion coefficient mapping for sinonasal diseases: differentiation of benign and malignant lesions. AJNR Am J Neuroradiol 2011;32(6):1100–6.
9. Sasaki M, Sumi M, Eida S, et al. Multiparametric MR imaging of sinonasal diseases: time-signal intensity curve- and apparent diffusion coefficient-based differentiation between benign and malignant lesions. AJNR Am J Neuroradiol 2011;32(11):2154–9.
10. Madani G, Beale TJ. Differential diagnosis in sinonasal disease. Semin Ultrasound CT MR 2009; 30(1):39–45.
11. Davide Farina RM. Neoplasms of the sinonasal cavities. In: Robert Hermans, editor. Head and Neck Cancer Imaging. 2nd edition. Berlin; Heidelberg (Germany): Springer-Verlag; 2012. p. 207–36.
12. Eisen MD, Yousem DM, Loevner LA, et al. Preoperative imaging to predict orbital invasion by tumor. Head Neck 2000;22(5):456–62.
13. Raghavan P, Phillips CD. Magnetic resonance imaging of sinonasal malignancies. Top Magn Reson Imaging 2007;18(4):259–67.
14. Maroldi R, Farina D, Battaglia G, et al. MR of malignant nasosinusal neoplasms. Frequently asked questions. Eur J Radiol 1997;24(3):181–90.
15. Eisen MD, Yousem DM, Montone KT, et al. Use of preoperative MR to predict dural, perineural, and venous sinus invasion of skull base tumors. AJNR Am J Neuroradiol 1996;17(10):1937–45.
16. Vural E, Hutcheson J, Korourian S, et al. Correlation of neural cell adhesion molecules with perineural spread of squamous cell carcinoma of the head and neck. Otolaryngol Head Neck Surg 2000; 122(5):717–20.
17. Gandour-Edwards R, Kapadia SB, Barnes L, et al. Neural cell adhesion molecule in adenoid cystic carcinoma invading the skull base. Otolaryngol Head Neck Surg 1997;117(5):453–8.
18. Ginsberg LE. MR imaging of perineural tumor spread. Magn Reson Imaging Clin N Am 2002; 10(3):511–25, vi.
19. van den Brekel MW, Castelijns JA, Stel HV, et al. Detection and characterization of metastatic cervical adenopathy by MR imaging: comparison of different MR techniques. J Comput Assist Tomogr 1990;14(4):581–9.
20. Som PM, Curtin HD. Inflammatory lesions and tumors of the nasal cavities and paranasal sinuses with skull base involvement. Neuroimaging Clin N Am 1994;4(3):499–513.
21. Jackson K, Donald PJ, Gandour-Edwards R. Pathophysiology of skull base malignancies. In: Donald PJ, editor. Surgery of the skull base. Philadelphia: Lippincott, Williams & Wilkins; 1998. p. 51–72.

Sinonasal Tumors
Computed Tomography and MR Imaging Features

Saugata Sen, MD*, Aditi Chandra, MD,
Sumit Mukhopadhyay, MD, Priya Ghosh, MD

KEYWORDS

• CT • MR imaging • Sinonasal • Tumors • Neoplasms

KEY POINTS

- Diverse tissue types in the sinonasal space give rise to a variety of tumors, most of which are malignant.
- Although pathologic diagnosis is not always possible, knowledge of the computed tomography (CT) and MR imaging features of individual is required to arrive at a working differential.
- Certain tumors behave in typical fashion. Hence, the review areas for these lesions need to be closely examined for proper staging.
- CT and MR imaging done together may give better overall information for staging and treatment.

INTRODUCTION

Sinonasal tumors are rare. Malignant lesions are more common than benign ones and prognosis is grave. A wide variety of lesions are possible. It is unlikely that CT and MR imaging would provide a pathologic diagnosis in most cases. Role of imaging is to:

1. Narrow down the imaging differential;
2. Distinguish benign from malignant lesions; and
3. Map the entire extent of a tumor with relations to adjacent vital structures and nerves.

This article describes the radiologic features of benign and malignant sinonasal tumors.

BENIGN AND MALIGNANT EPITHELIAL TUMORS
Papilloma

The ectodermally derived Schneiderian mucosa gives rise to 3 types of benign neoplastic papillomas in the sinonasal tract:

1. Fungiform or exophytic papillomas;
2. Inverted papillomas (IP); and
3. Oncocytic papillomas.

Overall, neoplastic papillomas constitute only 0.4% to 4.7 % of all sinonasal tumors. The fungiform and IP are commoner and some of their characteristics are summarized in **Box 1**:

Imaging Features (**Fig. 1**)
- Nonspecific, small polypoid lesions to large masses with significant enhancement.
- Expansion and remodeling of the nasal cavity with bowing of adjacent bony walls.[1]
- Thinning, sclerosis, intratumoral bony fragments.[2]
- Cerebriform or convoluted pattern in diffuse or partial form on T2-weighted images[3] and contrast enhanced T1-weighted images.
- Origin of IP is a focal bony hyperostosis seen on computed tomography (CT). Drilling and resection of this area leads to reduced rates of recurrence. Recurrence rates vary from 4% to 22%.[4]

Disclosures: Authors do not have any conflict of interest or financial disclosure to declare.
Department of Radiology and Nuclear Medicine, Tata Medical Center, 14, Main Arterial Road, Rajarhat, New Town, Kolkata 700156, India
* Corresponding author.
E-mail addresses: drsaugatasen@gmail.com; saugata.sen@tmckolkata.com

Neuroimag Clin N Am 25 (2015) 595–618
http://dx.doi.org/10.1016/j.nic.2015.07.006

Box 1
Comparative synopsis of Schneiderian papillomas

Type	Age (y)	Sex	Site of Origin	Malignant Potential	Incidence (%)
Fungiform	20–50	More common in males	Nasal septum	No	50
Inverted	40–70	More common in males	Lateral nasal wall near maxillary sinus, characteristic feature is extension into sinuses	Yes (2%–53%)	47
Oncocytic	40–70	More common in males	Lateral nasal wall	Yes (15%)	3

Both synchronous and metachronous malignant change can occur in IP leading to squamous cell carcinoma (**Box 2**). Dynamic contrast enhanced MR imaging has been shown to be useful in differentiating IP from malignant sinonasal tumors.[5] Malignant change is also possible in oncocytic papillomas.[2,6]

Squamous Carcinomas and Adenocarcinomas

Squamous cell carcinoma and adenocarcinoma of the sinonasal space are uncommon. The maxillary antrum is most commonly involved (**Fig. 2**).

Radiologic features are generally nonspecific for the carcinomas.

Squamous cell carcinomas are the commonest, accounting for 80% of all sinonasal tumors. They are a disease of elderly (6th to 7th decades) males.

Imaging Features[7] (**Fig. 3**).
- Site: Maxillary sinus.
- Large soft tissue mass with heterogeneous enhancement, necrosis, and bone destruction. Invasion of adjoining compartments.
- Intermediate signal on T2-weighted imaging.
- Perineural spread.

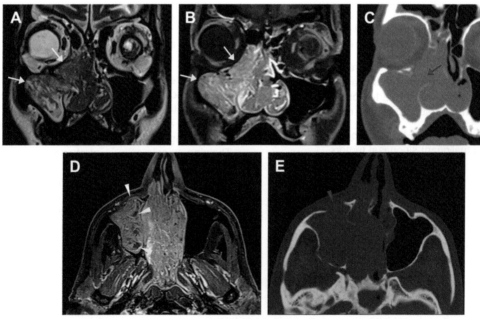

Fig. 1. Inverted papilloma. Classical convoluted cerebriform pattern is seen in the mass involving right maxillary antrum and nasal cavity (*yellow arrow*), both in T2-weighted imaging (*A*) and in postgadolinium T1-weighted imaging (*B*). Widening of maxillary ostium (*red arrow*) is noted in the coronal computed tomography (CT; *C*). Presence of areas of necrosis (*yellow arrowheads* in *D*: axial postgadolinium T1-weighted imaging), bone destruction (*red arrowhead* in *E*: axial CT scan image), and extrasinonasal extension (*white arrowhead* in *D*) indicate malignant transformation.

- Partial cerebriform pattern.[2]
- Destructive bony changes.
- Necrosis.
- Extrasinonasal extension.

- Less than 15% show nodal disease at presentation despite locally advanced disease.[8]

Adenocarcinomas are of intestinal and nonintestinal variety and occur in the fifth to 6th decades of life. The intestinal type may be occupation related or sporadic. The ones that are occupation related occur more in males and are associated with wood and leather dust inhalation. The latent period is of several decades and the risk for woodworkers is increased by 900 times. Because inhalation is the route of insult, ethmoidal region and nasal vault are the common sites. Early onset of clinical features at these sites leads to better prognosis. The sporadic forms are common in women and maxillary sinus is frequently involved. They present late and prognosis is poor.[1]

Imaging Features
- Site: occupation related: nasal vault and ethmoid sinus.
- Site: sporadic: maxillary sinus.
- Large soft tissue mass with or without bony destruction, nonspecific.
- Intermediate signal on T2-weighted imaging.
- Mucous producing; the mucous causes mixed solid and fluid signals. Diffusion-weighted and

contrast images help to differentiate from inspissated collection in adjacent blocked sinus.[9]

Staging of carcinomas are site specific according to the American Joint Committee on Cancer (AJCC) staging system manual 7th edition published in 2010. Separate staging systems exist for maxillary sinus (Box 3) and nasoethmoidal region. Owing to rarity, frontal and sphenoid sinus carcinomas do not have a staging system.

Nasal and ethmoidal carcinomas are staged together in the AJCC staging system (Box 4). Primary lesions as well as secondary extensions are seen in the ethmoidal sinuses. The nasoethmoid lesions are subdivided into several subsites for the benefit of staging. The 2 sides of the ethmoid sinus are taken as 2 subsites separated by the perpendicular plate of the ethmoid, which is a part of the nasal septum. The septum, floor, lateral wall, and vestibule are the 4 subsites proposed in the nasal cavity.

Salivary Gland Neoplasms

There are many minor salivary glands in the sinonasal tract and palate. The most common benign salivary gland neoplasm of the sinonasal space is pleomorphic adenoma.

Imaging Features
- Site: nasal septum and lateral nasal wall, maxillary sinus.[1,10]
- Spherical, bone remodeling.
- Cellular tumors, intermediate signals on T2-weighted imaging.

Adenoid cystic carcinomas are, overall, the most common salivary gland neoplasm in the

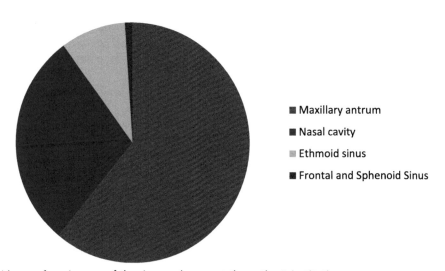

Fig. 2. Incidence of carcinomas of the sinonasal space at the author's institution.

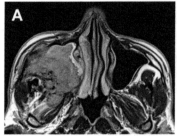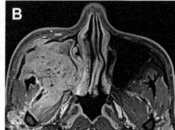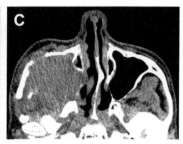

Fig. 3. Squamous cell carcinoma. Destructive mass with intermediate signal in T2-weighted imaging (*A*) and heterogeneous contrast enhancement (*B*) is seen in right maxillary sinus, with extrasinonasal spread to the pterygopalatine fossa, infratemporal fossa, and pterygoid muscles. Destruction of walls of maxillary sinus is seen in a corresponding computed tomography image (*C*).

sinonasal space. Common in the fifth decade of life, they are slow growing, with a propensity to recur after a long latent period. Recurrence rates are usually in the range of 60%.

Imaging Features (Figs. 4 and 5)
- Site: palate with secondary invasion of sinonasal space is commonest. Maxillary antrum, nasal cavity.
- Low grade: polypoidal, bone remodeling, high signal on T2-weighted imaging (paucicellular).
- High grade: locally aggressive, bone destruction, intermediate signal on T2-weighted imaging (highly cellular).
- Perineural spread is characteristic; submucosal and subperiosteal spread.[9]

Mucoepidermoid carcinomas and adenocarcinomas not otherwise specified are the other lesions arising from the minor salivary glands in the sinonasal space. They have no specific imaging features and may mimic squamous cell carcinoma.

NEUROENDOCRINE, NEUROECTODERMAL, NERVE SHEATH, AND NEURONAL TUMORS

The spectrum of the neuroendocrine tumors of the sinonasal tract has at 1 end the well-differentiated form, olfactory neuroblastoma (OLNB). At the other end are the undifferentiated forms called the sinonasal undifferentiated carcinomas. Sinonasal neuroendocrine carcinoma is somewhere between the 2 with more carcinomatous features and less differentiation than OLNB. All of these lesions usually affect the superior nasal cavity, ethmoids and nasal fossa.[1]

Olfactory Neuroblastoma

Also called esthesioneuroblastoma, these are rare and account for 2% of all sinonasal tumors. The lesions have a bimodal age incidence occurring in the 2nd and 6th decade with a slight male predilection.[11]

Imaging Features (Fig. 6)
- Site: olfactory epithelium at roof of ethmoidal sinus and adjoining cribriform plate, upper part of nasal septum, superior turbinates.
- Large soft tissue mass with intense enhancement.
- Intermediate signal on T1-weighted imaging. Hyperintense on T2-weighted imaging.[12]
- Calcification, bone destruction, and intracranial and intraorbital extension.[13]
- Cysts at interface between brain and tumor.[14]

Box 3	
T staging of maxillary sinus carcinomas according to the 7th edition of the AJCC Staging Manual, 2010	
Stage	**Description**
Tis	Carcinoma in situ
T1	Carcinoma limited to mucous lining
T2	Bone erosion or destruction limited to the hard palate and middle meatus
T3	Bone erosion or destruction of the posterior wall of maxillary sinus, floor and medial wall of orbit; tumor growth into the pterygoid fossa or ethmoid sinus
T4a	Tumor growth into the anterior orbit, pterygoid plates, infratemporal fossa, cribriform plate, frontal sinus, sphenoid sinus, or skin of cheek
T4b	Tumor growth into the orbital apex, dura, brain, middle cranial fossa, cranial nerves other than V2, nasopharynx and clivus

Box 4
T staging of nasal and ethmoidal sinus carcinomas according to the 7th edition of the AJCC Staging Manual, 2010

Stage	Description
Tis	Carcinoma in situ
T1	Tumor restricted to a single subsite, with or without bone erosion
T2	Tumor involving 2 subsites in a single region within the nasoethmoidal complex, with or without bone erosion
T3	Tumor invades medial wall or floor of orbit, maxillary sinus, palate or cribriform plate
T4a	Tumor growth into the anterior orbit, skin of nose or cheek, minimal invasion onto anterior cranial fossa, pterygoid plates, sphenoid or frontal sinuses
T4b	Tumor invades any of the following: orbital apex, dura, brain, middle cranial fossa, cranial nerves other than V2, nasopharynx or clivus

Craniofacial surgical management is among the preferred modalities in cases of intracranial disease without brain involvement. On imaging, the involvement of the dura needs careful assessment. A small dural postoperative defect can usually be covered by pericranial sheath. If a large dural defect is anticipated, a free flap needs to be harvested. The radiologist needs to alert the surgeon, because free flap harvest is a major undertaking. Staging of OLNB is by the Kadish system and is enumerated in **Box 5**. Dulgerov proposed a new staging system for OLNB, which takes in to account the nodal status.[15] This system seems to correlate better with survival and recurrence.[16]

Sinonasal Neuroendocrine Carcinoma and Sinonasal Undifferentiated Carcinoma

The relatively more undifferentiated forms of neuroendocrine carcinomas are classified under sinonasal neuroendocrine carcinoma and sinonasal undifferentiated carcinoma. As the name suggests, sinonasal undifferentiated carcinomas are the most undifferentiated and aggressive form. These lesions have a slight male preponderance and are seen in the fifth and 6th decades of life.[9]

Imaging Features (**Fig. 7**)
- Site: upper nasal cavity, ethmoids.
- Large soft tissue mass, destruction of sinonasal skeleton, invasion of skull base and orbits. No calcification, unlike OLNB.[17]
- Isointense on T1-weighted imaging, isointense to hyperintense on T2-weighted imaging.[18]
- Heterogenous enhancement.
- May have nodal disease and secondaries at presentation.

Early local recurrence and general aggressiveness are the reasons for poor prognosis of these neoplasms.

Melanoma

The primary malignant melanomas of the sinonasal tract are of the mucosal variety, contrary to the cutaneous ones found elsewhere, which are associated with sun exposure. The precursor melanocytes of the nasal mucosa migrate from the neural crest during embryologic development. The other sites for the development of the primary malignant mucosal melanomas (PMMM) are upper aerodigestive tract, anorectal region, and genitourinary tract.

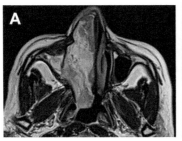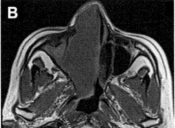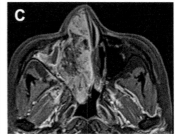

Fig. 4. Low-grade adenoid cystic carcinoma. High signal intensity is seen in T2-weighted image (*A*), suggesting a low grade tumor. T1-weighted image (*B*) shows hypointense mass with heterogeneous enhancement in postgadolinium image (*C*).

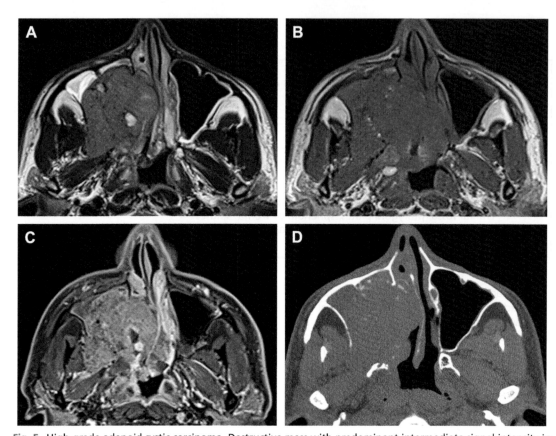

Fig. 5. High-grade adenoid cystic carcinoma. Destructive mass with predominant intermediate signal intensity in T2-weighted imaging (*A*) is seen in right maxilla and right nasal cavity. The mass is isointense to muscles in T1-weighted imaging (*B*), shows marked enhancement in postgadolinium T1-weighted imaging (*C*), and extensive bone destruction in axial computed tomography image (*D*).

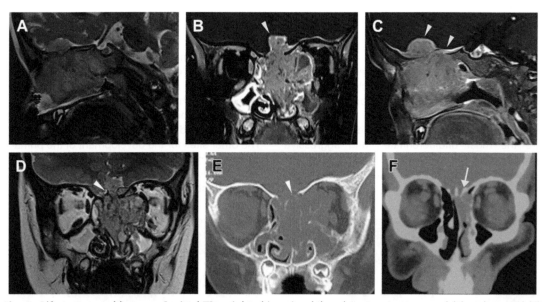

Fig. 6. Olfactory neuroblastoma. Sagittal T2-weighted imaging (*A*) and postcontrast coronal (*B*) and sagittal (*C*) T1-weighted imaging in a 3-year-old boy show a lobulated, well-defined, heterogeneously enhancing mass involving both nasal cavities, left ethmoidal air cells, extending into left maxillary antrum, clivus, and with dural involvement (*yellow arrowhead*). Breach of cribriform plate (*white arrowhead*) and intraorbital extension (*red arrowhead*) are seen in coronal T2-weighted imaging (*D*). Destruction of the cribriform plate, nasal septum, left lamina papyracea and orbital floor, and widening of left maxillary ostium are well demonstrated in the coronal computed tomography (CT) image (*E*). Coronal CT scan (*F*) in another 14-year-old boy shows an early tumor demonstrated by filling up of left olfactory recess and ethmoidal air cells (*yellow arrow*).

Box 5
The Kadish staging system for olfactory neuroblastoma

Stages	Description	5-y Survival (%)
Stage A	Lesions confined to nasal cavity	75
Stage B	Lesions confined to nasal cavity and ≥1 paranasal sinuses	68
Stage C	Lesions beyond nasal cavity and paranasal sinuses	41.2
Stage D	Distant metastasis at diagnosis	—

From Raghavan P, Phillips CD. Magnetic resonance imaging of sinonasal malignancies. Top Magn Reson Imaging. 2007;18(4):259–67; and Kadish S, Goodman M, Wang CC. Olfactory neuroblastoma. A clinical analysis of 17 cases. Cancer. 1976;37(3):1571–6.

PMMM are rare and account for only 3.5% of all sinonasal malignancies.[19] They carry a grave prognosis with 40% presenting with nodal disease at diagnosis.[20] The 5-year survival varies between 25% and 40%.[21] Local recurrence is up to 64% in 1 year after surgery.[22] Distant metastasis is also a common cause for treatment failure. Most of the sinonasal PMMM are melanotic; however, 10% to 30% can be amelanotic as well.[23]

Imaging Features (Fig. 8)
- Site: mucocutaneous junction of the anterior nasal septum, lateral nasal wall, inferior turbinate and maxillary sinus.
- Polypoidal with well-defined margins. Bone remodeling or destruction.
- Intermediate to hypointense on T2-weighted imaging. Hyperintense on T1-weighted imaging owing to melanin or hemorrhage.

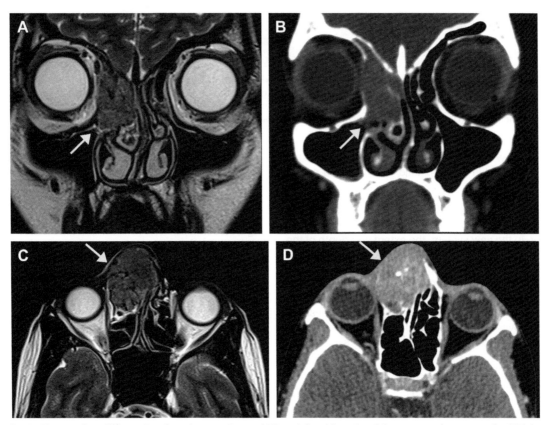

Fig. 7. Sinonasal undifferentiated carcinoma. Coronal T2-weighted imaging (A), computed tomography (CT) image (B), axial T2-weighted imaging (C), and CT scan image (D) show a mass (*yellow arrows*) in right anterior ethmoidal air cells and nasal cavity, with bone destruction.

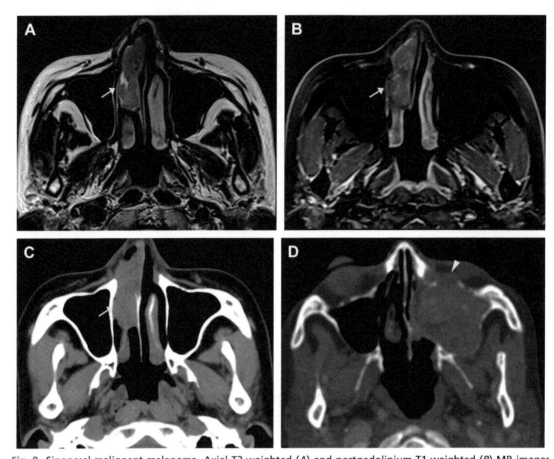

Fig. 8. Sinonasal malignant melanoma. Axial T2-weighted (*A*) and postgadolinium T1-weighted (*B*) MR images show a homogeneously enhancing soft tissue mass arising from the anterior right nasal cavity. Axial computed tomography (CT) in the same patient (*C*) shows bone remodeling (*yellow arrow*). CT scan in another patient with melanoma (*D*) shows bone destruction (*yellow arrowhead*).

- Flow voids, intense enhancement, perineural spread in desmoplastic variety after a period of latency.[24]

The AJCC 7th edition has included PMMM in the TNM classification and staging as a separate chapter. In the new system, the extent and depth of the disease has been taken into account rather than the site, as is the case with other sinonasal tumors. In the new system, there is no T1 or T2 disease and hence no stage I or stage II (Box 6). Nodal disease qualifies the lesion as stage IV in the new system. However, no significant survival benefit was observed using the new classification system.[21]

Ewing's Sarcoma Family of Tumors

Ewing's sarcoma family of tumors are derived from pluripotent neural crest cells. The members of this common and single neoplastic entity are Ewing's sarcoma, primitive neuroectodermal tumor, and Askin's tumors of the chest wall. They are distinguished by the tumor cell differentiation only.[25] Ewing's sarcoma family of tumors are common in the second decade of life. In the craniofacial region, the commonest site is mandible followed by the maxilla. Sinonasal Ewing's sarcoma can be a rare complication of radiation therapy for retinoblastoma.

Imaging Features (Fig. 9)
- Site: maxilla.
- Large soft tissue mass with varying degrees of bone involvement and aggressive periosteal reaction on CT[1]
- Hyperintense on T2-weighted imaging.
- Heterogeneous enhancement.

Peripheral Nerve Sheath Tumors

Peripheral nerve sheath tumors consist of Schwannoma, neurofibroma, and malignant peripheral nerve sheath tumor.

Box 6
Staging of primary malignant mucosal melanomas, 7th edition of the AJCC Staging Manual, 2010

Stage	Description
Primary Tumor (T)	
TX	Primary tumor cannot be assessed
T3	Mucosal disease
T4a	Moderately advanced disease: Tumor involving deep soft tissue, cartilage, bone, or overlying skin
T4b	Very advanced disease: Tumor involving brain, dura, skull base, lower cranial nerves (IX, X, XI, XII), masticator space, carotid artery, prevertebral space, or mediastinal structures
Regional lymph nodes (N)	
NX	Regional lymph nodes cannot be assessed
N0	No regional lymph node metastases
N1	Regional lymph node metastases present
Distant metastasis (M)	
M0	No distant metastasis
M1	Distant metastasis

Stage	T	N	M
III	T3	N0	M0
IVA	T4a	N0	M0
	T3	N1	M0
	T4a	N1	M0
IVB	T4b	N Any	M0
IVC	T any	N Any	M1

Schwannomas are benign neoplasms arising from Schwann cells of the nerve sheath.

Imaging Features (**Fig. 10**)

- Site: rare in sinonasal space,[26] Vth nerve commonly involved. Usually benign.
- Hyperintense signal on T2-weighted imaging.
- Bone remodeling. Bone destruction suggests malignant change.[27]
- Homogenous enhancement.[28] Cystic change and necrosis leads to heterogeneous enhancement.

Neurofibromas[1] are also benign neoplasms of the nerve sheath, but are interspersed with the nerve. When multiple or large (plexiform type), they are usually a part of Neurofibromatosis syndrome.

Imaging Features

- Well-defined ovoid.
- Hyperintense on T2-weighted imaging, heterogeneous enhancement.
- May remodel bone.

Malignant peripheral nerve sheath tumor mainly complicate neurofibromatosis syndrome. These lesions can be aggressive with bone destruction and can involve cranial nerves.[1]

Meningioma

Meningioma of the sinonasal space is rare and can occur in 4 distinct circumstances.[29,30]

1. Direct extension of an intracranial meningioma into the sinonasal space.
2. Metastasis to sinus from intracranial tumor.
3. Originating from arachnoid cells sequestered around suture lines, cranial nerves or vessels exiting foramina.
4. Isolated extracranial lesions with no intracranial component or association with cranial nerve or foramina also designated as ectopic meningioma.

These lesions are benign and slow growing lesions, found more commonly in middle aged females.

Imaging Features (**Fig. 11**)

- Site: nasal vault.
- Hyperdense on CT with brilliant enhancement.
- Hypointense on T1-weighted imaging and hyperintense on T2-weighted imaging.
- Bone changes are hyperostosis, sclerosis, remodeling, and erosive changes.

HEMATOLYMPHOID NEOPLASMS
Lymphoma

Although the head and neck region is uncommon for the development of extranodal lymphoma, the lesions present with interesting radiologic characteristics. There are 3 histologic types of sinonasal lymphomas, natural killer (NK)/T-cell, B-cell, and T-cell types. The NK/T-cell type is more common

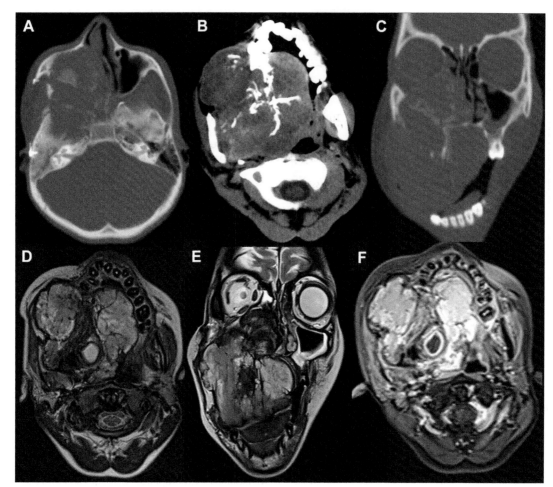

Fig. 9. Primitive neuroectodermal tumor. A 14-year old child presented with hemifacial swelling. Aggressive bone destruction with a large associated soft tissue mass is seen in axial (*A, B*) and coronal (*C*) computed tomography scan images, heterogeneous and predominantly high signal intensity is seen in T2-weighted axial (*D*) and coronal (*E*) MR images. The tumor is intensely enhancing in postgadolinium T1-weighted imaging (*F*).

in Asians, Central and South Americans and Mexicans. The B-cell type is more common in Europe and the United States.[31]

The 'NK/T-cell lymphoma of the nasal type' is a separate clinicopathologic entity in the World Health Organization classification of T-cell and NK cell neoplasms. There is a strong association with Epstein–Barr virus.[32]

Imaging Features (Fig. 12)
- Site: nasal space. May extend to nasopharynx and maxillary antrum.
- Not associated with cervical adenopathy, hence 'primary.'
- Plaquelike or sheetlike. Diffuse mass formation also seen.
- Hypointense on T1-weighted imaging and hypointense or intermediate signal on T2-weighted imaging.

- Bone erosion and destruction without sclerosis.

Prognosis of NK/T-cell lymphoma is poor with an aggressive clinical course.[32] Imaging differentials include Wegeners granulomatosis, granulomatous infections and carcinomas.

The B-cell lymphoma of sinonasal space occurs as a part of systemic disease.

Imaging Features (Fig. 13)
- Site: maxillary sinus.
- Large polyps or polypoidal masses.
- Bone remodeling.[7]
- Intermediate signal on T2-weighted imaging.
- Moderate enhancement.

Burkitt's lymphoma is a B-cell non-Hodgkin's lymphoma, which is highly aggressive and is endemic to the African continent involving facial

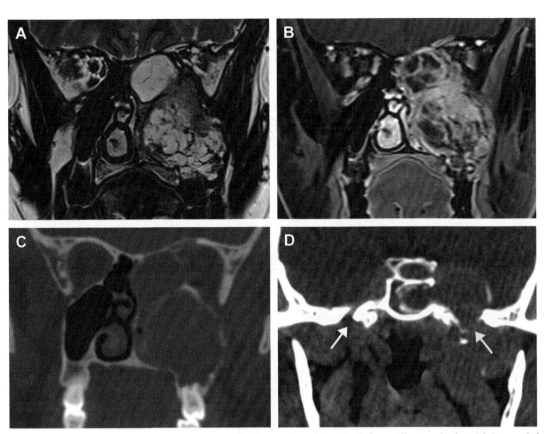

Fig. 10. Schwannoma. MR imaging shows an expansile mass involving the left maxillary and ethmoid sinuses, left nasal cavity, and infratemporal fossa. The mass is hyperintense with internal hypointense septations on T2-weighted imaging (A) and shows septal and nodular enhancement in postgadolinium T1-weighted imaging (B). Slow growing nature is evident in coronal computed tomography image (C) as bone remodeling and limited destruction is present. Involvement of the left foramen ovale (*yellow arrow*) indicates mandibular nerve pathology (D). Compare with normal opposite foramen ovale (*white arrow*).

skeleton apart from other parts of the lymphoretic-ular system (**Fig. 14**).

The role of imaging in the sinonasal lymphomas is to identify the primary site of disease, localize area for biopsy[33] and mapping the lesion in its entirety, should radiotherapy be contemplated.

Plasma Cell Neoplasm

Plasma cell neoplasm of the sinonasal space may occur as a local bony manifestation of multiple myeloma, or a solitary plasmacytoma involving bone or as extramedullary plasmacytoma, which is essentially a soft tissue lesion without bony involvement.[34]

Imaging Features
- Multiple myeloma: multiple punched out bony lesions with or without soft tissue component.
- Solitary plasmacytoma: lytic bony lesion with soft tissue component.

- Extramedullary plasmacytoma: soft tissue lesion without bony component, but may remodel bone.[35]
- Soft tissue component: intermediate signal on T2-weighted imaging, moderate enhancement (**Fig. 15**).

Chloroma

Chloroma or granulocytic sarcoma is a soft tissue lesion that develops as a part of myeloproliferative disorder, commonly acute myeloid leukemia.

Imaging Features (**Fig. 16**)
- Site: orbit, sinonasal tract and nasopharynx are commonly involved.
- Intermediate to hyperintense on T2-weighted imaging. Homogenous enhancement.
- Slightly infiltrative margins.[36]

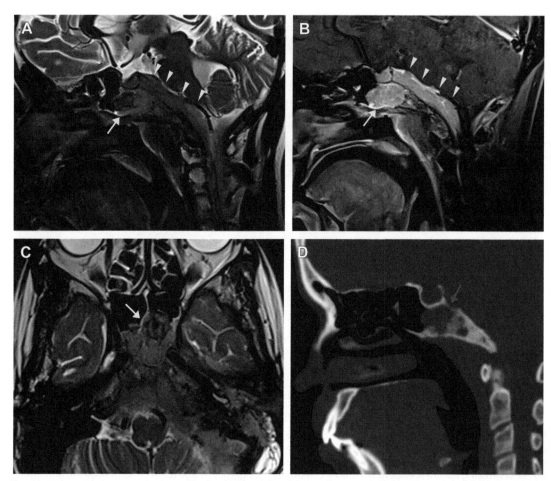

Fig. 11. Sphenoid sinus meningioma. Sagittal T2-weighted (*A*) and postgadolinium T1-weighted (*B*) MR images reveal a homogeneous plaquelike enhancing dural mass dorsal to clivus (*arrowheads*) and a nodular mass in sphenoid sinus, which is hyperintense on T2-weighted imaging and shows homogeneous enhancement (*yellow arrow*). Axial T2-weighted imaging (*C*) demonstrates the location of the mass precisely (*yellow arrow*). Erosive change in the clivus (*red arrow*) by the skull base meningioma and involvement of sphenoid sinus is well seen in the sagittal computed tomography image (*D*).

Langerhan's Cell Histiocytosis

Langerhan's Cell Histiocytosis is a disorder that is characterized by overproduction of histiocytes. There are 3 components to this disease, which is common in children. The Eosinophilic granuloma is a localized form, whereas Letterer–Siwe and Hand–Schuller–Christian's diseases are disseminated diseases.

Imaging Features[37] (**Fig. 17**)
- Site: facial bones.
- Lytic bony lesions.
- Intermediate to high signal on T1-weighted imaging. Hyperintense on T2-weighted imaging. Marrow involvement.
- Homogeneous intense enhancement.

PRIMARY SOFT TISSUE TUMORS

Mesenchymal tissue of the sinonasal region gives rise to various types of primary tumors. The lesions are uncommon and are enumerated in **Box 7**.

Juvenile Nasopharyngeal Angiofibroma

Juvenile nasopharyngeal angiofibroma is a benign but locally aggressive mesenchymal tumor with a very rich vascular supply. The typical presenting feature is profuse epistaxis in a young adolescent boy.[38] Some authors have suggested that these lesions are vascular malformations rather than tumors and arise from testosterone sensitive cells.[39] If this lesion occurs in females, studies should be performed to ascertain the genotype of the

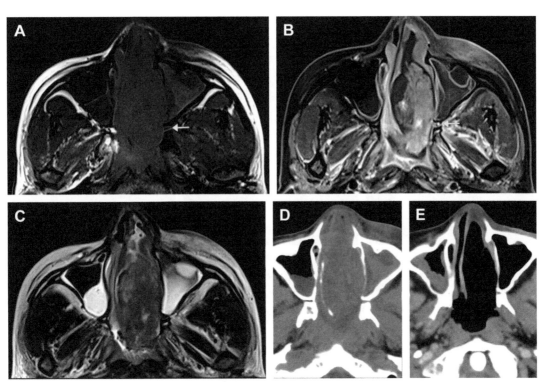

Fig. 12. Natural killer–T-cell lymphoma. This patient presented with a nasal mass expanding the left nasal cavity, remodeling the nasal septum and medial wall of maxillary antrum (D). Heterogeneous signal intensity soft tissue is noted in T2-weighted imaging (C). T1-weighted imaging (A) shows extension of the tumor into the left pterygopalatine fossa (*yellow arrow*) and infratemporal fossa, evidenced by replacement of fat signal. Marked enhancement of the tumor is seen (B). Resolution of the mass after therapy is seen in an axial computed tomography image (E). Note that destructive bony changes are usually encountered.

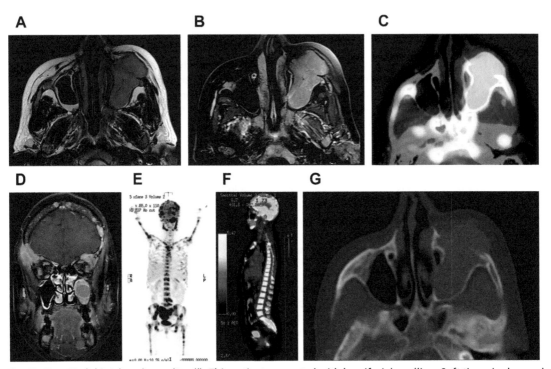

Fig. 13. Non-Hodgkin's lymphoma (B cell). This patient presented with hemifacial swelling. Soft tissue is observed in left maxillary antrum, showing mild hyperintense signals in T2-weighted imaging (A) and homogeneous enhancement (B), with destruction of anterior wall, better seen in axial computed tomography (CT) image (G). Numerous similar enhancing lesions were seen in the calvarium, skull base, and mandible (D). Maximum intensity projection image of PET scan (E) and axial (C) and sagittal (F) images of PET-CT scan show increased metabolic activity in almost all bones of the body.

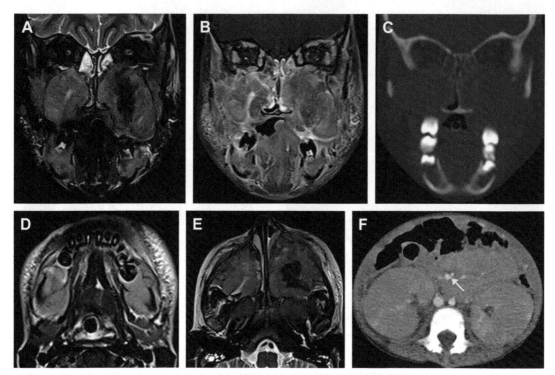

Fig. 14. Burkitt's lymphoma. Coronal T2-weighted (*A*) and postcontrast T1-weighted (*B*) images in a 14-year-old child with swelling of face and gums, and systemic symptoms, demonstrate extensive enhancing soft tissue mass involving both maxilla and nasal cavities, obliterating the maxillary and ethmoid sinuses. Axial T2-weighted images (*D, E*) show medullary expansion and marrow replacement involving the entire mandible, with cortical destruction and extraosseous soft tissue, a common finding in Burkitt's lymphoma. Coronal computed tomography (CT) image of the face (*C*) shows destruction of both maxilla, including orbital floors as well as cortical breach in the mandible. Axial postcontrast CT of the abdomen (*F*) shows bilateral renal and lymph nodal disease (*yellow arrow*: encased mesenteric vessels).

individual. The lesion is uncommon with incidence of less than 0.5% of all nasopharyngeal neoplasms.[38]

Imaging Features[40] (**Fig. 18**)
- Site: sphenopalatine foramen and pterygopalatine fossa. Secondary involvement of sinonasal space. Orbital and intracranial extensions.
- Heterogeneous signals on T1- and T2-weighted images with strong enhancement.
- Widened pterygopalatine fossa and bowed posterior maxillary sinus wall.
- Supply from internal maxillary artery and ascending pharyngeal artery.

Mainstay of treatment is surgery, both open and endoscopic resection may be performed.[41] Preoperative embolization is commonly performed for juvenile nasopharyngeal angiofibroma to reduce tumor bleed.[42]

Rhabdomyosarcoma

Rhabdomyosarcoma is the most common malignant sinonasal neoplasm in the pediatric

population with a very aggressive behavior and early metastasis to nodes and distant sites such as lungs.[7] At presentation, they are usually locally advanced with multicompartmental involvement of the sinonasal space, bone destruction, and frequent invasion of the orbit and deep neck spaces.

Imaging features (**Fig. 19**)
- Bone destruction on CT with invasion onto adjacent compartments.
- Isointense to hyperintense on T1-weighted imaging, heterogeneous signals on T2-weighted imaging.
- Moderate heterogeneous enhancement.
- Ring like enhancement in botyroid variety of embryonal rhabdomyosarcoma.[43]

FIBROOSSEOUS LESIONS AND BONE SARCOMA

A spectrum of fibroosseus lesions are possible in the sinonasal skeleton varying from osteoma which has the maximum bony content to the

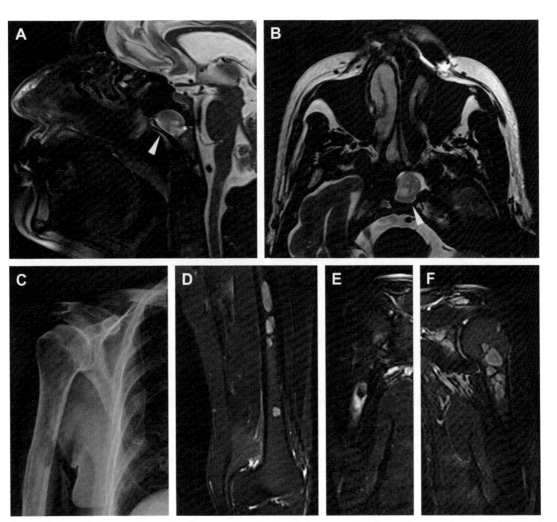

Fig. 15. Sphenoid sinus myeloma. An 83-year-old patient with known multiple myeloma underwent whole body MR imaging screening. In addition to multiple lesions throughout the body, a lobulated soft tissue (*arrowheads*) surrounded by collection was discovered in the sphenoid sinus, which showed mild hyperintense signals in T2-weighted imaging (*A, B*). Lytic lesion in rib and right humerus are seen in the radiograph (*C*), and multiple soft tissue lesions replacing the marrow signals are seen in the T2 turbo inversion recovery magnitude coronal MR images (*D–F*) of both humeri and left femur.

ossifying fibroma and fibrous dysplasia where there is more of fibrous content.[44]

Osteoma

Osteomas are the most common benign tumors of the sinonasal space. They are generally incidentally detected on imaging, but 37% lesions are associated with sinonasal pathologic findings.[45] They can block sinonasal or lacrimal drainage pathways and cause pent up collection, which may need surgical attention. Rarely, they may erode the skull base to cause cerebrospinal fluid rhinorrhea.

Imaging features (**Fig. 20**)
- Site: ethmoid,[45] frontal sinus.

- Broad base or pedicle may be seen.
- Well-defined lesions on CT with matrix density varying from 'ground glass' to 'bonelike' depending on consistency, which can vary from compact bone, spongy bone, or fibrous component.
- Hypointense or isointense on T2-weighted imaging.

Fibrous Dysplasia

Fibrous dysplasia is a nonneoplastic disorder that affects the craniofacial bones as well as other parts of the body. They can be monoostotic or polyostotic. Rarely, they can be a part of McCune–Albright syndrome where they are associated with autonomous

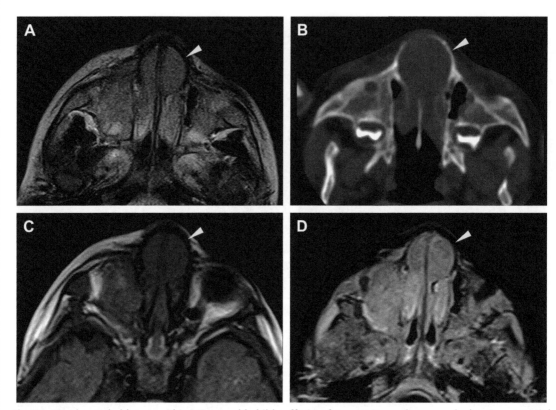

Fig. 16. Nasal septal chloroma. This 1.5-year-old child suffering from acute myelogenous leukemia presented with nasal swelling and noisy breathing. A well-defined soft tissue mass (*arrowhead*) was observed on either side of the cartilaginous part of nasal septum, which showed mild hyperintense signals in T2-weighted imaging (*A*), mild hypointense signals in T1-weighted imaging (*C*), and homogeneous contrast enhancement (*D*). Remodeling of nasal bones is seen in the axial computed tomography image (*B*).

endocrine dysfunction and cafe-au-lait skin lesions. Pathologically, the medulla of the involved bone is replaced by immature tissue, which varies between a spectrum of osseous and fibrous tissue. 0.5% of polyostotic forms and 4% of McCune–Albright syndrome patients develop malignant transformation.[46]

Imaging Features (**Fig. 21**)
- Site: any craniofacial bone, more in polyostotic form. If involvement is profuse, called 'leontiasis ossea.'
- Involved bone is expanded with thinned out cortex, ill-defined margins.
- Matrix varies from 'cotton wool' to 'ground glass' reflecting pathologic composition.[46]
- Intermediate to low signal on T2-weighted imaging; intermediate on T1-weighted imaging.
- Significant enhancement.

Ossifying Fibroma

Ossifying fibroma is an expansile well-circumscribed benign tumor that is, commonly seen in the mandible. They are notorious for local

recurrence and hence wide local excision is advocated.

Imaging Features (**Fig. 22**)
- Site: mandible, maxilla, lateral nasal wall, ethmoidal complex.
- Well-defined lesion on CT, egg shell–like calcified margins.[44]
- Varying matrix density, depending on composition, maximum with cement-ossifying form.
- Locally destructive, bone erosion.[47] MR imaging displays soft tissue extent better.

Even on histology, the differentiation of fibrous dysplasia from ossifying fibroma can be difficult.[9] Few radiologic features can aid in arriving at a conclusive diagnosis (**Box 8**).

Osteosarcoma

Only 8.6% osteosarcomas occur in the craniofacial region. They are prevalent in the third decade that is, a decade later than when it is common in other areas of the body.[48] Secondary OS have

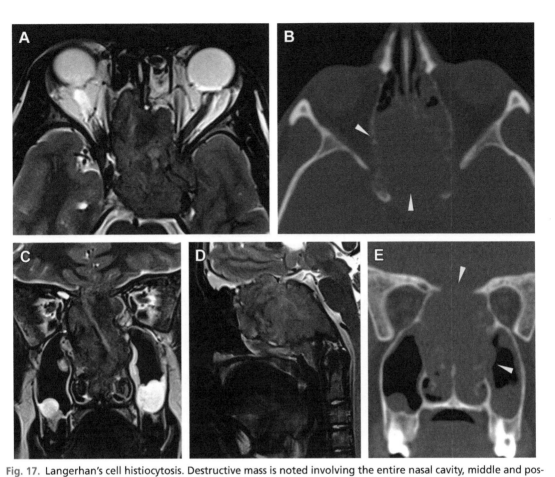

Fig. 17. Langerhan's cell histiocytosis. Destructive mass is noted involving the entire nasal cavity, middle and posterior ethmoidal air cells, with intermediate signals in T2-weighted imaging (axial, *A*; coronal, *C*; sagittal, *D*). The mass is seen to extend into the sphenoid sinus and clivus in (*D*). Extensive bone destruction (*arrowheads*) is demonstrated in axial (*B*) and coronal (*E*) computed tomography images.

been associated with several conditions, namely Paget's disease, previous radiotherapy and retinoblastoma.[49] The lesions are usually high grade with poor prognosis.

Box 7
Primary soft tissue tumors of the sinonasal space

Component	Description
Vascular	Hemangioma, angiofibroma, angiomatous polyp, angiosarcoma, hemangiosarcoma, Kaposi's sarcoma
Muscle	Leiomyoma, leiomyosarcoma, rhabdomyosarcoma
Lipoblastic	Lipoma, liposarcoma
Fibroblastic	Fibrosarcoma, fibrous histiocytoma (benign and malignant)

Imaging Features
- Site: maxilla.[48]
- Large soft tissue mass lesion with aggressive periosteal reaction and new bone formation on CT.
- Intermediate signals on T2-weighted imaging, calcified matrix, and new bone formation appears hypointense.

Chondrosarcoma

Primary chondrosarcomas of the craniofacial region are infrequent. Secondary CS are associated with Maffucci syndrome, Ollier disease, and prior radiation therapy.[50] The lesions are high grade[51] and show a large soft tissue mass lesion with typical stippled areas of chondroid calcification and bone erosion.

Imaging features
- Site: maxilla (alveolar process), nasal septum.
- Chondroid matrix is best seen on CT.

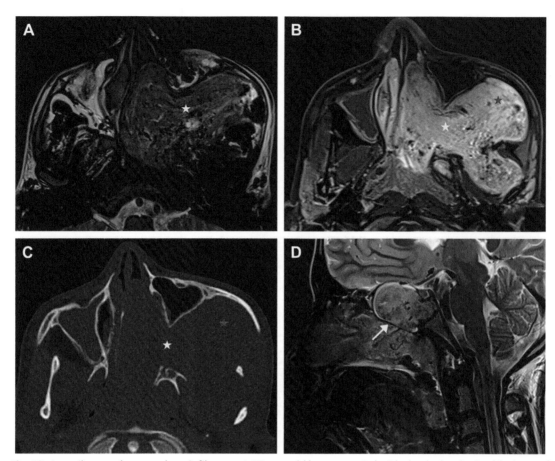

Fig. 18. Juvenile nasopharyngeal angiofibroma. A 16-year-old boy presented with slowly developing blockage of nose and episodes of epistaxis. T2-weighted imaging (*A*) shows prominent flow voids in the intermediate signal intensity mass involving nasopharynx, left nasal cavity, pterygopalatine fossa (PPF; *yellow star* in *A, B, C*) and infratemporal fossa (*red star* in *A, B, C*). Prominent enhancement is seen on postcontrast T1-weighted axial image (*B*). Widening of PPF and smooth anterior bowing of the posterior and lateral maxillary antral wall is seen on the axial computed tomography image (*C*). Clival involvement is noted in sagittal T2-weighted imaging (*yellow arrow* in *D*).

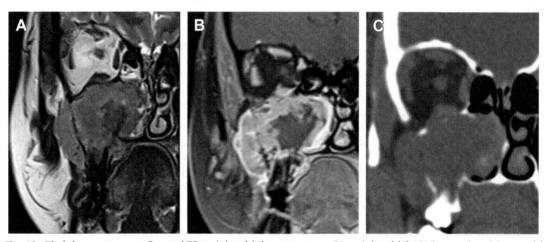

Fig. 19. Rhabdomyosarcoma. Coronal T2-weighted (*A*), postcontrast T1-weighted (*B*) MR images in a 26-year-old woman shows a heterogeneous signal intensity enhancing mass with necrotic areas in right maxillary sinus. Destruction of orbital floor, alveolus, hard palate, medial wall of maxilla is seen in coronal computed tomography (*C*).

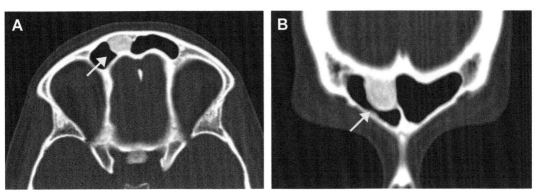

Fig. 20. Frontal sinus osteoma. Axial (*A*) and coronal (*B*) computed tomography images show a well-circumscribed dense bony mass (*yellow arrows*) arising from the wall of frontal sinus and growing into the sinus cavity.

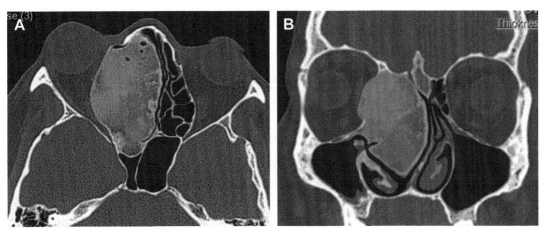

Fig. 21. Fibrous dysplasia. Axial (*A*) and coronal (*B*) computed tomography images (bone window) show expansile lesion of ground glass density involving the right ethmoidal air cells and nasal cavity, with thinned out overlying bones.

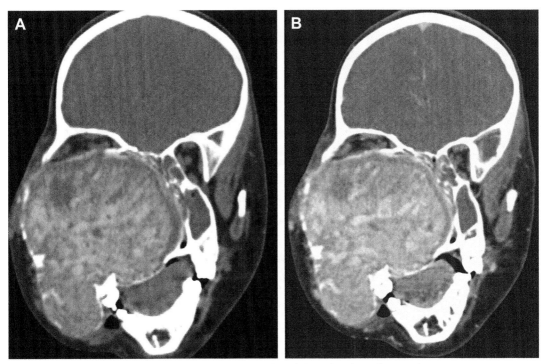

Fig. 22. Ossifying fibroma. A 10-year-old girl presented with hemifacial swelling and proptosis. In noncontrast coronal computed tomography image (*A*), a well-circumscribed expansile lesion is noted occupying the right maxilla with cortical thinning. Matrix consists of lamellated ossification and background soft tissue is seen to enhance mildly in postcontrast image (*B*).

Box 8
Radiologic features to differentiate fibrous dysplasia from ossifying fibroma

Fibrous Dysplasia	Ossifying Fibroma
Ill-defined border	Well-defined border with calcified wall
Indolent disease, burnt out by puberty	Aggressive disease, local bone destruction[47]
Encompass teeth roots	Absorb teeth roots[46]

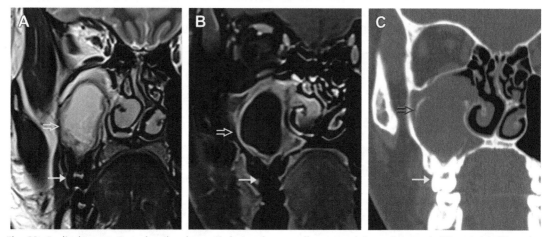

Fig. 23. Radicular cyst. Round unilocular cystic lesion (*open yellow arrow*), hyperintense in T2-weighted imaging (*A*), with uniform enhancement of walls in postgadolinium T1-weighted imaging (*B*) is seen in right maxillary antrum, centered on the apex of a tooth (*thin yellow arrow* in *A, B, C*). The lesion is bordered by thin rim of cortical bone (*red open arrow* in computed tomography image, *C*), separating it from the maxillary antrum, unlike a mucocele.

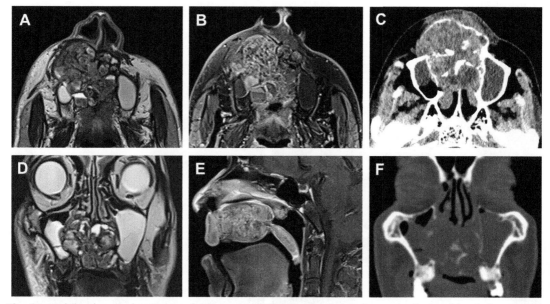

Fig. 24. Multilocular nasal septal ameloblastoma. Well-defined lobulated mass having multicystic honeycomb appearance and fluid-fluid levels in T2-weighted axial (*A*) and coronal (*D*) images is seen involving the hard palate, lower part of nasal septum, and medial walls of maxilla. Postgadolinium T1-weighted axial (*B*) and sagittal (*E*) images show enhancing septations and solid areas. Axial (*C*) and coronal (*F*) computed tomography images show expansile lesion with bone destruction and soft tissue component.

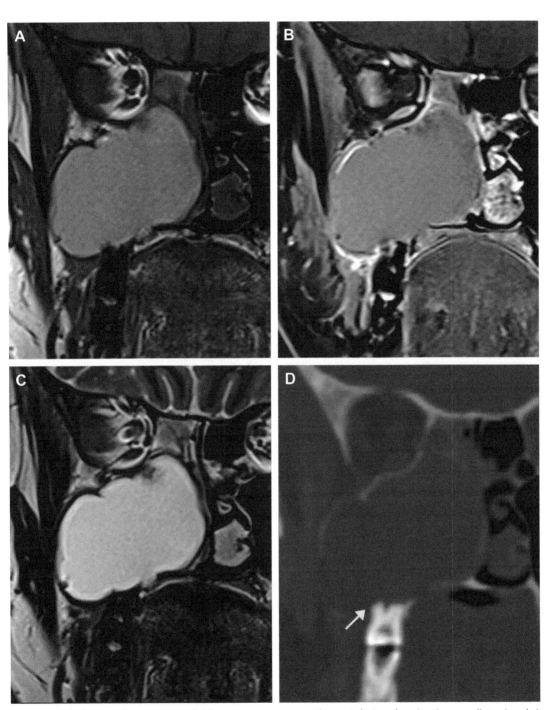

Fig. 25. Unilocular maxillary sinus ameloblastoma. Large expansile cystic lesion showing intermediate signals in T1-weighted imaging (*A*), hyperintense signals in T2-weighted imaging (*C*), and with a thin rim of enhancement in postgadolinium T1-weighted imaging (*B*) is seen to occupy the entire right maxillary antrum. Expansion of the walls of maxillary antrum and resorption of roots of an adjacent tooth is demonstrated in coronal computed tomography (*arrow* in *D*).

- Hyperintense on T2-weighted imaging owing to high water content of chondroid matrix.
- Enhancement of fibrovascular core, nonenhancement of chondroid and mucoid matrix, leading to heterogenous enhancement pattern.[52]

ODONTOGENIC TUMORS
Periodontal Cyst (Radicular Cyst)

Radicular cysts are the commonest jaw cysts. The lesions arise in carious teeth in the periapical region as a result of repeated infection and granuloma formation. They are common in the middle age and are painless.[53]

Imaging features (Fig. 23)
- Site: upper jaw, related tooth resorbed or displaced, erode into sinus.[53]
- Unilocular lucent cyst, hyperintense on T2-weighted imaging, thin calcified rim appreciated on CT.

Ameloblastoma

They are uncommon slow growing painless benign epithelial neoplasms affecting individuals from third to the fifth decade and constitute only 10% of all odontogenic tumors.[53] They are much more common in the mandible (80%) compared with the maxilla. Maxillary ameloblastomas manifest at a later age group and are more aggressive compared with those in the mandible.[9]

Imaging Features (Figs. 24 and 25)
- Site: maxillary sinus.
- Unilocular or multilocular cysts, thin calcified wall, no mineralization.
- Locally aggressive with destruction or remodeling of sinus on CT.[1]
- Intermediate signal on T1-weighted imaging and hyperintense on T2-weighted imaging.[1]

METASTASIS

Metastasis to the paranasal sinuses is very rare, the commonest primary being renal cell carcinoma. Other primary sites are lung, breast, thyroid, and prostate. Metastatic lesions may be single or multiple.

Imaging Features[54] (Fig. 26)
- Site: maxillary sinus.
- Soft tissue lesion, bone destruction.
- Variable enhancement, vascular metastasis in renal cell carcinoma and thyroid cancer show significant enhancement.

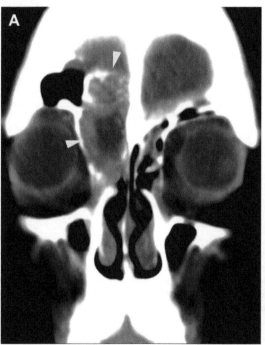 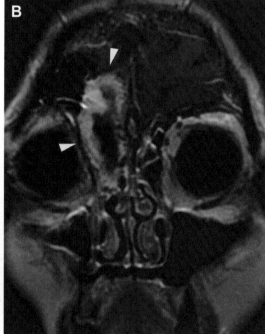

Fig. 26. Frontoethmoidal sinus metastasis from renal cell carcinoma. Coronal computed tomography (CT; *A*) and coronal postgadolinium T1-weighted MR imaging (*B*) show expansile soft tissue lesion (*yellow arrowheads*) in right frontal sinus and ethmoidal air cells with bone destruction, periosteal reaction evident in CT images and heterogeneous enhancement with central necrosis in MR images.

SUMMARY

A diverse nature of neoplastic diseases is possible in the sinonasal space. Although a specific pathologic diagnosis may not always be possible, the radiologist's role is to offer a realistic differential. Both CT and MR imaging play synergistic roles in this endeavor.

REFERENCES

1. Som PM, Brandwein-Gensler MS, Kassel EE, et al. Tumors and tumor-like conditions of the sinonasal cavities. In: Curtin DC, editor. Head and neck imaging. 5th edition. St Louis (MO): Mosby; 2011. p. 253–408. Tumors and tumor-like conditions of sinonasal cavities. 5th ed. St Louis, MO: Mosby; 2011.
2. Jeon TY, Kim HJ, Chung SK, et al. Sinonasal inverted papilloma: value of convoluted cerebriform pattern on MR imaging. AJNR Am J Neuroradiol 2008;29(8):1556–60.
3. Ojiri H, Ujita M, Tada S, et al. Potentially distinctive features of sinonasal inverted papilloma on MR imaging. AJR Am J Roentgenol 2000;175(2):465–8.
4. Lombardi D, Tomenzoli D, Butta L, et al. Limitations and complications of endoscopic surgery for treatment for sinonasal inverted papilloma: a reassessment after 212 cases. Head Neck 2011;33(8):1154–61.
5. Wang X, Zhang Z, Chen X, et al. Value of magnetic resonance imaging including dynamic contrast-enhanced magnetic resonance imaging in differentiation between inverted papilloma and malignant tumors in the nasal cavity. Chin Med J 2014; 127(9):1696–701.
6. Barnes L, Bedetti C. Oncocytic Schneiderian papilloma: a reappraisal of cylindrical cell papilloma of the sinonasal tract. Hum Pathol 1984;15(4):344–51.
7. Madani G, Beale TJ, Lund VJ. Imaging of sinonasal tumors. Semin Ultrasound CT MR 2009;30(1):25–38.
8. Cantu G, Bimbi G, Miceli R, et al. Lymph node metastases in malignant tumors of the paranasal sinuses: prognostic value and treatment. Arch Otolaryngol Head Neck Surg 2008;134(2):170–7.
9. Davide Farina RM. Neoplasms of the sinonasal cavities. In: Robert Hermans, editor. Head and Neck Cancer Imaging. 2nd edition. Berlin: Springer-Verlag; 2012. p. 207–36.
10. Compagno J, Wong RT. Intranasal mixed tumors (pleomorphic adenomas): a clinicopathologic study of 40 cases. Am J Clin Pathol 1977;68(2):213–8.
11. Thompson LD. Olfactory neuroblastoma. Head Neck Pathol 2009;3(3):252–9.
12. Derdeyn CP, Moran CJ, Wippold FJ 2nd, et al. MRI of esthesioneuroblastoma. J Comput Assist Tomogr 1994;18(1):16–21.
13. Regenbogen VS, Zinreich SJ, Kim KS, et al. Hyperostotic esthesioneuroblastoma: CT and MR findings. J Comput Assist Tomogr 1988;12(1):52–6.
14. Som PM, Lidov M, Brandwein M, et al. Sinonasal esthesioneuroblastoma with intracranial extension: marginal tumor cysts as a diagnostic MR finding. AJNR Am J Neuroradiol 1994;15(7):1259–62.
15. Dulguerov P, Allal AS, Calcaterra TC. Esthesioneuroblastoma: a meta-analysis and review. Lancet Oncol 2001;2(11):683–90.
16. Bachar G, Goldstein DP, Shah M, et al. Esthesioneuroblastoma: The Princess Margaret Hospital experience. Head Neck 2008;30(12):1607–14.
17. Raghavan P, Phillips CD. Magnetic resonance imaging of sinonasal malignancies. Top Magn Reson Imaging 2007;18(4):259–67.
18. Phillips CD, Futterer SF, Lipper MH, et al. Sinonasal undifferentiated carcinoma: CT and MR imaging of an uncommon neoplasm of the nasal cavity. Radiology 1997;202(2):477–80.
19. Conley JJ. Melanomas of the mucous membrane of the head and neck. Laryngoscope 1989;99(12):1248–54.
20. Franquemont DW, Mills SE. Sinonasal malignant melanoma. A clinicopathologic and immunohistochemical study of 14 cases. Am J Clin Pathol 1991;96(6):689–97.
21. Gal TJ, Silver N, Huang B. Demographics and treatment trends in sinonasal mucosal melanoma. Laryngoscope 2011;121(9):2026–33.
22. Yoshioka H, Kamada T, Kandatsu S, et al. MRI of mucosal malignant melanoma of the head and neck. J Comput Assist Tomogr 1998;22(3):492–7.
23. Yousem DM, Li C, Montone KT, et al. Primary malignant melanoma of the sinonasal cavity: MR imaging evaluation. Radiographics 1996;16(5):1101–10.
24. Chang PC, Fischbein NJ, McCalmont TH, et al. Perineural spread of malignant melanoma of the head and neck: clinical and imaging features. AJNR Am J Neuroradiol 2004;25(1):5–11.
25. Khoury JD. Ewing sarcoma family of tumors. Adv Anat Pathol 2005;12(4):212–20.
26. Younis RT, Gross CW, Lazar RH. Schwannomas of the paranasal sinuses. Case report and clinicopathologic analysis. Arch Otolaryngol Head Neck Surg 1991;117(6):677–80.
27. George KJ, Price R. Nasoethmoid schwannoma with intracranial extension. Case report and review of literature. Br J Neurosurg 2009;23(1):83–5.
28. Dublin AB, Dedo HH, Bridger WH. Intranasal schwannoma: magnetic resonance and computed tomography appearance. Am J Otolaryngol 1995; 16(4):251–4.
29. Rushing EJ, Bouffard JP, McCall S, et al. Primary extracranial meningiomas: an analysis of 146 cases. Head Neck Pathol 2009;3(2):116–30.
30. Thompson LD, Gyure KA. Extracranial sinonasal tract meningiomas: a clinicopathologic study of 30

cases with a review of the literature. Am J Surg Pathol 2000;24(5):640–50.

31. King AD, Lei KI, Ahuja AT, et al. MR imaging of nasal T-cell/natural killer cell lymphoma. AJR Am J Roentgenol 2000;174(1):209–11.

32. Lee HJ, Im JG, Goo JM, et al. Peripheral T-cell lymphoma: spectrum of imaging findings with clinical and pathologic features. Radiographics 2003; 23(1):7–26 [discussion: 28].

33. Borges A, Fink J, Villablanca P, et al. Midline destructive lesions of the sinonasal tract: simplified terminology based on histopathologic criteria. AJNR Am J Neuroradiol 2000;21(2):331–6.

34. Bachmeyer C, Levy V, Carteret M, et al. Sphenoid sinus localization of multiple myeloma revealing evolution from benign gammapathy. Head Neck 1997; 19(4):347–50.

35. Kondo M, Hashimoto S, Inuyama Y, et al. Extramedullary plasmacytoma of the sinonasal cavities: CT evaluation. J Comput Assist Tomogr 1986;10(5): 841–4.

36. Pomeranz SJ, Hawkins HH, Towbin R, et al. Granulocytic sarcoma (chloroma): CT manifestations. Radiology 1985;155(1):167–70.

37. De Schepper AM, Ramon F, Van Marck E. MR imaging of eosinophilic granuloma: report of 11 cases. Skeletal Radiol 1993;22(3):163–6.

38. Carrillo JF, Albores O, Ramirez-Ortega MC, et al. An audit of nasopharyngeal fibromas. Eur J Surg Oncol 2007;33(5):655–61.

39. Eggesbo HB. Imaging of sinonasal tumours. Cancer Imaging 2012;12:136–52.

40. Ludwig BJ, Foster BR, Saito N, et al. Diagnostic imaging in nontraumatic pediatric head and neck emergencies. Radiographics 2010;30(3):781–99.

41. Godoy MD, Bezerra TF, Pinna Fde R, et al. Complications in the endoscopic and endoscopic-assisted treatment of juvenile nasopharyngeal angiofibroma with intracranial extension. Braz J Otorhinolaryngol 2014;80(2):120–5.

42. Mortazavi S, Tummala R, Grande A, et al. E-068 dual lumen balloon assisted pre-operative embolization with onyx for hypervascular head and neck tumors. J Neurointerv Surg 2014;6(Suppl 1):A70–1.

43. Hagiwara A, Inoue Y, Nakayama T, et al. The "botryoid sign": a characteristic feature of rhabdomyosarcomas in the head and neck. Neuroradiology 2001;43(4):331–5.

44. Eller R, Sillers M. Common fibro-osseous lesions of the paranasal sinuses. Otolaryngol Clin North Am 2006;39(3):585–600, x.

45. Erdogan N, Demir U, Songu M, et al. A prospective study of paranasal sinus osteomas in 1,889 cases: changing patterns of localization. Laryngoscope 2009;119(12):2355–9.

46. MacDonald-Jankowski DS. Fibro-osseous lesions of the face and jaws. Clin Radiol 2004;59(1):11–25.

47. Melroy CT, Senior BA. Benign sinonasal neoplasms: a focus on inverting papilloma. Otolaryngol Clin North Am 2006;39(3):601–17, x.

48. Lee YY, Van Tassel P, Nauert C, et al. Craniofacial osteosarcomas: plain film, CT, and MR findings in 46 cases. AJR Am J Roentgenol 1988;150(6): 1397–402.

49. Galera-Ruiz H, Sanchez-Calzado JA, Rios-Martin JJ, et al. Sinonasal radiation-associated osteosarcoma after combined therapy for rhabdomyosarcoma of the nose. Auris Nasus Larynx 2001;28(3):261–4.

50. Hyde GE, Yarington CT Jr, Chu FW. Head and neck manifestations of Maffucci's syndrome: chondrosarcoma of the nasal septum. Am J Otolaryngol 1995; 16(4):272–5.

51. Yamamoto S, Motoori K, Takano H, et al. Chondrosarcoma of the nasal septum. Skeletal Radiol 2002;31(9):543–6.

52. Momeni AK, Roberts CC, Chew FS. Imaging of chronic and exotic sinonasal disease: review. AJR Am J Roentgenol 2007;189(6 Suppl):S35–45.

53. Scholl RJ, Kellett HM, Neumann DP, et al. Cysts and cystic lesions of the mandible: clinical and radiologic-histopathologic review. Radiographics 1999;19(5):1107–24.

54. Prescher A, Brors D. Metastases to the paranasal sinuses: case report and review of the literature. Laryngorhinootologie 2001;80(10):583–94 [in German].

The Skull Base in the Evaluation of Sinonasal Disease
Role of Computed Tomography and MR Imaging

Steve E.J. Connor

KEYWORDS

- Imaging • Computed tomography • MR imaging • Skull base pathology • Sinonasal pathology
- Anatomy

KEY POINTS

- Computed tomography (CT) helps assess the cortical bone changes of the anterior skull base (ASB) whereas MR imaging is superior for evaluating the bone marrow and foramina of the central skull base (CSB).
- The paranasal sinuses contribute to the median ASB and CSB, and important variant anatomy should be recorded to help prevent surgical complications.
- MR imaging is useful in delineating sinonasal malignancy by demonstrating direct extension through the ASB, perineural extension through the CSB and involvement of intracranial structures.
- Intrinsic bone lesions are most frequently benign in the ASB whereas primary or secondary malignant intrinsic bone lesions may also feature in the CSB.
- Endocranial tumors and contents may traverse the skull base into the sinonasal region. Cephalocele is an important consideration when imaging demonstrates a sinonasal mass with a skull base defect.

INTRODUCTION

The median ASB and CSB form an interface between the sinonasal and intracranial compartments. Because clinical and endoscopic assessment is limited, the cross-sectional imaging modalities of CT and MR imaging play a key role in addressing the origin, nature, and extent of disease within the ASB and CSB. Advances in endoscopic surgical approaches, image-guided surgery, and targeted radiotherapy have expanded therapeutic possibilities, and the radiologist is central within the multidisciplinary team when deciding on treatment planning.

This review briefly describes the appropriate CT and MR imaging techniques, and the pertinent anatomy of the median ASB and CSB relevant to the spread of disease and surgical planning. It then focuses on the imaging appearances of pathologic processes that involve and traverse the skull base between the sinonasal and intracranial compartments.

TECHNIQUES

CT and MR imaging are frequently complementary in characterizing and demonstrating the extent of

Disclosure: None.
Neuroradiology Department, King's College Hospital, Denmark Hill, London SE5 9RS, UK
E-mail address: steve.connor@nhs.net

Neuroimag Clin N Am 25 (2015) 619–651
http://dx.doi.org/10.1016/j.nic.2015.07.007
1052-5149/15/$ – see front matter © 2015 Elsevier Inc. All rights reserved.

neuroimaging.theclinics.com

pathologic processes within the median ASB and CSB.

CT is excellent at detecting cortical bone erosion or deficiency and hence is particularly useful for assessing the thin bony structures of the ASB or the foramina of the CSB. CT is also used to provide a bony roadmap for surgery. It may help differentiate pathologies by demonstrating calcific or ossific elements (eg, fibrous dysplasia [FD] and osteoma), adjacent bony sclerotic reactions (eg, meningioma, olfactory neuroblastoma, inverted papilloma, and chronic inflammation), bony destruction (eg, high-grade carcinoma or neuroendocrine tumor) or bony remodeling (eg, low-grade tumors, including sarcoma, lymphoma, melanoma, and olfactory neuroblastoma).

Multidetector CT is performed with a single axial volume acquired at submillimetric slice collimation, with generation of multiplanar 1-mm reformats (including a bone algorithm). If concurrent MR imaging is not available, then increased milliampere-seconds (>50 mAs), intravenous contrast, and 3-mm thick reconstructions help optimize the soft tissue appearances. If only bone detail is required, then cone-beam CT may also be used to evaluate the skull base[1] at a lower radiation dose. CT angiography and CT cisternography are additional techniques that may be indicated for evaluation of skull base pathology.

MR imaging is superior for detecting infiltration of the bone marrow and perineural extension of disease, so it is valuable for imaging the CSB. MR imaging also provides superior mapping of the intrasinus extent of lesions (and hence contact with the skull base) while better delineating any intracranial extension.

MR imaging requires a combination of T1W, T2W, and gadolinium-enhanced T1W images. Sagittal sequences supplement routine coronal and axial planes for the assessment of midline pathology. Imaging is generally performed with 3- to 4-mm slice thickness and no gap, with an optimal field of view of 16 to 18 cm. Occasionally, volumetric sequences are used for image-guided surgery and radiotherapy planning and (with 3-D heavily T2W sequences) to demonstrate a cerebrospinal fluid (CSF) leak or cephalocele. T1W sequences are particularly useful for assessing bone marrow abnormality, whereas gadolinium enhancement delineates pathologic meningeal and perineural extension. Higher-resolution (eg, 512×512 matrix) sequences may be used to evaluate the integrity of bone and periosteum at the ASB or to assess for perineural spread (PNS). Fat-suppressed sequences are often included for imaging the CSB. Failure of fat suppression at the interface of the skull base and the paranasal sinuses is a problem with sequences based on frequency selective pulses, but this may be overcome by using short tau inversion recovery (STIR) or 3-point Dixon techniques.[2] Diffusion imaging of the paranasal sinuses and the skull base is feasible and can be optimized with parallel imaging, readout segmented techniques, multishot acquisition, and turbo spin-echo techniques; however, there is little data on the diagnostic impact of diffusion-weighted imaging (DWI) in the setting of skull base and sinonasal pathology.[3–5]

Intraoperative image guidance is frequently required to aid surgical approaches to the skull base. A tracking system (eg, optical or electromagnetic) simultaneously references a sensor on a surgical instrument with the patient and a preoperative or intraoperative imaging data set (using CT or MR imaging) (**Fig. 1**).[6]

ANATOMY

The paranasal sinuses contribute to the ASB and CSB in the midline and paramidline. Thus, the median ASB comprises the posterior wall of the frontal sinus, the roof of the nasoethmoid region, and the planum sphenoidale, whereas more posteriorly, the median CSB houses the sphenoid sinus. A coronal projection through the chiasmatic sulcus, tuberculum sella, and anterior clinoids separates the median ASB from the CSB (**Fig. 2**). The wide range of variant anatomy within this part of the skull base should be recognized to distinguish it from pathologic processes and to prevent complications of sinonasal surgical approaches (**Table 1**).[8,18,19]

Median Anterior Skull Base: Applied Anatomy

The median ASB is formed by the paired orbital plates of the frontal bone, the cribriform plate of ethmoid, and the lesser wing of sphenoid (see **Fig. 2**). Unlike the lateral ASB, which forms the roofs of the orbits, the median ASB it is directly related to the sinonasal region.

The orbital plate of frontal bone contributes to the ipsilateral posterior wall of frontal sinus and the fovea ethmoidalis (or roof of ethmoid). It generally consists of resistant compact bone, although there are multiple diploic valveless veins that traverse its walls with the potential to transmit infection. A large frontal sinus (pneumosinus) should be distinguished from abnormal expansion that encroaches on other structures, which is termed a pneumosinus dilatans (with a normal thickness wall) or a pneumocele (with thinned or deficient wall) (**Fig. 3**).[20] The fovea ethmoidalis slopes inferiorly at an angle of 15° as it extends posteriorly to the planum sphenoidale.

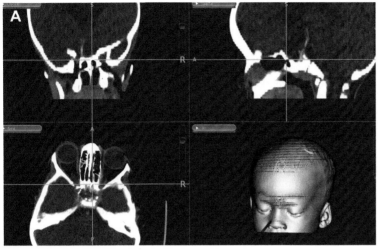

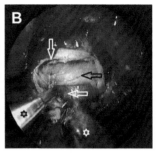

Fig. 1. Intraoperative image guidance used for transsphenoidal resection. Screenshot from an intraoperative CT guidance system, which uses electromagnetic triangulation and tracking to localize instruments within the surgical field. Multiplanar CT image (*A*) complements the endoscopic image (*B*) for anatomic localization during sinonasal approaches to the skull base. (*B*) Note the edge of the resected sellar floor (*vertical white arrow*), the dura (*black arrow*), and the contents of a craniopharyngioma seen through a defect in the tumor capsule (*horizontal white arrow*). The tip of the probe (*black star* [*B*]) corresponds to the location of the cross hairs (*A*). The endoscope and probe are held by one operator while another operator uses a sucker (*white star* [*B*]) through the opposite nasal cavity. (*Courtesy of* Sinan Barazi, Nicholas Thomas, Christopher Chandler, and Bassel Zebian).

The fronto-cribriform suture represents the junction between the fovea ethmoidalis and the more medial cribriform plate (or roof of the nasal cavity). These structures converge at the vertically orientated lateral lamella of the cribriform plate (Fig. 4). Sinonasal variant anatomy predisposes

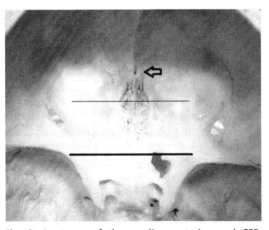

Fig. 2. Anatomy of the median anterior and CSB. Photograph of a dry skull (base) visualised from superiorly, demonstrates the demarcation of the ASB from CSB (*thick line*). The thin line corresponds to a coronal plane (see Fig. 4) through the crista galli and the perforations of the cribriform plate. The foramen caecum (*open arrow*) is also seen more anteriorly.

to surgical ASB injury. The Keros classification grades the length of the lateral lamella, with the longest (>7 mm or type III) present in 8% of individuals and most prone to surgical injury.[7,9] The lateral lamella is attached to the vertical lamella of the middle turbinate and this may be damaged by turbinate manipulation (see Fig. 4; Fig. 5). The lateral lamella is also traversed by the anterior ethmoidal artery and this is a site of particular bony weakness (see Figs. 4 and 5).[11] The cribriform plate itself is a delicate structure, which is susceptible to injury and erosion. It demonstrates multiple perforations through which pass the olfactory nerves. Small defects in the cribriform plate and lateral lamella are a normal finding on CT.[21] The olfactory nerves form a potential pathway for tumor spread as they extend superiorly to the olfactory bulbs (see Fig. 4). The bulbs sit on the cribriform plate and beneath the frontal lobes with decreased bulb volume noted in patients with congenital or acquired olfactory dysfunction (see Fig. 4). The dura is tightly adherent to the bone of the cribriform plate and ethmoid roof, so it is often disrupted by adjacent fractures and is also prone to tumor invasion.

The midline portion of the ASB is largely unossified at birth, with variable rates of subsequent ossification (Fig. 6). It may be judged to be complete on CT at between 14 months and 4 years.[22,23] The crista galli is the triangular process of the

Table 1
Anatomic variants of surgical relevance within the median anterior and central skull base: what the referring clinician needs to know

Median ASB	
Angulated or low fovea ethmoidalis	A steeper sagittal skull base angle and a lower position of the fovea ethmoidalis relative to the orbit is associated with an increased incidence of surgical damage.[7]
Deep cribriform plate or asymmetric lateral lamellae (see Fig. 5)	A deep cribriform plate relative to the fovea ethmoidalis (hence, longer lateral lamella as graded by the Keros classification) or an asymmetric configuration increases the risk of penetration at surgery.[8–10]
Anterior ethmoid artery dehiscence (see Fig. 5)	It should be noted whether the anterior ethmoid artery lies immediately adjacent to the skull base before it enters the cribriform plate or whether it is suspended by a mesentery (as is present in 30% of cases) where it may be vulnerable to injury.[11]
Median CSB	
Extent of sphenoid sinus pneumatization	Presellar or conchal type pneumatizations are less favorable for transsphenoidal surgical approaches to the pituitary fossa.[12]
Variations in sphenoid sinus septae (see Fig. 10)	There are challenges to sphenoid sinus surgery posed by the considerable variation in the configuration of intersphenoid sinus septations. An asymmetric septation inserting on the (possibly dehiscent) carotid canal should be communicated to the surgeon.[13]
Dehiscent bone overlying the optic nerve or carotid artery (see Fig. 10)	The optic nerves indent or course through the sphenoid sinus in 24% of cases. Dehiscence of the optic nerves is also often associated with a pneumatized anterior clinoid. Bulging and dehiscence of the ICA is seen in 4% of individuals and this should also be documented to prevent surgical complications.[14]
Onodi (sphenoethmoidal) cell (see Fig. 10)	This posterior ethmoid air cell extends superior to the sphenoid sinus. The surgeon may anticipate that the posterior wall of this air cell will access the sphenoid sinus; however, it will potentially breach the optic nerve canal.[15]
Protrusion and dehiscence of the vidian and maxillary nerves (see Fig. 10)	Extension of the sphenoid sinus between the vidian canal and foramen rotundum occurs in 40% of sinuses, with nerve protrusion and dehiscence having been associated with iatrogenic injury.[16,17]

ethmoid on the superior surface of the cribriform plate, which attaches the dura of the anterior falx (see Fig. 2). T1W high signal from the yellow marrow of the crista galli should not be misinterpreted as pathology, such as a dermoid, on MR imaging. The foramen caecum is located just anterior to the cribriform plate and crista galli at the frontoethmoid suture (see Fig. 2).[24,25] It corresponds to the site of a temporary dural diverticulum, which extends to the nasal bridge in embryogenesis and hence it is the origin of various ASB developmental anomalies. The foramen caecum is usually 3 mm or less in size in children[24] and 2 mm in adults.[25] It is usually blind ended; however, it may transmit an emissary vein. A wide foramen caecum (see Fig. 6) and bifid crista galli may, but does not necessarily indicate that a midline developmental lesion extends intracranially.[24]

Median Central Skull Base: Applied Anatomy

The sphenoid sinus is contained within the body of the sphenoid bone, which is the principle median structure of the CSB.[26,27] It variably occupies the midline sagittal compartment of the CSB, which is formed by the body of sphenoid, including the upper clivus (basisphenoid), and is bordered laterally by the petro-occipital fissures (Fig. 7).[28,29] The sphenoid largely consists of medullary bone, which makes it a focus for hematogenous spread of pathology. The MR imaging signal of the basisphenoid marrow varies considerably. Although more homogenously increased T1W signal yellow marrow is seen with age, 30% to 60% of healthy adults demonstrate heterogenous signal in the basisphenoid marrow.[30,31] A more focal benign variation in the imaging appearances of the bone adjacent to the sphenoid sinus is seen with

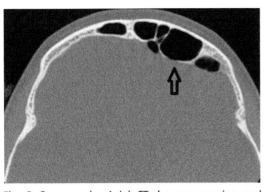

Fig. 3. Pneumocele. Axial CT shows expansion and thinning of the dorsal wall of the left frontal sinus (*open arrow*) with associated pneumocephalus. It was probably secondary to chronic raised intracranial pressure in early life.

arrested pneumatization (Fig. 8).[32] It is proposed that this is a consequence of failed sinus formation, despite preparation for pneumatization by earlier marrow conversion.[33] Foci of T1W high signal (fatty) and T1W low-signal/T2W high-signal (microcystic) change are seen on MR imaging, with characteristic curvilinear calcification and fat density, but without expansion or foraminal distortion demonstrated on CT (see Fig. 8).[32]

A corticated defect extending from the floor of the sellar within the central sphenoid bone is thought to be associated with a Rathke pouch remnant and has been termed the *craniopharyngeal canal*. This may be an incidental variant when small, or may contain ectopic adenohyphysis, cephaloceles, and tumors when larger (Fig. 9).[34] Sphenoid ossification occurs in numerous centers

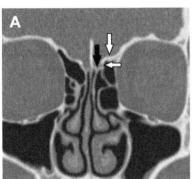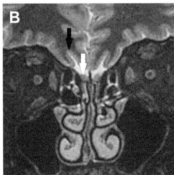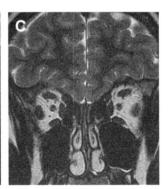

Fig. 4. Coronal anatomy of the ASB and olfactory bulbs. (A) Coronal CT demonstrates the fovea ethmoidalis (*vertical white arrow*). The vertical lamella of the middle turbinate inserts on the cribriform plate (*black arrow*). The lateral lamella (*horizontal white arrow*) joins the fovea ethmoidalis to the cribriform plate: note the small defects in lateral lamella due to anterior ethmoidal artery. (B) Coronal MR imaging demonstrates the olfactory bulbs (*white arrow*) sitting on the cribriform plate. Note the olfactory sulci of the inferior frontal lobes (*black arrow*), the depth of which is related to the development of the olfactory tract. (C) MR imaging in a patient with congenital anosmia with hypoplastic/aplastic olfactory bulbs and blunted olfactory sulcation.

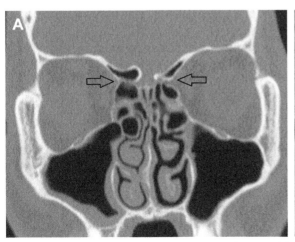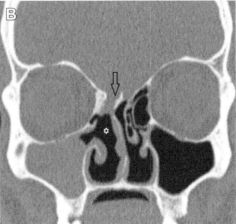

Fig. 5. Variant anatomy of the ASB and surgical injury. (A) Coronal CT shows inferiorly situated and partially dehiscent ethmoidal artery canals (*arrows*). (B) Coronal CT performed post–middle turbinectomy (*star*) in a different patient reveals a defect in the ASB (*arrow*) and reactive sclerosis. Adjacent soft tissue within the superior nasoethmoid cavity corresponds to graft rather than cephalocele.

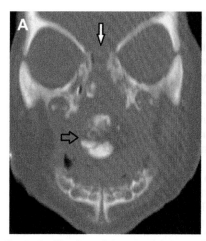

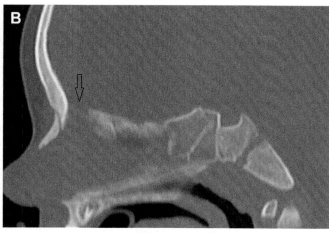

Fig. 6. Ossification of the ASB. (A) Coronal CT shows the normal lack of ossification within the ASB in a neonate. There is a large midline facial teratoma (*horizontal open arrow*) but the skull base was intact. The lack of ossification at the midline ASB (*white arrow*) and nasal capsule is an expected finding in the neonate. (B) Sagittal CT shows an enlarged foramen caecum (*open arrow*) in a patient with a nasal dermoid. (*From [A] Connor SEJ. Imaging of skull-base cephaloceles and cerebrospinal fluid leaks. Clin Radiol 2010;65:835; with permission.*)

and is not complete until the spheno-occipital synchondrosis fuses at 12 to 16 years (see Fig. 9). Pneumatization of the sphenoid progresses inferiorly and posteriorly. It develops most rapidly between the ages of 1 and 5 and is generally thought to reach its full extent by age 12 to 14,[35] although it may continue until adulthood.[36] Pneumatization is most frequently postsellar in configuration, whereby it extends below or more posterior to the sellar floor and hence is directly related to the inferior pituitary gland. Other forms of presellar (10%–25%) or rudimentary conchal-type (2%)

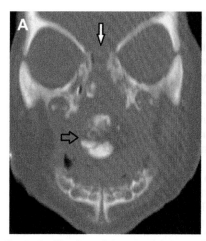

Fig. 7. Anatomy of the median CSB. Photograph of a dry skull (base) as visualised from superiorly demonstrates the division of the midline from the paramidline sagittal compartments of the CSB (*vertical line*). This is demarcated by the petro-occipital fissure (*large vertical open arrow*). Close proximity of the vidian canal (posterior aspect [*small vertical open arrow*]), foramen rotundum (*vertical black arrow*), and optic canal (*horizontal black arrow*) are demonstrated.

pneumatizations are less frequent[37,38] but less favorable for transsphenoidal surgery.

There may be further challenges to sphenoid sinus surgery posed by the considerable variation in the configuration of intersphenoid sinus septations. Although a simple configuration is present in a majority of individuals, up to 30% of sphenoid sinuses demonstrate 2 or more asymmetric or additional horizontal septae (Fig. 10).[12,39] When a horizontal septation is demonstrated, the radiologist should consider whether this represents an Onodi (sphenoethmoidal) cell extending superior to the sphenoid sinus, because this is a surgically important variation (see Fig. 10).

The lateral walls are thin bony layers that are related to the orbits and superior orbital fissures anteriorly as well as the optic nerves, medial cavernous sinuses, and internal carotid arteries (ICAs) posteriorly.[13,15] Dehiscence of the optic nerves[14] may predispose to inflammatory complications or iatrogenic injury (see Fig. 10). A further critical lateral relationship of the sphenoid sinus is the neurovascular structures of cavernous sinus, which may be a source, pathway of spread, or a target for paranasal sinus pathology. The cavernous carotid artery and the VI nerve are contained within the cavernous sinus itself, whereas the III, IV, VI, and V2 nerves are interposed between the inner and outer dural layers along its lateral wall. Foci of fat density and signal within the cavernous sinuses are more common in obese patients or those with high corticosteroid levels. Variable contrast opacification on CT venography studies may also be a normal imaging feature, depending on the relative inflow of the ophthalmic veins, pterygoid plexi, and sylvian veins.

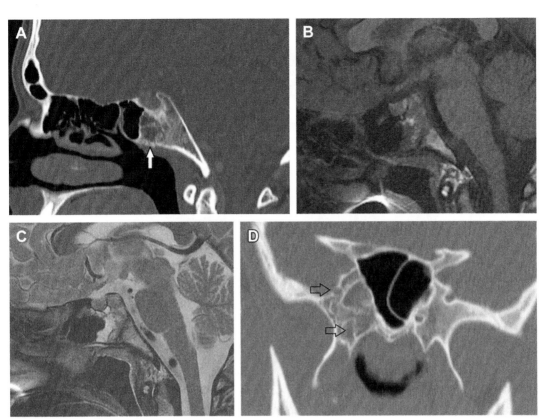

Fig. 8. Arrested pneumatization of the sphenoid. (*A*) sagittal CT shows heterogeneity to the sphenoid (*arrow*) with curvilinear calcification and fat density. Corresponding T1W (*B*) and T2W (*C*) sagittal MR images show foci of T1W high-signal (fatty) and T2W high-signal (microcystic) change. (*D*) In a different patient a coronal CT shows heterogeneity to the right sphenoid and pterygoid base, but without foraminal expansion or narrowing demonstrated (*open arrows*).

When there is extensive anterolateral sinus pneumatization, the sphenoid sinus may also occupy the greater wing of sphenoid and pterygoid base, abutting the structures of the parasagittal CSB compartment. Sternberg's canal (or lateral

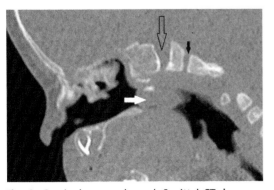

Fig. 9. Craniopharyngeal canal. Sagittal CT shows an enlarged craniopharyngeal canal (*open arrow*) related to an extracerebral neuro-glial hamartoma (*white arrow*) in the nasopharynx. The unossified spheno-occipital synchondrosis (*small black arrow*) is also noted.

craniopharyngeal canal) is a potential bony defect, resulting from incomplete fusion between the basisphenoid and greater wing of sphenoid. It has been proposed to be the origin of cephaloceles, which extend into the lateral recesses of the sphenoid sinus,[40] although this has been disputed.[41] Extension of the sphenoid sinus between the vidian canal and foramen rotundum (containing the maxillary nerve) occurs in 40% of sinuses, with nerve protrusion and dehiscence having been associated with iatrogenic injury and neuritis secondary to sphenoid sinusitis (see **Fig. 10**).[16,17]

SINONASAL PATHOLOGY EXTENDING TO THE SKULL BASE
Neoplastic

Malignant
Imaging may depict the intracranial extension of malignancy, either directly through the bone of the skull base or via foramina and fissures (**Table 2**). It helps predict the involvement of structures, such as the dura, cisternal cranial nerves,

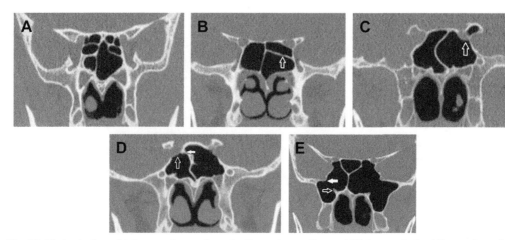

Fig. 10. Variant sphenoid sinus anatomy of surgical importance. Coronal CT demonstrates (*A*) complex sphenoid sinus septations, (*B*) horizontal septation at the site of an Onodi cell (*arrow*), (*C*) a dehiscent optic nerve canal related to a pneumatized anterior clinoid (*arrow*), (*D*) a dehiscent carotid artery (*open arrow*) adjacent to the insertion of the intersphenoid sinus septum (*white arrow*), and (*E*) prominent pneumatization of the sphenoid sinus inferolateral recesses with dehiscent foramen rotundum (*white arrow*) and pedunculated vidian canal (*open arrow*).

brain parenchyma, cavernous sinus, and carotid artery, and thus plays a critical role in the staging, treatment planning, and prediction of clinical outcome (see **Table 2**).[42]

Sinonasal carcinomas are the most frequent malignant tumor and are usually of advanced stage at the time of diagnosis.[43] The importance of skull base involvement by carcinoma is reflected by the TNM classification,[44] which stages such maxillary and nasoethmoid carcinomas as T3 or T4 (**Table 3**). Skull base or intracranial extension are also features of staging systems for other malignant neoplasms, such as olfactory neuroblastoma (Kadish stage C)[45] and melanoma (T4).[46]

Direct extension Direct skull base extension of malignant tumor usually involves the ASB and is most frequently seen in the context of squamous cell carcinoma or sinonasal undifferentiated carcinoma (SNUC). When such patients undergo surgery, they require endoscopic resection with reconstruction or craniofacial resection to gain tumor clearance. The radiologist must first assess whether there is contact of tumor with the skull base, which requires the intrasinus delineation of tumor from inflammatory changes or sinonasal secretions (**Fig. 11**). Fortunately, most malignant high-grade tumors tend to be intermediate T2W signal due to the high cellularity, and they may be delineated from the T2W hyperintensity of inflammatory change and secretions (see **Fig. 11**),[10,11,47] although there are pitfalls (see **Table 2**).

Having established skull base contact, it is important to determine whether there is direct extension through the bone and infiltration of the dura or brain. The breaching of the cortical bone of the ASB is well shown by CT (**Fig. 12**). MR imaging is effective in demonstrating both the cortical bone and the periosteum of the skull base, which are seen together as a hypointense interface on all sequences. The nonmineralized periosteum is potentially more important because it may demonstrate greater resistance to tumor spread,[48] and this layer is only visualized on MR imaging. The interruption of this hypointense line implies there is intracranial (extradural) extension of tumor and the potential for dural invasion (**Fig. 13**).

Dural tumor infiltration must be distinguished from reactive dural inflammation. To achieve this, MR imaging criteria for dural invasion are proposed. These include the presence of dural nodularity, marked dural thickening (which is variably stated as >2 mm or >5 mm) (see **Fig. 13**),[49,50] or leptomeningeal enhancement.[49] The presence of dural involvement has implications for treatment planning, because it requires resection and reconstruction to prevent CSF leak and generally requires postoperative radiotherapy. When dural invasion is extensive, or it extends laterally over the orbital roofs, then an open surgical approach is preferred to an endoscopic approach. There is also an impact on outcome with a reduction in disease specific and overall 5-year survival.[51]

There may be further direct intracranial extension to involve the brain, which is characterized on MR imaging by effacement of the CSF signal and parenchymal edema (**Fig. 14**). Limited brain invasion may be addressed with craniofacial resection with a nonsignificant decrease in survival compared with dural invasion alone.[52] More

Table 2
Skull base extension of sinonasal malignancy: imaging appearances, pearls, and pitfalls

Imaging Appearance	Implications	Pitfalls in Imaging Assessment
Sinonasal tumor extending to skull base (see Fig. 11): Tissue abutting skull base is of similar signal (usually T2W intermediate signal) and enhancement characteristics to the sinonasal tumor.	Endoscopic resection with reconstruction or craniofacial resection is required to obtain tumor clearance.	1. T2 hyperintense tumor (eg, salivary gland malignancy due to increased mucin content) at the skull base may mimic inflammatory change. 2. T2 isointense proteinaceous secretions at the skull base may mimic tumor.
ASB cortical bone destruction (see Fig. 12): Deficiency of bone on CT and loss of the low signal (bone and periosteum) on high-resolution coronal MR imaging.	Indicates there is intracranial (extradural) extension of tumor and potential for dural invasion. Impacts on T staging.	1. Numerous neurovascular perforations at the nasoethmoid roof should not be misinterpreted as erosive change. 2. Other non-neoplastic processes (eg, associated mucocele) may cause cortical bone pressure deossification. 3. Nasoethmoid mass with ASB defect may also be secondary to a cephalocele.
CSB marrow involvement (see Fig. 16): Replacement of high-signal yellow marrow by intermediate T1 signal with enhancement on fat-saturated T1W sequences.	Impacts on resectability and T staging	If no pregadolinium or fat-saturated postgadolinum T1W imaging is performed, then (enhancing) tumor may appear similar to the normal marrow signal and not be detected.
Dural involvement (see Fig. 13): Dural nodularity and marked dural thickening or the presence of leptomeningeal enhancement on MR imaging	Impacts on T staging and outcome. Dural resection and reconstruction will be required. When dural invasion is extensive or extends laterally over the orbital roofs, then an open surgical approach is preferred to an endoscopic approach.	Dural inflammation may result in a thin rim of dural enhancement and should not be misinterpreted as tumor invasion.
Perineural extension (see Fig. 17): Neural foraminal enlargement and destruction on CT. MR imaging demonstrates effacement of adjacent fat planes on T1W as well as neural enlargement and enhancement with gadolinium.	Impacts on T staging and radiotherapy planning and it is important for prognosis (with a reduction in the local control).	1. Neural enhancement may also be secondary to postoperative change, radiotherapy or inflammation. Enhancement of the maxillary nerve (in the foramen rotundum) may occasionally be seen in normal subjects, due to the perineural vascular plexus. 2. Denervation changes in the masticator muscles may be demonstrated as a consequence of trigeminal nerve PNS, so muscle T2W high signal and enhancement due to subacute denervation must not be misinterpreted as tumor extension.
Involvement of intracranial structures (see Fig. 14): MR imaging criteria for brain, cavernous sinus, Meckel cave, optic pathways, ICA involvement	Impacts on T staging, resectability, and outcome	Resectability depends on tumor histology and local surgical protocols.

Table 3
Impact of skull base extension on T staging of sinonasal carcinoma

Imaging Feature	T Stage
Invading the bone of the cribriform plate	T3 nasoethmoid carcinoma T4a maxillary carcinoma
Minimally invades the anterior cranial fossa	T4a nasoethmoid carcinoma
Invading the dura, brain, clivus, and middle cranial fossa	T4b nasoethmoid and maxillary carcinoma

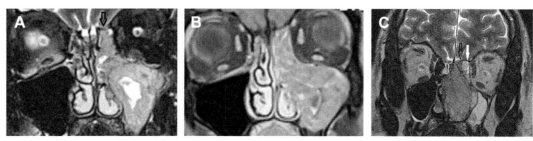

Fig. 11. Carcinoma extending to the ASB with an intact ASB. Coronal MR imaging (A) T2W and (B) gadolinium-enhanced, fat-saturated T1W MR imaging show an intermediate T2W enhancing maxillary sinus carcinoma extending to abut the ASB (open arrow in [A]) but with intact signal void at the ASB. (C) Coronal T2W MR imaging in a different patient with nasoethmoid carcinoma shows the tumor T2W signal abutting the skull base medially (open arrow) but with T2W high-signal inflammatory change (white arrow) more laterally.

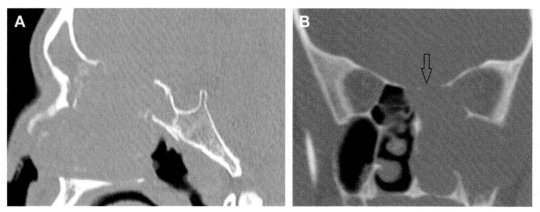

Fig. 12. ASB cortical erosion on CT. (A) Coronal and (B) Sagittal CT show a maxillary carcinoma with ASB cortical bony destruction (arrow [B]) of aggressive-type.

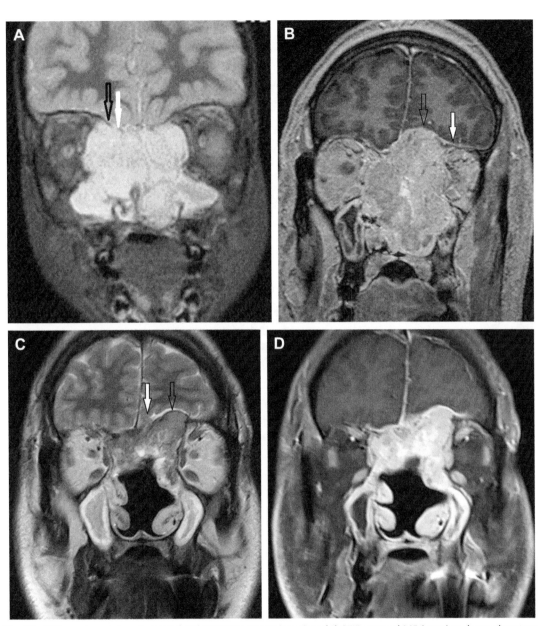

Fig. 13. ASB erosion and malignant dural invasion on MR imaging. (*A*) STIR coronal MR imaging shows the attenuation of the low signal bone/periosteal complex (*white arrow*) by a rhabdomyosarcoma compared with the intact layer more laterally (*black arrow*). (*B*) Metastatic sinonasal carcinoma in a different patient, attenuates the enhancing dura medially (*open arrow*) with normal thin reactive enhancing dura more laterally (*white arrow*). (*C*) T2W and (*D*) gadolinium-enhanced, fat-saturated T1W coronal MR imaging in a further patient, shows nodularity and thickening of the dura medially, with attenuation of the low T2w signal at the ASB (*white arrow* in [*C*]). Distinguish this from the intact ASB (*open arrow* in [*C*]) with reactive dural enhancement more laterally in (*D*).

extensive frontal lobe involvement by high-grade malignancy usually precludes surgical treatment and portends a poor outcome.[53] Lower-grade malignant tumors, such as olfactory neuroblastoma, may be suitable for surgical intervention despite extensive intracranial involvement. The intracranial extension of olfactory neuroblastoma is characterized by peritumoural cysts on imaging studies (**Fig. 15**).[54]

Extension of tumor by direct extension through the lateral walls or roof of the sphenoid sinus is generally deemed inoperable,[55] although specific criteria for resectability vary between surgeons. Primary sphenoid sinus malignancy is rare[56,57]

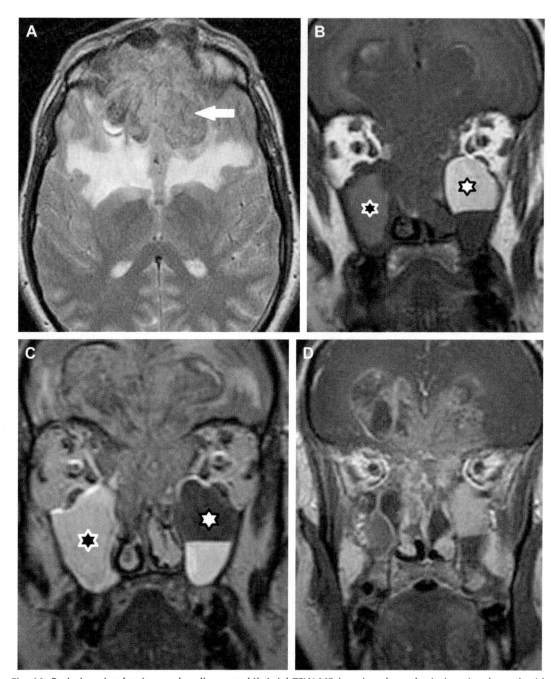

Fig. 14. Brain invasion by sinonasal malignancy. (A) Axial T2W MR imaging shows brain invasion (arrow) with parenchymal edema. (B) T1W, (C) T2W, and (D) gadolinium-enhanced T1W MR imaging demonstrate intracranial extent of the tumor. Note the differing signal of the maxillary sinus proteinaceous secretions (T1w high signal/T2W low signal [white star] and T1W high signal/T2W high signal [black star]), which can be confused with tumor on postgadolinium images (D).

and sphenoid sinus erosion is normally seen in the context of large multisite sinonasal tumors or nasopharyngeal carcinoma. MR imaging with T1W sequences is particularly useful for assessing bone marrow abnormality within the basisphenoid

(Fig. 16). When tumor has extended through the CSB, the cavernous sinus, Meckel cave, anterior visual pathways, and the ICA are further critical structures that should be evaluated for tumor involvement. Cavernous sinus tumor extension

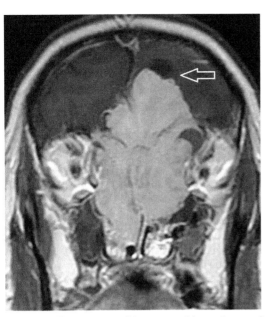

Fig. 15. Olfactory neuroblastoma with peritumoral cysts. Gadolinium-enhanced T1W coronal MR imaging demonstrates peritumoural cysts (*open arrow*) adjacent to the intracranial component.

may be seen as encasement and stenosis of the ICA together with a lateral convexity. Cavernous sinus involvement usually precludes surgery.[58] Although imaging features of ICA involvement at the skull base have not been validated, it may be possible to extrapolate those criteria established for the infracranial ICA; these include tumor encroachment exceeding 270° of the arterial

perimeter,[59] compression of the artery, and ill definition of the carotid wall.[60] Reduced survival rates are predicted when there is ICA tumor encasement.[58] Although there are palliative surgical options, such as carotid resection after balloon test occlusion, endoscopic approaches are generally avoided, and nonoperative approaches are favored.[61]

Perineural extension Tumor may also access the intracranial structures by extending through neurovascular foramina and fissures, often by PNS. Although direct extension usually involves the ASB, the focus of PNS is on the CSB.[62] PNS comprises the extension of malignancy along the scaffolding of a nerve or nerve plexus[63] either within the perineural space or within the nerve fascicles. It is distinct from perineural or neural tumor invasion, which is a microscopic feature portending a poor prognosis but which is not appreciated on imaging.[64] Neurotropic cancers, such as adenoid cystic carcinoma, squamous cell carcinoma, SNUC,[65] and lymphoma, have a propensity to PNS. It is important to carefully analyze for PNS in all cases, because up to 50% of patients do not have associated symptoms.[66–68] Most patients with extension of PNS to the skull base, and certainly those with extension beyond the skull base foramina (including extension to the cavernous sinus) are not amenable to curative resection. The mapping of PNS is also important for radiotherapy planning and influences prognosis, with a reduction in the local control by more than 30%.[66] Sinonasal malignancy most frequently gains access to the maxillary nerve

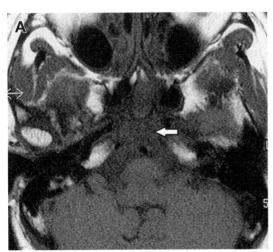
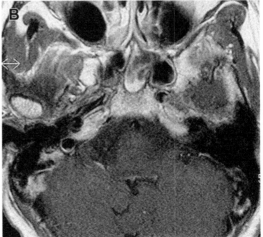

Fig. 16. Importance of pregadolinium images at the CSB. (*A*) Axial T1W and (*B*) postgadolinium axial T1W images show how the postgadolinium images (without fat saturation) may mask the CSB signal abnormality (*arrow* in [*A*]) secondary to invasion by carcinoma.

(foramen rotundum) and vidian nerve (vidian canal) within the CSB via the pterygopalatine fossa. Infratemporal fossa extension of tumor may also allow for mandibular nerve (foramen ovale) PNS. Due to the multiple trigeminal nerve/facial nerve connections within the face and skull base, the course of the facial nerves should also be carefully inspected.

CT and MR imaging may again be complementary in the demonstration of PNS; however, MR imaging is generally superior, with the sensitivity for detection reported to be more than 95%.[66–68] Imaging features include asymmetric neural enhancement (although other causes should be considered[69]) (see Table 2) and enlargement (Fig. 17). A further imaging feature of PNS is the loss of the perineural fat planes, which is well demonstrated on thin-section T1W images within the pterygopalatine fossa (see Fig. 17), the retromaxillary region, the orbital fissures, and the exocranial openings of the neurovascular foramina.

Benign
A range of benign epithelial, neuroectodermal, vascular, and connective tissue sinonasal tumors may also extend to the skull base. Some benign tumors (eg, schwannoma, meningioma, and pituitary adenomas) are usually intracranial but can rarely have a sinonasal origin, so may potentially traverse the skull base in either direction.[70,71] Similar to low-grade malignant tumors, the slower growth rate of these neoplasms generally results in a pattern of thinning and pressure remodeling of bone on CT studies; however, a simulated aggressive appearance of bony destruction is occasionally demonstrated.[72] Juvenile angiofibromas have a characteristic pattern of skull base erosion and intracranial extension. Intracranial extension most frequently occurs via the inferior and superior orbital fissures or other foramina within the CSB, which lead to finger-like projections and potential

invasion of the cavernous sinus (Fig. 18). They also have a particular tendency to invade the cancellous bone of the pterygoid base, and this is a common site for recurrent tumor.[73] A key imaging issue in terms of planning endoscopic resection relates to whether tumor extends medial to the cavernous carotid artery, because this indicates a midline surgical approach as opposed to an infratemporal fossa approach.[74]

Inflammatory and Infectious
Acute and chronic infective and inflammatory sinonasal processes may extend to the skull base and involve intracranial structures.

Acute suppurative rhinosinusitis
Endocranial complications of acute suppurative rhinosinusitis are usually associated with frontoethmoid or sphenoid infection. Infection may extend directly across the skull base, with bony destruction due to osteomyelitis, and this is often associated with an epidural abscess. When this develops in the frontal sinus and extends to the anterior table of the frontal bone, it may result in a subgaleal abscess or Pott puffy tumor (Fig. 19).[75] Indirect spread via the valveless veins allows infection to traverse the skull base without evidence of bony erosive change, and such venous propagation of infection may also extend to the orbits and cavernous sinus (Fig. 20). Rarely there may be ascending transcranial infection due to acquired and congenital skull base defects.[76] Other intracranial septic complications include epidural abscess, subdural empyema, intracerebral abscess (Fig. 21), meningitis, and venous thrombosis. These are reported to occur in 3.7% of patients hospitalized with sinusitis and approximately half of these also have orbital complications.[77,78] Sphenoid sinusitis represents only 3% of all acute sinusitis, but it is the commonest sinogenic source of meningitis. It may lead to visual

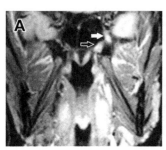 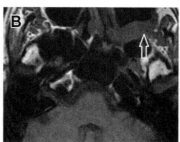 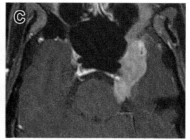

Fig. 17. PNS at the CSB. (A) Coronal gadolinium-enhanced, fat-saturated T1W MR imaging demonstrates enlargement and enhancement of the left vidian nerve (open arrow) and maxillary nerve (white arrow) due to PNS of adenoid cystic carcinoma. (B) T1W and (C) fat-saturated postgadolinium axial MR imaging demonstrate PNS from lymphoma extending posteriorly to the cisternal portion of the trigeminal nerve. Note the effacement of the T1W hyperintense fat plane within the pterygopalatine fossa and retro-maxillary fat (arrow [B]).

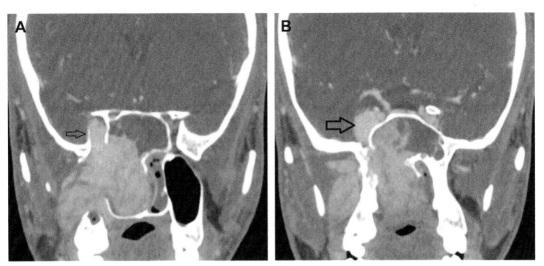

Fig. 18. Juvenile angiofibroma extension to the CSB. Coronal images from a CT angiography study demonstrate the finger-like insinuation of tumor through the superior orbital fissure (*arrow* [*A*]) to the cavernous sinus (*arrow* [*B*]).

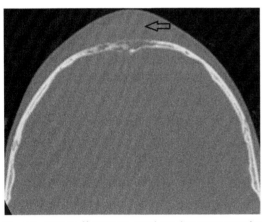

Fig. 19. Pott puffy tumor. Axial CT demonstrates the osteomyelitis of the frontal bone with associated subgaleal abscess (*arrow*).

loss or cranial nerve palsies due to the close proximity of the neural structures.[79] MR imaging is generally considered the imaging of choice for the detection and delineation of intracranial septic complications, although CT may be indicated in the emergency setting.

Acute invasive fungal rhinosinusitis

Acute fulminant fungal rhinosinusitis is a rapidly progressive infection with a high morbidity and mortality. It is generally associated with the immunocompromised state but may also occur in immunocompetent individuals.[80] Both CT and MR imaging may demonstrate sinonasal soft tissue, which is characteristically of low T2W signal (Fig. 22) but which is often nonspecific and may be of small volume. Although there may be adjacent osseous erosion on CT,[80–82] the infection

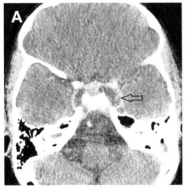
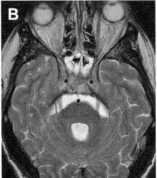
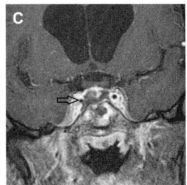

Fig. 20. Cavernous sinus septic thrombophlebitis/thrombosis. (*A*) Axial contrast-enhanced CT shows expansion and nonenhancement of the cavernous sinuses (*arrow*). (*B*) Axial T2W and (*C*) gadolinium-enhanced, fat-saturated T1W MR imaging show heterogenous signal abnormality and enhancement with expansion of the cavernous sinuses. Note the narrowing of the right ICA flow void (*open arrow* in [*C*]), the enhancing CSB osteomyelitis and the congestive stranding within the orbital fat in (*B*).

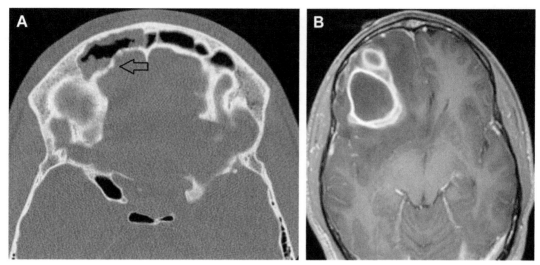

Fig. 21. Frontal sinusitis with frontal lobe abscess. (A) Axial CT demonstrates thinning and erosion of the dorsal wall of the frontal sinus (*open arrow*) with associated frontal sinus soft tissue. (B) Axial T1W postgadolinium MR imaging shows a ring-enhancing, multiloculated, right frontal lobe abscess.

can also traverse the skull base by vascular channels. The complications of intracranial extension are again better depicted with MR imaging. In addition to those previously discussed, fungal infection has a propensity for vascular invasion leads to an increased risk of cerebral infarcts (see **Fig. 22**), hemorrhages, and pseudoaneurysm formation.

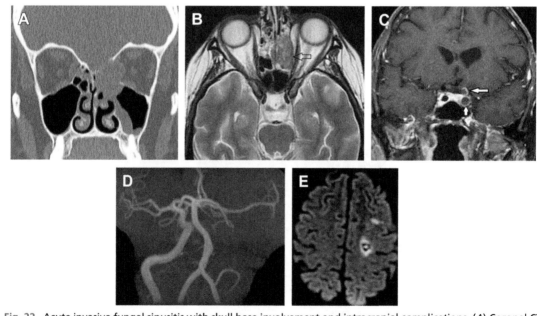

Fig. 22. Acute invasive fungal sinusitis with skull base involvement and intracranial complications. (A) Coronal CT and (B) axial T2W MR imaging shows left-sided T2W intermediate signal nasoethmoid soft tissue (*arrow*) with associated sinonasal and ASB bony destruction. (C) T1W postgadolinium coronal, (D) magnetic resonance angiography frontal maximum intensity projection, and (E) DWI axial images in a different patient, demonstrate a small volume of poorly enhancing tissue invading the left cavernous sinus (*small vertical white arrow* in [C]) with thrombosis and rim enhancement (*horizontal white arrow* in [C]) of the left ICA. There are watershed-type left hemispheric acute infarcts shown in (E).

Chronic sinonasal inflammation and infection

A range of chronic infectious and inflammatory sinonasal processes may involve the skull base. Chronic osteomyelitic destruction of the ASB occasionally occurs secondary to chronic invasive fungal sinusitis (Fig. 23). Although chronic CSB osteomyelitis is typically secondary to necrotising otitis externa, there are some cases thought secondary to sinonasal gram-positive bacterial (see Fig. 23) or chronic invasive fungal infection.[83,84] Additional noninfectious sinonasal chronic inflammatory or vasculitic processes may invade the skull base, for instance, granulomatosis with polyangiitis (GPA), sarcoid, and IgG4-related disease. Sinonasal sarcoid and GPA may directly extend through the ASB[85–88]; and diffuse and extensive skull base erosion is also a rare presentation.[89] These pathologic processes may also primarily arise from the skull base or intracranial structures.[90] Such patients may present with nonspecific clinical features, such as headache and cranial neuropathies, so the radiologist plays a key role in detecting pathology and assessing the disease extent. Although the diagnosis is typically made on the basis of any multisystem clinical features and pathologic features, the imaging features may be contributory.

CT may demonstrate sclerosis, rarefaction, fragmentation, and sequestration of the bone with chronic osteomyelitis. Advanced GPA involving the skull base is associated with CT evidence of extensive sinonasal erosive change with possible autorhinectomy; however, such a combination of imaging features is also associated with other angioinvasive processes, such as lymphoma,[87] invasive fungal disease,[81] and cocaine abuse.[91] All these pathologies are characterized by low T2W signal on MR imaging and there may be overlapping imaging features with lymphoma. Sarcoid, IgG4-related disease, and GPA also have a propensity to PNS (Fig. 24) and may be seen to access the CSB along the trigeminal nerve divisions or the vidian nerves.[92,93]

Mucoceles, polyps, and noninvasive fungal disease

There are further noninvasive, non-neoplastic sinonasal processes that may penetrate the skull base through a process of expansion and pressure deossification. Mucoceles most frequently develop within the frontal sinuses (60%–65%) and are least commonly seen within the sphenoid sinus (2%–5%).[94–96] Supraorbital frontoethmoidal mucoceles may remodel the adjacent ASB and the thinning of the bony margins of the airless expanded sinus is appreciated on CT (Fig. 25).[97] Sphenoid mucoceles occasionally have a pattern of more aggressive bony destruction, particularly when associated with mycetoma. They also have a propensity to present with visual impairment due to pressure or inflammation of the adjacent optic nerves.[97] An associated mycetoma is suggested by central hyperdensity with linear and round calcifications (Fig. 26) and decreased T2W signal.

Advanced benign sinonasal polyps (with or without mucoceles) may also remodel the skull base.[98] They can extend within the extradural space and may become adherent to or penetrate the dura (Fig. 27).[96] Sinonasal polyps are sometimes associated with respiratory epithelial adenomatoid hamartoma, which is a benign malformation of tissue that may expand the olfactory clefts adjacent to the ASB.[99]

Finally, allergic fungal rhinosinusitis represents a noninvasive process, which may develop

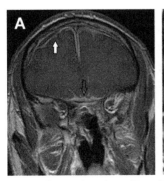
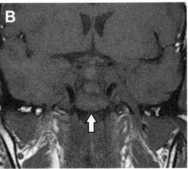
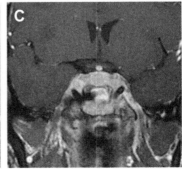

Fig. 23. Chronic invasive ASB and CSB extension of sinonasal infection. (A) Postgadolinium coronal MR imaging shows dural and leptomeningeal enhancement adjacent to the ASB (*open arrow*) with a frontal subdural rim enhancing collection (*white arrow*) in a case of chronic invasive aspergillus infection. (B) T1W and (C) gadolinium-enhanced, fat-saturated T1W coronal MR imaging demonstrates CSB extension (*arrow*) of sinonasal actinomycosis with cavernous sinus extension.

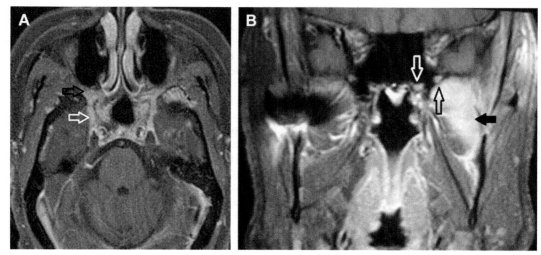

Fig. 24. GPA with PNS to the skull base. Gadolinium-enhanced, fat-saturated T1W MR imaging (*A*) axial and (*B*) coronal images demonstrate PNS of GPA. Enhancement is seen in the pterygopalatine fossa (*black open arrow*) and foramen rotundum (*white open arrow* [*A*]) as well as the vidian canal (*black open arrow*) and foramen rotundum (*white open arrow* [*B*]). Note the enhancement related to left masticator muscle denervation, which should not be misinterpreted as disease spread (*black arrow* [*B*]).

alongside sinonasal polyposis, typically in immunocompetent individuals with atopy.[100] Typical imaging findings include multiple sinuses opacified with hyperattenuating material on CT and low T2W signal on MR imaging. Advanced disease may erode both the anterior and CSB and this is reported to occur in up to 30% of cases.[8]

SKULL BASE PATHOLOGY EXTENDING TO THE SINONASAL REGION

There are additional lesions that arise from the bone of the skull base or from intracranial structures but which may extend into the nasal cavity or paranasal sinuses.

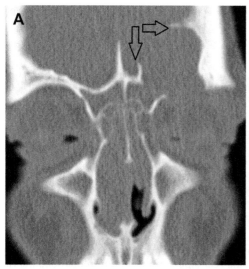
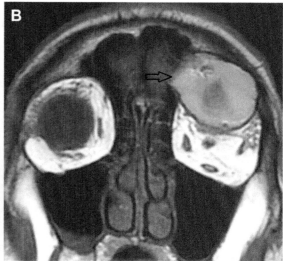

Fig. 25. Frontal mucocele. (*A*) Coronal CT shows an expanded left frontal sinus with a benign pattern of bony molding and pressure deossification (*arrows*). (*B*) T1W MR imaging demonstrates the mucocele contents to be of increased T1W signal.

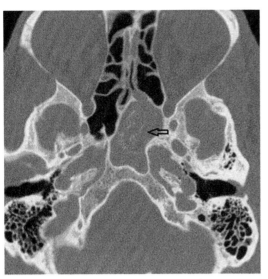

Fig. 26. Sphenoid sinus mucocele and mycetoma. Axial CT shows mild expansion of the left sphenoid sinus with speckled central calcification (*open arrow*).

Intrinsic (Bony) Skull Base

A range of primary (including osteogenic, chondrogenic, fibrogenic and hematopoietic) or secondary bone neoplasms may arise from the skull base. Many of these processes may also originate from the sinonasal region, so larger lesions may encompass both skull base and other sinonasal bony structures. Some of these pathologies may occur at any skull base location but have a prediction

for either the ASB (eg, benign osteoid lesions) or the CSB (eg, chondroid lesons or hematogenous metastases). Other lesions (eg, chordoma) are more site specific. The imaging appearances of those pathologies intrinisic to the skull base are shown in **Table 4**.[101–119]

Benign neoplasms

The commonest benign bone pathologies are osteoma and FD. Osteomas are most commonly seen within the fronto-ethmoid region and may involve the ASB, with CSB involvement being rare.[110] They are most frequently incidental benign proliferations of bone; however, they may be associated with deformity and ocular disturbance, or may be complicated by mucocele formation and pneumocephalus (**Fig. 28**).[111]

FD is an idiopathic replacement of medullary bone by fibrous and osteoid tissue, which may occur either in the ASB or CSB. Craniofacial and skull base involvement is present in 10% to 25% of mono-ostotic and 50% of polyostotic FD.[112] It may be complicated by mucocele formation and rarely by malignant degeneration. Sphenoid FD results in optic canal narrowing in 50% to 90% of cases,[101,102,113] with endonasal decompression considered for symptomatic patients (**Fig. 29**).[101] A better demarcated, focal expansile, fibro-osseous lesion indicates an ossifying fibroma.

Fluid-fluid levels are useful diagnostic feature of some benign chondroid tumors, giant cell tumors, and (rarely) ossifying fibromas in the skull base (**Fig. 30**).

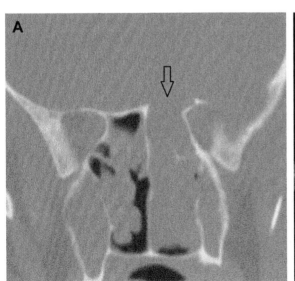
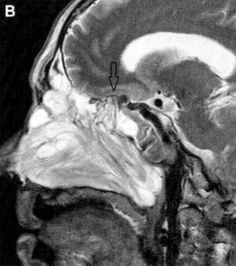

Fig. 27. Intracranial extension of sinonasal polyposis. (*A*) Coronal CT shows a breach in the ASB (*arrow*). (*B*) T2W sagittal shows the minor extradural extension of sinonasal polyps (*arrow*).

Table 4
Imaging appearances of intrinsic bone lesions within the median anterior and central skull base: differential diagnosis

	Imaging Appearances	Notes
Osteoma (see Fig. 28)	Well-defined sclerotic lesion (compact) with possible trabeculae (cancellous) and lucent (fibrous) areas on CT. Signal void on MR imaging.	Consider Gardner syndrome if multiple. Other benign osteoid lesions, such as osteoid osteoma (central lucent zone) and osteoblastoma (larger lesion in younger patient) are rare.
FD (see Fig. 29)	Intact cortical bone. Most frequently ground glass (56%) but also sclerotic and lytic patterns on CT.[101,102] T2W low signal in mineralized areas and high signal in cystic areas. May be marked enhancement on MR imaging if active.	Usually younger patients but may present later. Look for stenosis of neurovascular foramina. MR imaging may misleadingly suggest an aggressive process; however, CT is usually diagnostic.
Chondrosarcoma (see Fig. 32)	Expansile lytic and hyperdense lesion on CT with central calcification in lower-grade lesions. Chondroid matrix is of increased T2W signal and there is septal enhancement on MR imaging.	Usually paramedian CSB although midline (from spheno-occipital synchondrosis or attachment of vomer) variants occur. Generally indolent although 10% are the rarer aggressive subtypes.[103,104]
Chordoma (see Fig. 31)	Hypodense lytic, sharply demarcated lesion with internal dispersed fragments of bone on CT. Heterogenous honeycomb enhancement. T2W hyperintense (unless a high-grade tumor) with foci of low T2W signal (dirty cauliflower). A thumbprint of tissue may point toward pons on the sagittal images.	The clivus is the site of 32% of cordomas[105,106] and more common in younger patients. Distinguish from an invasive pituitary lesion by looking for superior displacement of pituitary gland.
Metastasis	Lytic or sclerotic on CT depending on primary tumor. Variable MR signal. Some metastases (eg, kidney and thyroid carcinoma) show marked vascularity and enhancement.	Lung, breast, and prostate are most frequent primary tumors. There is a predeliction for CSB, with spread hematogenous or via Batson venous plexus. Consider neuroblastoma metastasis in the infant.
Myeloma/plasmacytoma	Expansile lytic lesion with hyperdensity on CT. May cross sutures into petrous apex (see Fig. 32). Often marked increase T2W signal and enhancement on MR imaging.	Isolated plasmacytoma is rare, and those with lesions in the CSB often subsequently develop multiple myeloma.
Rarer lesions		
Benign chondrogenic (condroma, chondroblastoma, chondromyxoid fibroma)	Expansile and lytic with a thin shell and possible chondroid calcification. Variable T2W signal and heterogenous enhancement. Chondroblastoma may have a fluid-fluid level.	Often related to CSB syncochondroses. May be difficult to distinguish from a well-differentiated chondrosarcoma on imaging criteria (see Fig. 32).

(continued on next page)

Table 4
(continued)

	Imaging Appearances	Notes
Giant cell lesions (giant cell tumor [GCT], aneurysmal bone cyst [ABC], giant cell reparative granuloma, Brown tumor)	Expansile with bony remodeling and hyperdense on CT. May be low T2/T2* components due to hemosiderin content. Fluid-fluid levels in ABC and GCT (see Fig. 30).	ABC may develop secondary to other bone lesions. Suggest a parathormone assay[107] if a giant cell lesion is considered.
Langerhans cell histiocytosis (see Fig. 35)	Punched out lytic lesion without marginal sclerosis on CT. Variable T2W signal and may be markedly enhancing.	Consider in younger patients, with a single skull lesion the most frequent presentation. Sphenoid is the commonest site within the midline skull base.[108] May mimic a sarcoma in a child.
Lymphoma	Lytic, sclerotic, or permeative patterns on CT. There are bulky extraosseous soft tissue masses with T2W isointense and markedly enhancing tissue.	Skull base lymphoma is generally B-cell non- Hodgkin lymphoma. Does not always demonstrate restricted diffusion.
Other sarcomas (osteosarcoma, Ewing sarcoma, and fibrosarcoma)	Aggressive patterns of bony destruction (see Fig. 35) with sunburst (osteosarcoma) or onion-peel (Ewing) periosteal reaction. Heterogenous signal and enhancement on MR imaging.	Sarcomas account for majority of malignant skull base tumors in childhood[109] but are rare. Maybe secondary to radiotherapy or Paget disease in the adult.

Malignant neoplasms

Malignant skull base bony lesions are most commonly seen in the CSB. Chordomas originate in the midline clivus from remnants of notochord (Fig. 31),[105] whereas chondrosarcomas more commonly arise in an off-midline/paramedian location, developing from embryonic remnants of cartilage in the spheno-occipital synchondrosis or adjacent endochondral bone (Fig. 32). Both tumors usually present between 30 and 50 years of age. A majority of chondrosarcomas are of conventional subtype and they are indolent lesions with a greater than 90% progression-free 5-year survival.[103,104] This compares with chordoma,

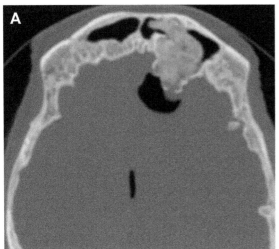
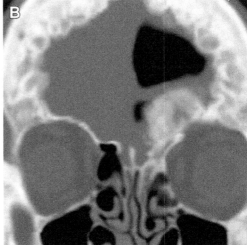

Fig. 28. Frontal sinus osteoma with complicating pneumocephalus. (*A*) Axial and (*B*) coronal CT reveal a left frontal sinus osteoma with an associated breach in the dorsal wall of the frontal sinus and pneumocephalus.

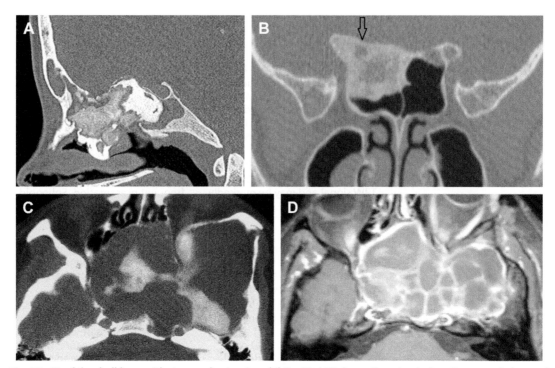

Fig. 29. FD of the skull base with sinonasal extension. (*A*) Sagittal CT shows the mixed sclerotic, ground glass and lytic sphenoethmoid skull base FD. (*B*) Coronal CT reveals right sphenoid dysplasia to constrict the right optic nerve canal (*arrow*). (*C*) Axial CT and (*D*) postgadolinium T1W MR imaging shows extensive CSB FD with signal heterogeneity and enhancement on MR imaging, mimicking a more aggressive process.

which has a 50% 5-year survival.[106] Metastasis and myeloma or plasmacytoma[114] are key differential diagnoses for a CSB mass. Metastasis is considered less likely than chordoma or chondrosarcoma in the absence of a known primary lesion.[115] Chordomas, chondrosarcomas, and

Fig. 30. CSB aneurysmal bone cyst. Axial CT demonstrates a fluid-fluid level (*arrow*).

plasmacytomas may all demonstrate markedly increased T2W signal (see **Figs. 31** and **32**; **Fig. 33**), which is less frequently a feature of metastasis. Invasive nasopharyngeal (infracranial) and pituitary adenomas (intracranial) lesions may appear centered in the clivus and so mimic primary lesions of the CSB (**Fig. 34**). These and other (eg, lymphoma)[116,117] pathologies may require nonoperative therapy, so such diagnostic possibilities should be highlighted by the radiologist to prompt biopsy rather than surgical debulking. The principle differential diagnoses of a destructive skull base and sinonasal bony lesion in the pediatric population includes neuroblastoma metastases, lymphoma, sarcoma (**Fig. 35**), and Langerhans cell histiocytosis (see **Fig. 35**), although a primary CSB osteomyelitis is a potential non-neoplastic mimic (see **Fig. 35**).[108,109,118]

Others
Finally, there may be bony expansion and sinonasal encroachment secondary to diffuse dysplasia, dysostosis, or metabolic abnormalities, such as osteopetrosis, Paget, and Gaucher disease.[120,121] Diffuse marrow disorders, such as leukemia and hyperplasia, can also result in paraosseous sinonasal soft tissue extension (**Fig. 36**).[122]

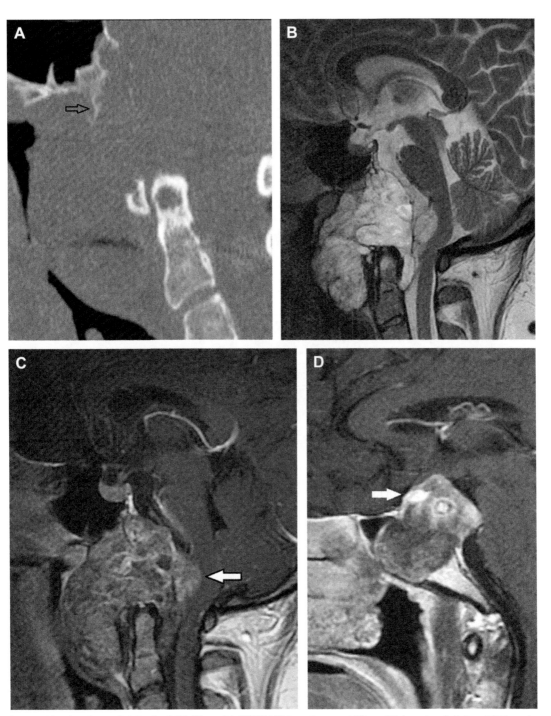

Fig. 31. CSB chordoma. (A) Sagittal CT, (B) sagittal T2W MR imaging, and (C) sagittal postgadolinium MR imaging demonstrates a clival chordoma extending to the sphenoid sinus. Note the spicules of residual bone (arrow [A]), the marked T2W high signal, and the thumbprinting of the pons (arrow [C]). (D) A more superiorly located CSB chordoma elevates the enhancing pituitary gland (arrow), a feature distinguishing it from a pituitary mass.

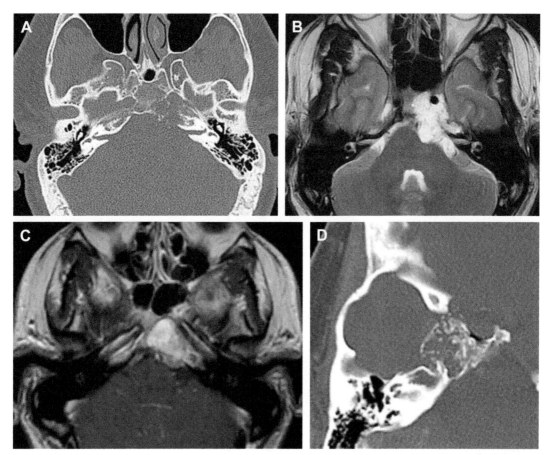

Fig. 32. CSB chondrosarcoma. (*A*) Axial CT, (*B*) axial T2W MR imaging, and (*C*) postgadolinium axial MR imaging demonstrate a chondrosarcoma with lytic destruction, marked T2W high signal and enhancement. It is centered on the petro-occipital fissure. (*D*) Axial CT in a different patient with chondrosarcoma shows a well-defined lesion with chondroid calcification, and it would be difficult to distinguish these appearances from a benign chondroid lesion.

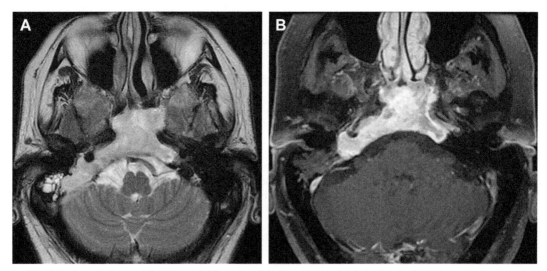

Fig. 33. CSB plasmacytoma. (*A*) T2W and (*B*) postgadolinium T1W axial fat-saturated MR imaging images show the characteristic extension of a plasmacytoma across the petro-occipital fissure to the petrous apex.

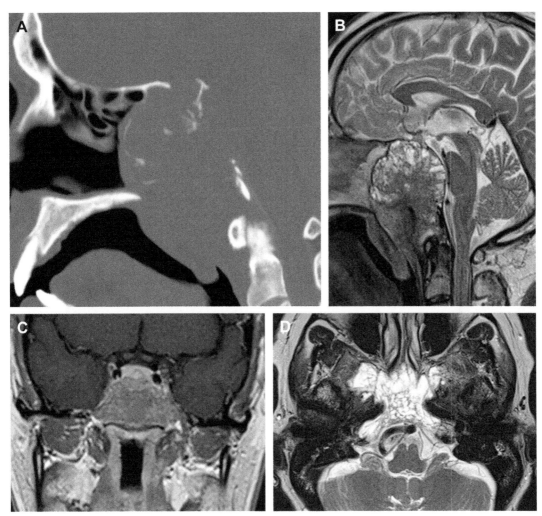

Fig. 34. Primary CSB lesion mimics. (*A*) Sagittal CT and (*B*) T2W MR imaging demonstrate a destructive lesion to be centered on the CSB and displacing bone anteriorly. This was nasopharyngeal carcinoma on biopsy (with no mucosal abnormality noted within the nasopharynx). (*C*) Coronal postgadolinium T1W and (*D*) axial T2W MR imaging shows a prolactinoma with virtually no sellar involvement and with marked CSB extension.

Intracranial

Sinonasal masses may also develop secondary to the extension of intracranial tumors (eg, meningioma, schwannoma, and pituitary tumors) or tissues (cephaloceles).

Intracranial tumors

Intracranial meningiomas extend through the skull base into the sinonasal region in 3% of cases[123] so can present with symptoms of nasal obstruction (**Fig. 37**).[124] ASB (tuberculum sella, planum sphenoidale, and olfactory groove) and CSB (sphenocavernous and petroclival) meningiomas both account for 10% to 20% of all intracranial meningiomas.[10,125,126] They may traverse the skull

base directly, with associated remodeling and hyperostosis of bone, or extend by transforaminal spread (see **Fig. 37**). Meningiomas are typically broad-based, intensely enhancing lesions that show high density and possible calcification on CT with gray matter isointensity with restricted diffusion on MR imaging. Pneumosinus dilatans is occasional demonstrated adjacent to the meningioma.[127] The CSB meningiomas are particularly challenging to manage due to the proximity of the ICA (which may be constricted on imaging), cavernous sinus and cranial nerves.

CSB schwannomas usually arise from cranial nerve V and its divisions[11,128] (and more rarely from III, IV, VI, and vidian nerves), whereas ASB olfactory groove schwannomas are of uncertain

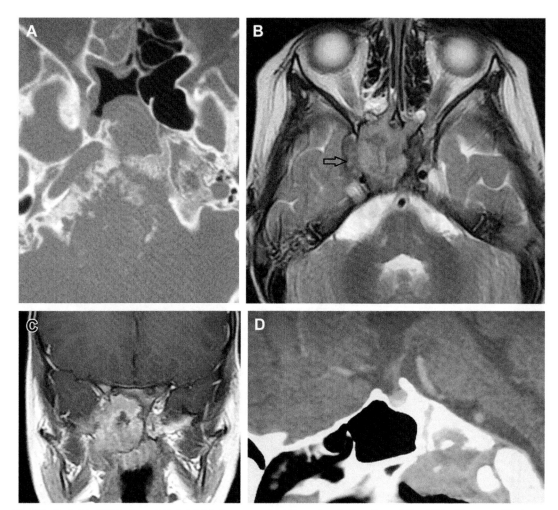

Fig. 35. Pediatric CSB lesions. (*A*) Axial CT shows marked irregular destruction of the CSB with an ossified mass lesion proving to be osteosarcoma. (*B*) T2W and (*C*) postgadolinium coronal T1W MR imaging demonstrate a right CSB and sphenoid sinus mass (*arrow* [*B*]) due to LCH. (*D*) Contrast-enhanced sagittal CT of a pimary clival osteomyelitis possibly arising from lymphoid extension through a fossa navicularis.

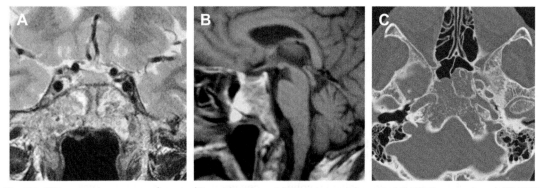

Fig. 36. CSB systemic marrow abnormality with sphenoid sinus encroachment. (*A*) T2W coronal and (*B*) T1W sagittal MR imaging shows heterogeneous signal and expansion of the CSB with sphenoid sinus extension due to Gaucher disease. (*C*) Axial CT demonstrates expansion and heterogeneity of the CSB in a patient with chronic thalassemia and soft tissue extension into the sphenoid sinus, with suspected (unproved) extramedullary hematopoiesis.

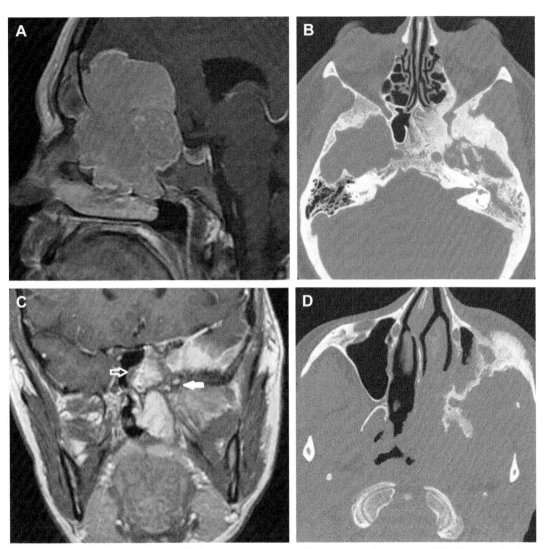

Fig. 37. Transcranial meningioma with sinonasal extension. (A) Postgadolinium sagittal T1W image of a large transcranial ASM meningioma with marked sinonasal extension. (B) Axial CT (C) postgadolinium axial T1W MR imaging at a similar level and (D) more inferior axial CT, demonstrate a CSB, facial, and sinonasal meningioma. There is marked hyperostosis of the CSB and the midface (including the maxillary sinus). Arrows in (C) indicate sphenoid sinus extension (*open arrow*) and perineural extension through the CSB (*white arrow*).

origin.[129] Schwannomas are circumscribed lesions that are isodense to hyperdense on CT, although isointense on T1W and hyperintense on T2W.[124,128] They are usually homogenous enhancing, although larger schwannomas are more heterogenous, and cystic changes may also be seen. When schwannomas traverse the skull base foramina, they result in smooth expansion and bony scalloping on CT. Sinonasal encroachment may result from remodeling and expansion of the pterygopalatine fossa, foramen rotundum, or vidian canal (Fig. 38).

Pituitary adenomas develop an infrasellar component in 28% of cases.[130,131] Sellar-based tumors, such as pituitary adenomas or craniopharyngiomas, may have an inferior vector of growth such that they present as a predominantly sphenoethmoid mass (Fig. 39). Remodeling of the sphenoid sinus may also result from the arterial pulsation of giant aneurysms of the cavernous carotid artery, so it is important for the radiologist to evaluate for imaging evidence of arterial enhancement, flow and thrombosed blood degradation products.[10,11] Other intracranial pathologies, such as granulomatous disease,[90] lymphoma, glial tumors,[132] metastases, and sarcoma are all described as invading the skull base[124] or extending through skull base foramina.

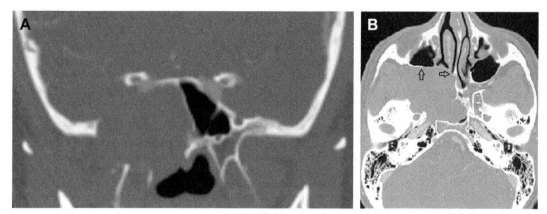

Fig. 38. CSB schwannoma with sinonasal extension. (A) Coronal and (B) axial contrast-enhanced CT show a benign pattern of bony molding and expansion (*arrows*) related to the schwannoma arising within the right sphenoid. The epicenter is on the vidian canal or foramen rotundum with marked enlargement of the pterygo-palatine fossa.

Cephaloceles

Skull base cephaloceles result from the herniation of intracranial contents (meninges with or without brain tissue) through bony defects, and may be spontaneous or secondary (posttraumatic or postsurgical).[133]

Spontaneous congenital skull base cephaloceles are sincipital (90%) or basal (10%).[40] Sincipital cephaloceles present with extranasal masses; however, some basal cephaloceles may extend through a midline anterior or CSB deficiency to present as a nasoethmoid or sphenoid sinus mass. In this context, the delayed ossification of the midline ASB in early life should not be misinterpreted as a defect on CT (see **Fig. 6**). Other sinonasal developmental lesions, such as heterotopic brain tissue (nasal glioma) or dermoids, may also be associated with bony defects.[134]

A group of spontaneous skull base cephaloceles are now recognized as secondary to acquired osseodural defects at the site of aberrant arachnoid granulations. These are frequently seen at the cribriform plate or within the lateral sphenoid sinus. These cephaloceles have an association with idiopathic intracranial hypertension, and there may be associated imaging features such as multiple arachnoid granulations, petrous apex cephaloceles, or an empty sella.[135,136] Cephaloceles should always be considered in a patient with a sinonasal polypoid lesion and a skull base defect on CT at any age. This should not be misinterpreted as an erosive lesion and hence prompt a potentially disastrous biopsy. MR imaging secures the diagnosis by demonstrating CSF in the sinonasal lesion, in continuity with that in the subarachnoid space (**Fig. 40**).

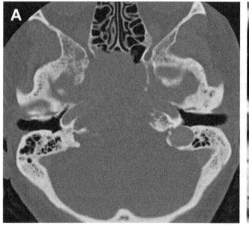
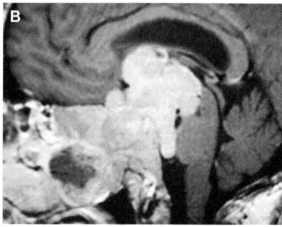

Fig. 39. Pituitary adenoma with sinonasal extension. (A) Axial CT and (B) postgadolinium sagittal T1W MR imaging show extensive nasoethmoid extension of a pituitary adenoma with bony destruction of the CSB and nasoethmoid region.

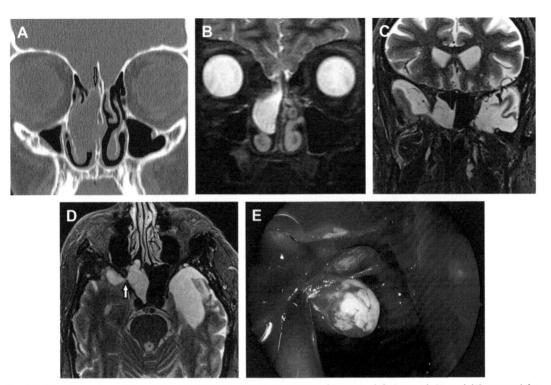

Fig. 40. Meningoceles of the ASB and CSB presenting as sinonasal masses. (A) Coronal CT and (B) coronal fat-saturated T2W MR imaging show a pedunculated polypoid right nasal mass arising from the ASB. The bony defect is not clearly shown on CT (arrow in [A]) but continuity with the subarachnoid space is revealed by the MR imaging. (C) Coronal and (D) axial STIR images demonstrate a CSF isointense lesion extending through a small defect in the right lateral sphenoid (arrow in [D]). Posttraumatic encephalomalacia is seen at the contralateral temporal pole. (E) Endoscopic image shows a sphenoid meningocele (yellow) bulging into the right sphenoid sinus. (Courtesy of Claire Hopkins FRCS, London.)

MR imaging also helps distinguish from other developmental lesions and (with gadolinium) evaluate for any infective complications.

SUMMARY

The paranasal sinuses contribute to the median ASM and CSB and thus form an interface with intracranial structures. Sinonasal disease may traverse the skull base to reach the intracranial structures, whereas intrinsic skull base or endocranial lesions may extend to the sinonasal region. Knowledge of the anatomy helps the radiologist understand the spread of disease, and variant anatomy should be recorded to help prevent surgical complications. CT and MR imaging are complementary imaging investigations, with CT useful for detecting cortical bone changes within the ASB and characterizing lesions by their pattern of bony involvement. MR imaging is superior at evaluating the bone marrow of the CSB as well as perineural or intracranial extension of sinonasal disease.

REFERENCES

1. Miracle AC, Mukherji SK. Conebeam CT of the Head and Neck, Part 2: clinical Applications. AJNR Am J Neuroradiol 2009;30:1285–92.
2. Barger AV, DeLone DR, Bernstein MA, et al. Fat signal suppression in head and neck imaging using fast spin-echo-IDEAL technique. AJNR Am J Neuroradiol 2006;27:1292–4.
3. Ginat DT, Mangla R, Yeaney G, et al. Diffusion-weighted imaging of skull lesions. J Neurol Surg B Skull Base 2014;75:204–13.
4. Wei XE, Li WB, Li YH, et al. Detection of brain lesions at the skull base using diffusion-weighted imaging with readout-segmented echo-planar imaging and generalized auto-calibrating partially parallel acquisitions. Neurol India 2011;59:839–43.
5. White ML, Zhang Y, Robinson RA. Evaluating tumors and tumorlike lesions of the nasal cavity, the paranasal sinuses, and the adjacent skull base with diffusion-weighted MRI. J Comput Assist Tomogr 2006;30:490–5.

6. Eggers G, Muhling J, Marmulla R. Image to patient registration techniques in head surgery. Int J Oral Maxillofac Surg 2006;35:1081.

7. Heaton CM, Goldberg AN, Pletcher SD, et al. Sinus anatomy associated with inadvertent cerebrospinal fluid leak during functional endoscopic sinus surgery. Laryngoscope 2012;122:1446–7.

8. Vaid S, Vaid N, Rawat S, et al. An imaging checklist for pre-FESS CT: framing a surgically relevant report. Clin Radiol 2011;66:459–70.

9. Ramakrishnan VR, Suh JD, Kennedy DW. Ethmoid skull-base height: a clinically relevant method of evaluation. Int Forum Allergy Rhinol 2011;1:396–400.

10. Keros P. On the practical value of differences in the level of the lamina cribrosa of the ethmoid. Z Laryngol Rhinol Otol 1962;41:809–13.

11. McDonald SE, Robinson PJ, Nunez DA. Radiological anatomy of the anterior ethmoidal artery for functional endoscopic sinus surgery. J Laryngol Otol 2008;122:264–7.

12. Zada G, Agarwalla PK, Mukundan S, et al. The neurosurgical anatomy of the sphenoid sinus and sellar floor in endoscopic transsphenoidal surgery. J Neurosurg 2011;114:1319–30.

13. Fernandez-Miranda JC, Prevedello DM, Madhok R, et al. Sphenoid septations and their relationship with internal carotid arteries: anatomical and radiological study. Laryngoscope 2009;119:1893–6.

14. DeLano MC, Fun FY, Zinreich SJ. Relationship of the optic nerve to the posterior paranasal sinuses: a CT anatomic study. AJNR Am J Neuroradiol 1996; 17:669–75.

15. Cho JH, Kim JK, Lee JG, et al. Sphenoid sinus pneumatisation and its relation to bulging of surrounding neurovascular structures. Ann Otol Rhinol Laryngol 2010;119:646–50.

16. Birsen U, Gulsah B, Yasemin K, et al. Risky anatomic variations of sphenoid sinus for surgery. Surg Radiol Anat 2006;28:195–201.

17. Citardi MJ, Gallivant RP, Batra PS, et al. Quantitative computer-aided computed tomography analysis of sphenoid sinus anatomical relationships. Am J Rhinol 2004;18:173–8.

18. Deutschmann MW, Yeung J, Bosch M, et al. Radiologic reporting for paranasal sinus computed tomography: a multi-institutional review of content and consistency. Laryngoscope 2013;123:1100–5.

19. Parmar H, Gujar S, Shah G, et al. Imaging of the anterior skull base. Neuroimaging Clin N Am 2009;19:427–39.

20. Urken ML, Som PM, Lawson W, et al. Abnormally large frontal sinus. II. Nomenclature, pathology and symptoms. Laryngoscope 1987;97:606–11.

21. Jang YJ, Park HM, Kim HG. The radiographic incidence of bony defects in the lateral lamella of the cribriform plate. Clin Otolaryngol Allied Sci 1999; 24:440–2.

22. Belden CJ, Mancuso AA, Kotzur IM. The developing anterior skull base: CT appearance from birth to 2 years of age. AJNR Am J Neuroradiol 1997;18:811–8.

23. Hughes DC, Kaduthodil MJ, Connolly DJA, et al. Dimensions and ossification of the normal anterior cranial fossa in children. AJNR Am J Neuroradiol 2010;31:1268–72.

24. Lewinska-Smialek B, Szao P, Ciszek B. Anatomy of the adult foramen caecum. Eur J Anat 2003;17: 142–5.

25. Hedlund G. Congenital frontonasal masses: developmental anatomy, malformations, and MR imaging. Pediatr Radiol 2006;36:647–62.

26. Chong VF, Fan YF, Lau DP. Imaging the sphenoid sinus. Australas Radiol 1994;29:47–54.

27. Chong VFH, Fan YF, Tng CH. Pictorial review: radiology of the sphenoid bone. Clin Radiol 1998;53: 882–93.

28. Borges A. Skull base tumours part II. Central skull base tumours and intrinsic tumours of the bony skull base. Eur J Radiol 2008;66:348–62.

29. Borges A. Imaging of the central skull base. Neuroimaging Clin N Am 2009;19:441–68.

30. Kimura F, Kim KS, Freiedman H, et al. MR imaging of the normal and abnormal clivus. AJR Am J Roentgenol 1990;155:1285–91.

31. Loevner LA, Tobey JD, Yousem DM, et al. MR imaging characteristics of cranial bone marrow in adult patients with underlying systemic disorders compared with healthy control subjects. AJNR Am J Neuroradiol 2002;23:248–54.

32. Welker KM, DeLone DR, Lane JI, et al. Arrested pneumatisation of the skull base: imaging characteristics. AJR Am J Roentgenol 2008;190:1691–6.

33. Aoki S, Dillon WP, Barkovich AJ, et al. Marrow conversion before pneumatization of the sphenoid sinus: assessment with MR imaging. Radiology 1989;172:373–5.

34. Abele TA, Salzman HR, Harnsberger HR, et al. Craniopharyngeal canal and spectrum of pathology. AJNR Am J Neuroradiol 2014;35:772–7.

35. Shah RK, Dhingra JK, Carter BL, et al. Paranasal sinus development: a radiographic study. Laryngoscope 2003;113:205–9.

36. Yonetsu K, Watanabe M, Nakamura T. Age related expansion and reduction in aeration of the sphenoid sinus: volume assessment by helical CT scanning. AJNR Am J Neuroradiol 2000;21:179–82.

37. Levine HL, Clemente MP. Sinus surgery: endoscopic and microscopic approaches. New York: Thieme; 2005. p. 6–12.

38. Sareen D, Agarwal AK, Kaul JM, et al. A study of sphenoid sinus anatomy in relation to endoscopic surgery. Int J Morphol 2005;23:261–6.

39. Hamid O, El Fiky L, Hassan O, et al. Anatomic variation of the sphenoid sinus and their impact on

trans-sphenoid pituitary surgery. Skull Base 2008; 18:9–16.

40. Bendersky DC, Landriel FA, Ajler PM, et al. Sternberg's canal as a cause of encephalocele within the lateral recess of the sphenoid sinus: a report of two cases. Surg Neurol Int 2011;2:171–5.

41. Settecase F, Harnsberger MA, Chapman MP, et al. Spontaneous lateral sphenoid cephaloceles: anatomic factors contributing to pathogenesis and proposed classification. AJNR Am J Neuroradiol 2014;35:784–9.

42. Patel SG, Singh B, Polluri A, et al. Craniofacial surgery for malignant skull base tumors: report of an international collaborative study. Cancer 2003;98: 1179–87.

43. Eggesbo H. Imaging of sinonasal tumours. Cancer Imaging 2012;12:136–52.

44. Sobin L, Gospodarowicz M, Wittekind C. Nasal cavity and paranasal sinuses. In: Sobin L, Gospodarowicz M, Wittekind C, editors. TNM classification of malignant tumours. 7th edition. West Sussex (United Kingdom): Wiley-Blackwell; 2010. p. 46–50.

45. Jethanamest D, Morris LG, Sikora AG, et al. Esthesioneuroblastoma a population-based analysis of survival and prognostic factors. Arch Otolaryngol Head Neck Surg 2007;133:276–80.

46. Michel J, Perret-Court A, Fakhry N. Sinonasal mucosal melanomas: the prognostic value of tumor classifications. Head Neck 2014;36:311–6.

47. Maroldi R, Farina D, Battaglia G, et al. MR of malignant nasosinusal neoplasms. Frequently asked questions. Eur J Radiol 1997;24:181–90.

48. Kimmelman CP, Korovin GS. Management of paranasal sinus neoplasms invading the orbit. Otolaryngol Clin North Am 1988;21:77–92.

49. Eisen MD, Yousem DM, Montone KT, et al. Use of preoperative MR to predict dural, perineural, and venous sinus invasion of skull base tumors. AJNR Am J Neuroradiol 1996;17:1937–45.

50. McIntyre JB, Perez C, Penta M, et al. Patterns of dural involvement in sinonasal tumors: prospective correlation of magnetic resonance imaging and histopathologic findings. Int Forum Allergy Rhinol 2012;2:336–41.

51. Bentz BG, Bilsky MH, Shah JP, et al. Anterior skull base surgey for malignant tumors: a multivariate analysis of 27 years of experience. Head Neck 2003;25:515–20.

52. Maroldi R, Ravanelli M, Borghesi A, et al. Paranasal sinus imaging. Eur J Radiol 2008;66:372–86.

53. Lund VJ, Stammberger H, Nicolai P, et al, European Rhinologic Society Advisory Board on Endoscopic Techniques in the Management of the Nose, Paranasal Sinus and Skull Base Tumors. European position paper on endoscopic management of tumours of the nose, paranasal sinuses and skull base. Rhinol Suppl 2010;22:1–143.

54. Som PM, Lidov M, Brandwin M, et al. Sinonasal esthesioneuroblastoma with intracranial extension: marginal tumour cysts as a diagnostic MR finding. AJNR Am J Neuroradiol 1994;15:1259–62.

55. Durden DD, Williams DW III. Radiology of skull base neoplasms. Otolaryngol Clin North Am 2001;34:1043–64.

56. Batra K, Chhabra A, Rampure J, et al. CT appearances of primary sphenoid melanoma. AJNR Am J Neuroradiol 2005;26:2642–4.

57. Esposito F, Kelly DF, Vinter HV, et al. Primary sphenoid sinus neoplasms: a report of four cases with common clinical presentation treated with transsphenoidal surgery and adjuvant therapies. J Neurooncol 2006;76:299–306.

58. Singh N, Eskander A, Huang S-H, et al. Imaging and resectability issues of sinonasal tumors. Expert Rev Anticancer Ther 2013;13:287–312.

59. Yousem DM, Gad K, Tufano RP. Resectability issues with head and neck cancer. AJNR Am J Neuroradiol 2006;27:2024–36.

60. Yu Q, Wang P, Shi H, et al. Carotid artery and jugular vein invasion of oro-maxillofacial and neck malignant tumors: diagnostic value of computed tomography. Oral Surg Oral Med Oral Pathol Oral Radiol Endod 2003;96:368–72.

61. Nayak UK, Donald PJ, Stevens D. Internal carotid artery resection for invasion of malignant tumors. Arch Otolaryngol Head Neck Surg 1995;121: 1029–33.

62. Ginsberg LE. MR imaging of perineural tumor spread. Neuroimaging Clin N Am 2004;14: 663–77.

63. Stambuk HE. Perineural tumor spread involving the central skull base region. Semin Ultrasound CT MR 2013;34:445–58.

64. Johnston M, Yu E, Kim J. Perineural invasion and spread in head and neck cancer. Expert Rev Anticancer Ther 2012;12:359–71.

65. Gil Z, Carlson DL, Gupta A, et al. Patterns and incidence of neural invasión in patients with cancers of the paranasal sinuses. Arch Otolaryngol Head Neck Surg 2009;135:173–9.

66. Nemec SF, Hemeth AM, Czemy C. Perineural tumor spread in malignant head and neck tumors. Top Magn Reson Imaging 2007;18:467–71.

67. Nemzek WR, Hecht S, Gandour-Edwards R, et al. Perineural spread of head and neck tumors: how accurate is MR imaging? AJNR Am J Neuroradiol 1998;19:701–6.

68. Gandhi MR, Panizza B, Kennedy D. Detecting and defining the anatomic extent of large nerve perineural spread of malignancy: comparing "targeted" MRI with histologic findings following surgery. Head Neck 2011;33:469–75.

69. Williams LS, Schmalfuss IM, Sistrom CL, et al. MR imaging of the trigeminal ganglion, nerve, and perineural vascular plexus: normal appearance and variants with correlation to cadaver specimens. AJNR Am J Neuroradiol 2003;24:1317–23.

70. Siqueira MG, Jennings E, Moraes OJS, et al. Nasoethmoid schwannoma with intracranial extensión. Arq Neuropsiquiatr 2001;59:421–3.

71. Thompson LDR, Gyure KA. Extracranial sinonasal tract meningiomas: a clinicopathologic study of 30 cases with a review of the literature. Am J Surg Pathol 2000;24:640–50.

72. Som PM, Lawson W, Lidov MW. Simulated aggressive skull base erosion in response to benign sinonasal disease. Radiology 1991;180:755–9.

73. Howard DJ, Lloyd G, Lund V. Recurrence and its avoidance in juvenile angiofibroma. Laryngoscope 2001;111:1509–11.

74. Snyderman CH, Pant H, Carrau RL, et al. A new endoscopic system for angiofibromas. Arch Otolaryngol Head Neck Surg 2010;136:588–94.

75. Babu RP, Tudor R, Kasoff SS. Pott's puffy tumor: the forgotten entity. Case report. J Neurosurg 1996;84:110–2.

76. Kriss TC, Kriss VM, Warf BC. Recurrent meningitis: the search for the dermoid or epidermoid tumor. Pediatr Infect Dis J 1995;14:697–700.

77. Clayman GL, Adams GL, Paugh DR, et al. Intracranial complications of paranasal sinusitis: a combined institutional review. Laryngoscope 1991;101:234–9.

78. Osborn Melissa K, Steinberg James P. Subdural empyema and other suppurative complications of paranasal sinusitis. Lancet Infect Dis 2007;7:62–7.

79. Lew D, Southwick FS, Montgomery WW, et al. Sphenoid sinusitis: a review of 30 cases. N Engl J Med 1983;19:1149–54.

80. Siddiqui AA, Bashir SH, Shah AA, et al. Diagnostic MR imaging features of craniocerebral Aspergillosis of sino-nasal orogin in immunocompetent patients. Acta Neurochir (Wien) 2006;148:155–66.

81. Aribandi M, McCoy VA, Bazan C 3rd. Imaging features of invasive and non-invasive fungal sinusitis: a review. Radiographics 2007;27:1283–96.

82. Fatterpekar G, Mukerji S, Arbealez A, et al. Fungal diseases of the paranasal sinuses. Semin Ultrasound CT MR 1999;20:391–401.

83. Chan L-L, Singh S, Jones D, et al. Imaging of mucormycosis skull base osteomyelitis. AJNR Am J Neuroradiol 2000;21:828–31.

84. Chang PC, Fischbein NJ, Holliday RA. Central skull base osteomyelitis in patients without otitis externa: imaging findings. AJNR Am J Neuroradiol 2003;24:1310–6.

85. Wold SM, Sinacori JT. Intracranial sarcoid granuloma as an extension of severe sinonasal sarcoidosis. Ear Nose Throat J 2012;91:e27–9.

86. Dessouky OY. Isolated sinonasal sarcoidosis with intracranial extension: case report. Acta Otorhinolaryngol Ital 2008;28:306–8.

87. Borges A, Fink J, Villablanca P, et al. Midline destructive lesions of the sinonasal tract: simplified terminology based on histopathological criteria. AJNR Am J Neuroradiol 2000;21:331–6.

88. Prabhu SM, Yadav V, Mani S, et al. IgG4-related disease with sinonasal involvement: a case series. Indian J Radiol Imaging 2014;24:117–20.

89. Suh JD, Ishiyama A, Bhuta S, et al. Radiology quiz case 1.Skull base osseous sarcoidosis. Arch Otolaryngol Head Neck Surg 2010;136:200.

90. Tobias S, Prayson RA, Lee JH. Necrotizing neurosarcoidosis of the cranial base resembling an en plaque sphenoid wing meningioma: case report. Neurosurgery 2002;51:1290–4.

91. Dubow JS, Singer S, Segal AZ. Rombencephalitis due to cocaine-induced bony erosion of skull base. Neurology 2011;77:1313.

92. Keni SP, Wiley EL, Dutra JC, et al. Skull base Wegener's granulomatoss resulting in multiple cranial neuropathies. Am J Otolaryngol 2005;26:146–9.

93. Mazziotti S, Gaeta M, Blandino A, et al. Perineural spread in a case of sinonasal sarcoidosis: case report. AJNR Am J Neuroradiol 2001;22:1207–8.

94. Mossa-Basha M, Blitz AM. Imaging of the paranasal sinuses. Semin Roentgenol 2013;48:14–34.

95. Capra GG, Carbone PN, Mullin DP. Paranasal sinus mucocele. Head Neck Pathol 2012;6(3):369–72.

96. Alsarraf R, Goldman ND, Kuntz C, et al. Isolated intracranial mucocele. Arch Otolaryngol Head Neck Surg 1999;125:1023–4.

97. Lee DH, Kim SK, Joo YE, et al. Fungus ball within a mucocele of the sphenoid sinus and infratemporal fossa: case report with radiological findings. J Laryngol Otol 2012;126:210–3.

98. Hao SP, Chang CN, Chen HC. Transbasal nasal polyposis masquerading as a skull base malignancy. Otolaryngol Head Neck Surg 1996;115:556–9.

99. Seol JG, Livolsi VA, O'Malley BW Jr, et al. Respiratory epithelial adenomatoid hamartoma of the bilateral olfactory recesses: a neoplastic mimic? AJNR Am J Neuroradiol 2010;31:277–9.

100. Marfani MS, Jawaid MA, Shaikh SM, et al. Allergic fungal rhinosinusitis with skull base and orbital erosion. J Laryngol Otol 2010;124:161–5.

101. Amit M, Fliss DM, Gil Z. Fibrous dysplasia of the sphenoid and skull base. Otolaryngol Clin North Am 2011;44:891–902.

102. Chong VFH, Khoo JBK, Fan YF. Fibrous dysplasia involving the base of skull. AJR Am J Roentgenol 2002;178:717–20.

103. Crockard HA, Cheeseman A, Steel T, et al. A multidisciplinary team approach to skull base chondrosarcomas. J Neurosurg 2001;95:184–9.

104. Brackmann DE, Teufert KB. Chondrosarcoma of the skull base: long term follow up. Otol Neurotol 2006;27:981–91.

105. Bag AK, Chapman PR. Neuroimaging: intrinsic lesions of the central skull base region. Semin Ultrasound CT MR 2013;34:412–35.

106. Maio SD, Temkin N, Ramanathan D, et al. Current comprehensive management of cranial base chordomas: 10 year meta-analysis of observational studies. J Neurosurg 2011;115:1094–105.

107. Al-Gahtany M, Cusimano M, Singer W, et al. Brown tumor of the skull base: case report and review of the literature. J Neurosurg 2003;98:417–20.

108. Prayer D, Grois N, Prosch H, et al. MR imaging presentation of intracranial disease associated with langerhans cell histiocytosis. AJNR Am J Neuroradiol 2004;25:880–91.

109. Hanbali F, Tabrizi P, Lang Demonte F. Tumors of the skull base in children and adolescents. J Neurosurg 2004;100:169–78.

110. Chen CY, Ying SH, Yao MS, et al. Sphenoid sinus osteoma at the sella turcica associated with empty sella: CT and MR imaging findings. AJNR Am J Neuroradiol 2008;29:550–1.

111. Rappaport JM, Attia EL. Pneumocephalus in frontal sinus osteoma: a case report. J Otolaryngol 1994; 23:430–6.

112. Abdel Razek AAK. Imaging appearance of bone tumors within the maxillofacial region. World J Radiol 2011;3:15–134.

113. Commins DJ, Tolley NS, Milford A. Fibrous dysplasia and ossifying fibroma of the paranasal sinuses. J Laryngol Otol 1998;112:964–8.

114. Wein RO, Popat SR, Doerr TD, et al. Plasma cell tumors of the skull base: four case reports and literature review. Skull Base 2002;12:77–86.

115. Pallini R, Sabatino G, Doglietto F, et al. Clivus metastases: report of seven patients and literature review. Acta Neurochir (Wien) 2009;151:291–6.

116. Wang L, Lin S, Zhang J, et al. Primary non-Hodgkin's lymphoma of the skull base: a case report and literature review. Clin Neurol Neurosurg 2013; 115:237–40.

117. Choi HK, Cheon JE, Kim IO, et al. Central skull base lymphoma in children: MR and CT features. Pediatr Radiol 2008;38:863–7.

118. Lui YW, Dasari SB, Young RJ. Sphenoid masses in children: radiologic differential diagnosis with pathologic correlation. AJNR Am J Neuroradiol 2011; 32:617–26.

119. Haygood TM, Herndon M, Chitkara P, et al. Chondromyxoid fibroma involving the sphenoid sinus: case report and literature review. Radiology Case Reports 2010;5:337.

120. Hamdan A-L, Nabulsi MM, Farhat FT, et al. When bone becomes marble: head and neck manifestations of ostepetrosis. Paediatr Child Health 2006;11:37–40.

121. Karabulut N, Ahmetoglu A, Ariyürek M, et al. Obliteration of maxillary and sphenoid sinuses in Gaucher's disease. Br J Radiol 1997;70:533–5.

122. Joseph M, Rajsekhar V, Chandy MJ. Haematopoietic tissue presenting as a sphenoid sinus mass. Neuroradiology 2000;42:153–4.

123. Keskin G, Ila K. Meningioma arising from the anterior skull base and filling the nasal cavity. J Craniofac Surg 2013;24:441–4.

124. Vattoth S, DeLappe S Jr, Chapman PR. Endocranial lesions. Semin Ultrasound CT MR 2013;34: 393–411.

125. Condra KS, Buatti JM, Meenhall WM, et al. Benign meningiomas: primary treatment selection affects survival. Int J Radiat Oncol Biol Phys 1997;39: 427–36.

126. Mendenhall WM, Friedman WA, Amdur RJ, et al. Management of benign skull base meningiomas: a review. Skull Base 2004;14:53–61.

127. Parizel PM, Carpentier K, Van Marck V, et al. Pneumosinus dilatans in anterior skull base meningiomas. Neuroradiology 2013;55:307–11.

128. Majoie CB, Hulsmans FJ, Castelijns JA, et al. Primary nerve sheath tumours of the trigeminal nerve: clinical and MR findings. Neuroradiology 1999;41: 100–8.

129. Figueiredo EB, Soga Y, Amorim RLO, et al. The puzzling olfactory groove schwannoma: a systematic review. Skull Base 2011;21:31–6.

130. Famini P, Maya MM, Melmed S. Pituitary magnetic resonance imaging for sellar and parasellar masses: ten-year experience in 2598 patients. J Clin Endocrinol Metab 2011;96:1633–41.

131. Chen X, Dai J, Ai L, et al. Clival invasion on multidetector CT in 390 pituitary macroadenomas: correlation with sex, subtype and rates of operative complication and recurrence. AJNR Am J Neuroradiol 2011;32:785–9.

132. Kwak R, Shatzkes D. Transdural spread of glioblastoma through the foramen ovale with presentation as a masticator space mass. AJNR Am J Neuroradiol 2009;30:808–10.

133. Connor SEJ. Imaging of skull-base cephaloceles and cerebrospinal fluid leaks. Clin Radiol 2010; 65:832–41.

134. Shah J, Patkar D, Krishnan A, et al. Pedunculated nasal glioma: MRI features and review of the literature. J Postgrad Med 1999;45:15–7.

135. Suryadevera AC, Fattal M, Woods CI. Non traumatic cerebrospinal fluid rhinorrhea as a result of benign intracranial hypertension. Ann Otol Rhinol Laryngol 2006;115:495–500.

136. Alorainy IA. Petrous apex cephalocele and empty sella: is there any relation? Eur J Radiol 2007;62: 378–84.

Posttreatment Imaging of the Paranasal Sinuses Following Endoscopic Sinus Surgery

Daniel Thomas Ginat, MD, MS

KEYWORDS

• Radiology • Paranasal sinuses • Surgery • Endoscopic • Imaging • Complications • Posttreatment

KEY POINTS

- Postoperative sinonasal diagnostic imaging techniques and protocols are reviewed.
- The different types of endoscopic sinus surgery techniques are described and the corresponding expected postoperative findings are presented.
- Complications resulting from endoscopic sinus surgery are summarized and selected examples of diagnostic imaging are presented.

INTRODUCTION

Endoscopic sinus surgery is a minimally invasive option for the treatment of several nonneoplastic indications, particularly for medically refractory sinusitis and polyposis. Numerous interventions can be performed through endoscopic sinus surgery (Box 1), many of which may be performed together during the same procedure. There are also a variety of complications that can result from endoscopic sinus surgery (Box 2).[1–10] Radiological imaging plays an important role in the evaluation of patients after endoscopic sinus surgery. Thus, it is important to be familiar with the expected and complicated imaging findings associated with endoscopic sinus surgery, which are reviewed in this article.

POSTOPERATIVE IMAGING TECHNIQUES AND PROTOCOLS

The main radiological imaging modalities available for evaluating patients following endoscopic sinus

surgery include computed tomography (CT), MR imaging, and angiography. High-resolution CT with multiplanar reconstructions is invaluable for a detailed depiction of the changes in bony anatomy and the presence of implants after surgery and can provide an overview of the extent of sinonasal opacification. CT can also be useful for screening orbital and intracranial complications. The administration of intravenous contrast with sinus CT is generally unnecessary, but can be helpful in cases of suspected orbital, facial, or intracranial infection. MR imaging often serves a complementary role to CT for optimal soft tissue characterization, particularly for delineating certain intracranial complications and further elucidating nonspecific findings on CT that are otherwise not readily amenable to endoscopic examination. Angiography, either in the form of CT angiography (CTA), MR angiography (MRA), or catheter angiography, is indicated for the evaluation of vascular complications. Notably, catheter angiography can serve as both a diagnostic and therapeutic modality in certain cases of

Disclosures: There are no conflicts of interest of relevant disclosures.
Department of Radiology, University of Chicago Medical Center, Pritzker Medical School, 5841 South Maryland Avenue, Chicago, IL 60637, USA
E-mail address: dtg1@uchicago.edu

Neuroimag Clin N Am 25 (2015) 653–665
http://dx.doi.org/10.1016/j.nic.2015.07.008
1052-5149/15/$ – see front matter © 2015 Elsevier Inc. All rights reserved.

postoperative hemorrhage. Fluoroscopy is mainly limited to guiding and verifying the completion of certain endoscopic procedures, such as balloon sinuplasty. Additional guidance for determining the appropriate imaging modalities can be found in the American College of Radiology Appropriateness Criteria for sinonasal disease.[11] Protocol details for sinonasal CT and MR imaging techniques in adults are listed in Table 1.

TYPES OF SURGERY AND IMAGING FINDINGS
Ostiomeatal Unit Endoscopic Sinus Surgery

The goal in treating an obstructed ostiomeatal unit via endoscopic surgery is to improve mucociliary clearance by removing anatomic obstacles. The procedure most typically involves uncinectomy and middle meatal antrostomy, which creates a wide neoinfundibulum that is best delineated on coronal CT images (Fig. 1). Variable degrees of ethmoidectomy and middle turbinectomy may also be performed, depending on the extent of disease; for example, medial deviation of the lamina papyracea with or without posterior repositioning of the globe frequently occurs after ethmoidectomy because of the loss of buttressing effects ordinarily provided by the ethmoid septations.[11] The medial bowing of the lamina papyracea can be observed on postoperative CT and is generally on the order of a 1-mm to 3-mm decrease in the interorbital distance (Fig. 2). Another less commonly implemented option for treating patients with ostiomeatal unit complex diseases is inferior antrostomy, which provides an alternate drainage pathway and can be useful in cases of severe disease that cannot be addressed through the usual uncinectomy and middle meatal antrostomy.[12] This procedure results in a defect in the inferior nasoantral wall that can mimic a secondary ostium (Fig. 3).

Frontal Sinusotomy and Stenting

Frontal sinusotomy is indicated when frontal sinus disease persists despite more conservative endoscopic approaches directed at the infundibulum and anterior ethmoid region. The Draf classification describes various types of endoscopic frontal sinusotomy based on the extent of surgical resection of the regional sinonasal skeleton (Table 2).[13] The postoperative status of the frontoethmoid recess is best delineated on sagittal and coronal CT images. For example, frontal sinus stenting is indicated if the neo-ostium measures less than 5 mm in width,[14] and CT can be useful for verifying the position of the stents (Fig. 4) and assessing surrounding anatomy if further surgery is contemplated.

Table 1
Sinonasal CT and MR imaging protocol parameters in adults

Modality	Parameters
CT	Helical acquisition with 0.6-mm collimation at 200 mAs and 120 kVp in axial plane with 1-mm axial, coronal, and sagittal reformatted images using bone algorithm, and 3-mm axial, coronal, and sagittal reformatted images using soft tissue algorithm
MR imaging	• Axial T1 (FOV, 240; slice thickness, 3 mm) • Coronal T1 (FOV, 160; slice thickness, 3 mm) • Axial T2 (FOV, 240; slice thickness, 3 mm) • Coronal T2 (FOV, 160; slice thickness, 3 mm) • Optional postcontrast axial and coronal T1 without or with fat suppression (if fat suppression is implemented, techniques such as mDIXON are useful for minimizing susceptibility artifacts) • Optional diffusion-weighted imaging (techniques such as FSE are useful for minimizing susceptibility artifacts)

Abbreviations: FOV, field of view; FSE, fast spin echo; kVp, kilovoltage peak.

Sphenoidotomy

Endoscopic sphenoidotomy is commonly performed to address disease that involves the sphenoid sinus and can be achieved without or with ethmoidectomy and other endoscopic sinus surgery.[15,16] The main approaches for accessing the sphenoid sinus include widening the natural ostium or creating a second opening through the posterior ethmoid sinuses. In either case, CT can show a widened communication between the sphenoid and ethmoid sinuses, which is most conspicuous on axial and sagittal reformatted images (Fig. 5). Marsupialization is another option for treating chronically infected sphenoid sinus and consists of exteriorizing the affected sinus.[17]

Furthermore, sphenoid drill-out may also be performed for chronic sinusitis and can be considered as an intermediate procedure between sphenoidotomy and sphenoid marsupialization.[18] Regardless of the technique that is implemented, the goal is improved aeration of the sphenoid sinus.

Balloon Sinuplasty

Balloon sinuplasty is a minimally invasive endoscopic treatment that involves dilating the paranasal ostia while minimizing mucosal damage. The inflated balloon delicately displaces, microfractures, and molds the bone surrounding the sinus outflow and may be used alone or in combination with conventional endoscopic surgery.[19,20]

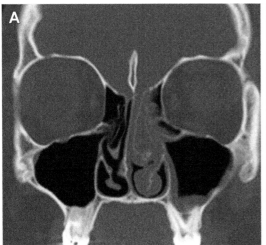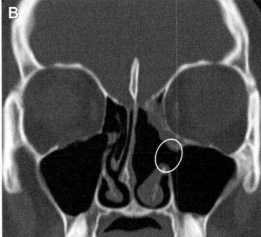

Fig. 1. Osteomeatal unit complex functional endoscopic surgery. Preoperative coronal CT image (*A*) shows opacification of the left osteomeatal unit complex. Postoperative coronal CT image (*B*) shows interval left uncinectomy and middle meatus antrostomy with a wide neoinfundibulum (*oval*), left ethmoidectomy, and left middle turbinectomy.

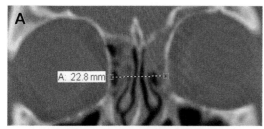

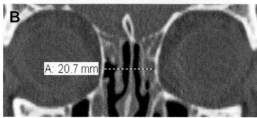

Fig. 2. Lamina papyracea medialization after ethmoidectomy. Preoperative coronal CT (*A*) shows an interlaminar distance of 22.8 mm. Postoperative coronal CT (*B*) shows interval partial bilateral internal ethmoidectomy with interval medial bowing of the lamina papyracea and a decreased interlaminar distance of 20.7 mm.

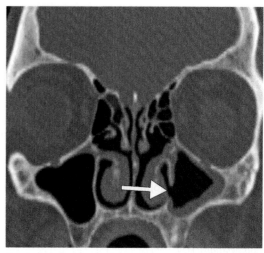

Fig. 3. Inferior meatal antrostomy. Coronal CT image shows a defect in the inferior nasoantral wall (*arrow*) in addition to uncinectomy and middle meatus antrostomy. There is mild mucosal thickening in the left maxillary sinus.

Fluoroscopic imaging guidance can be used to visualize the position and expansion of the contrast-filled balloon, which appears radiopaque (**Fig. 6**).

Mucocele Drainage

Endoscopic techniques can be effective for treating paranasal sinus mucocele, including those with orbital extension, thereby often obviating an trans-orbital approach.[21–23] In addition to clearing the affected paranasal sinus contents of the mucocele, packing material, stents, or spacers are sometimes placed and may be observed on imaging obtained soon after surgery (**Fig. 7**). Postoperative CT can be useful to evaluate for residual mucocele components and the status of the paranasal sinus walls, whereas MR imaging can

be appropriate for delineating intracranial or intraorbital extension. Following successful mucocele drainage, remineralization of the affected paranasal sinus walls can be observed and associated proptosis can diminish.

Sinonasal Debridement

Invasive fungal sinusitis can be successfully treated through endoscopic sinus surgery and nasal irrigation with antifungal agents. Endoscopic surgical intervention may consist of resecting necrotic sinonasal mucosa and bone in addition to fungal debris. Postoperative CT can be challenging to interpret following debridement for invasive fungal sinusitis when there is sinonasal opacification, because it can be can be difficult to distinguish postoperative hemorrhage, irrigation fluid, and packing material from residual fungal matter (**Fig. 8**). Under such circumstances, MR

Table 2
Draf classification for frontal sinusotomy

Category	Findings
Draf 1	Simple drainage: complete resection of the anterior ethmoid cells and uncinate process surrounding the frontal recess to the frontal ostium
Draf 2	Extended drainage: resection of the floor of the frontal sinus from the nasal septum medially to the lamina papyracea laterally (can be difficult to distinguish from Draf 1 on CT)
Draf 3 (modified Lothrop procedure)	Resection of the superior nasal septum and entire frontal sinus floor

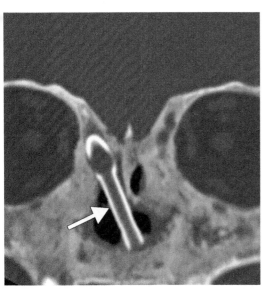

Fig. 4. Frontal sinus stent. Coronal CT image shows a right frontal sinus self-retaining stent (*arrow*) that empties into the nasal cavity. There is extensive sclerosis of the sinonasal region associated with the patient's underling Wegener granulomatosis.

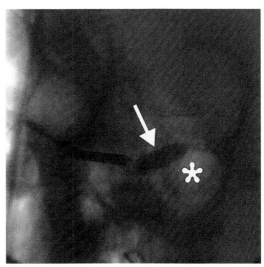

Fig. 6. Balloon sinuplasty. Fluoroscopic image shows an expanded radio-opaque contrast-filled balloon (*arrow*) that extends from the nasal cavity into the maxillary antrum (*asterisk*).

imaging may be more useful for characterizing the sinonasal contents, which can include neoplasms that sometimes coexist with fungal disease. MR imaging is also useful for early assessment of disease extension into the orbits and intracranial compartment.[24]

Septoplasty and Septorhinoplasty

The presence of a deviated nasal septum can contribute to nasal obstruction. This condition can be addressed at the time of fiberoptic endoscopic sinus surgery through septoplasty or septorhinoplasty. On CT, septoplasty produces a straightened appearance of nasal septum as well as reduction or absence of associated spurs (**Fig. 9**).[25] Silicone stents or nasopharyngeal airway tubes can be used to prevent contracture and may be encountered on imaging during the early postoperative period.[26,27] These stents appear as linear or tubular hyperattenuating structures on CT.

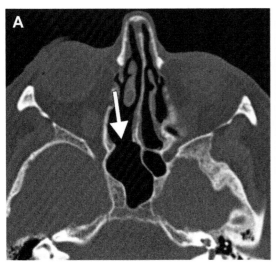

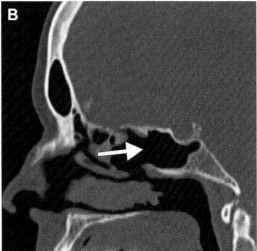

Fig. 5. Sphenoidotomy. Axial (*A*) and sagittal (*B*) CT images show a wide right sphenoid ostium (*arrows*).

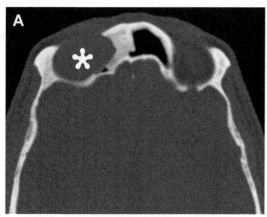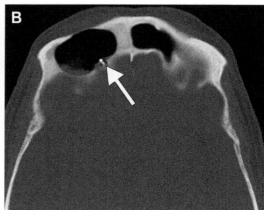

Fig. 7. Mucocele drainage. Preoperative axial CT (*A*) shows a right frontal sinus mucocele (*asterisk*). Postoperative axial CT (*B*) shows interval clearance of the right frontal sinus and insertion of a MicroFlow spacer (*arrow*).

Inferior Turbinate Reduction and Turbinoplasty

Hypertrophy of the inferior turbinates associated with allergic rhinitis can cause symptomatic obstruction of the nasal cavity. This condition can be treated via mucosal or submucosal resection. Mucosal volume can be reduced using a variety of techniques, such as coblation, radiofrequency ablation, or laser ablation. These procedures cause scarring and shrinkage of the mucosa.[28,29] Alternatively, submucosal resection typically involves resection of bone in the inferior

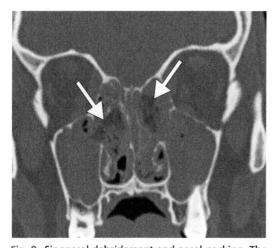

Fig. 8. Sinonasal debridement and nasal packing. The patient has a history of fungal sinusitis (*Fusarium* and *Scopulariopsis* spp). Coronal CT image obtained after recent surgery shows extensive sinonasal opacification, including nasal packing material (*arrows*) and other nonspecific contents, which may represent blood products, postoperative fluid, residual fungal debris, reactive mucosal thickening, inflammatory granulation tissue, or a combination thereof.

turbinate. In either case, the structural changes in the inferior turbinate volume can be delineated on CT (Fig. 10).[29] In addition, turbinoplasty or lateralization of the inferior turbinates can be performed along with reduction in order to further widen the nasal passage, and consists of inferior turbinate out-fracture.

Ophthalmic Indications for Endoscopic Sinus Surgery

Endoscopic sinus surgery can be used as an approach for treating several ophthalmic conditions, such as silent sinus syndrome, nasolacrimal duct obstruction, optic nerve compression, subperiosteal abscess, foreign bodies, and orbital wall fractures.[30,31] Consequently, alterations in sinonasal anatomy and associated complications may be encountered on postoperative orbital imaging. For example, following orbital decompression, the orbital contents can sometimes herniate to such an extent as to obstruct the passage of secretions from the adjacent paranasal sinuses (Fig. 11). In contrast, the orbital floor can gradually assume a more anatomic configuration after endoscopic widening of the infundibulum, although some cases require insertion of orbital implants in order to address enophthalmos.

SURGICAL COMPLICATIONS AND THEIR IMAGING FINDINGS
Skull Base and Intracranial Complications

Cerebrospinal fluid (CSF) leakage is a major complication of endoscopic sinus surgery that can result from disruption of the skull base by the surgical instruments. Thin-section noncontrast CT with multiplanar reformatted images is generally adequate for showing the site of CSF leakage

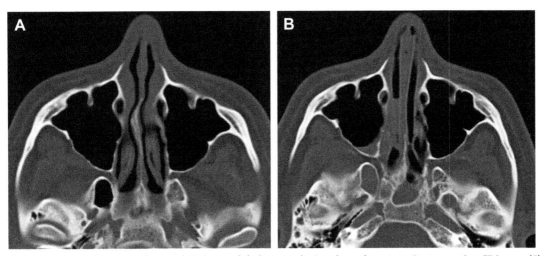

Fig. 9. Septoplasty. Preoperative axial CT image (A) shows a deviated nasal septum. Postoperative CT image (B) shows interval straightening of the nasal septum and Silastic stents within the nasal cavity.

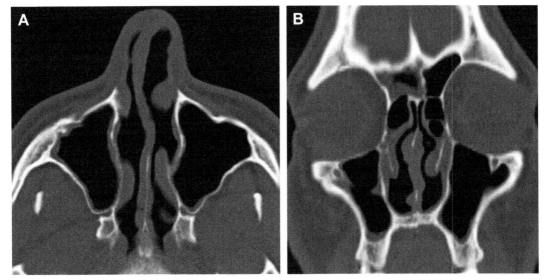

Fig. 10. Turbinate reduction. Axial (A) and coronal (B) CT images show truncation of portions of the bilateral inferior turbinates.

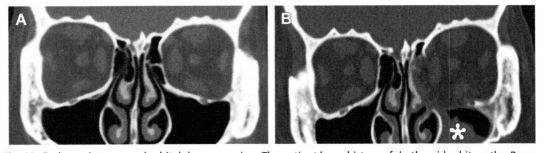

Fig. 11. Endoscopic transnasal orbital decompression. The patient has a history of dysthyroid orbitopathy. Preoperative coronal CT image (A) shows clear paranasal sinuses and intact sinonasal bony anatomy, as well as enlargement of the extraocular muscles, left greater than right. Postoperative coronal CT image (B) shows interval inferior and medial left orbital wall decompression with uncinectomy and antrostomy. The left orbital contents have prolapsed through the orbital wall defect and obstruct the neoinfundibulum with resultant obstructed secretions in the left maxillary sinus (asterisk).

and enabling accurate measurement of the skull base defect, as well as depicting associated complications, such as intracranial hemorrhage and brain laceration (**Fig. 12**).[32] However, CT has a limited ability to characterize sinonasal opacities that may be present adjacent to the skull base defect. In such cases, MR imaging may be useful for determining whether the opacities are secretions or cephaloceles, which is important to consider before surgical repair. Furthermore, MR imaging of the brain with contrast can be useful for evaluating suspected intracranial infections that may be predisposed by CSF leak. CT cisternography or MR imaging cisternography with intrathecal gadolinium and nuclear medicine scans are mainly reserved as options for attempting to localize the source of CSF leakage in patients with multiple defects, and implementing delayed scans can increase diagnostic sensitivity.[33] An unusual complication that may be associated with postoperative CSF leak is an intracranial gossypiboma, which forms from retained gauze and can resemble a mass with low T2 signal on MR imaging.[5]

Vascular Complications

Several critical vascular structures can be injured by surgical instrumentation during endoscopic sinus surgery, such as the ethmoid arteries, sphenopalatine artery, anterior cerebral arteries, and internal carotid arteries.[34,35] Injury to some of these vessels may be predisposed by preexisting dehiscences in the skull base and not only by iatrogenic defects, hence the importance of

preoperative sinus CT evaluation and/or intraoperative imaging guidance. Patients with postoperative epistaxis may warrant angiography in order to identify the source of hemorrhage, which can manifest as pseudoaneurysm. CTA is a reasonable option for evaluating such cases and identifying bony defects and the distribution of the associated hemorrhage. However, catheter angiography provides higher spatial resolution and dynamic imaging, as well as the possibility for endovascular treatment (**Fig. 13**). On the other hand, the spatial resolution of MRA for vascular structures is generally inferior to both CTA and catheter angiography and the modality can be impractical for emergent situations.

Ophthalmic Complications

Virtually any of the orbital contents can be affected by penetrating injury from surgical instruments used during endoscopic sinus surgery.[2,3,36] The most common site of entry into the orbit during endoscopic sinus surgery is the medial orbital wall, followed by the inferior orbital wall.[3] The orbital wall defects can be readily depicted on CT, particularly coronal images, and accompanying orbital hemorrhage may be apparent, manifesting as orbital fat stranding (**Fig. 14**). The presence of irregular contours to the optic nerve in the setting of vision loss is suggestive of optic nerve injury and MR imaging may reveal signal abnormality within the nerve itself. Injury to the extraocular muscles can lead to scarring and ocular dysmotility. Orbital MR imaging and CT findings correlate well with the clinical findings and can

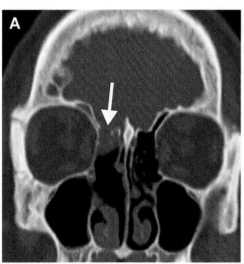
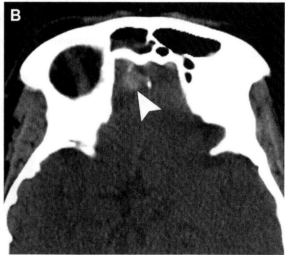

Fig. 12. Intracranial hemorrhage and CSF leak. Coronal CT image (*A*) shows postsurgical findings related to right-sided endoscopic sinus surgery, a defect in the right fovea ethmoidalis (*arrow*), and an adjacent opacity. Axial CT image (*B*) shows an area of acute hemorrhage in the right gyrus rectus (*arrowhead*).

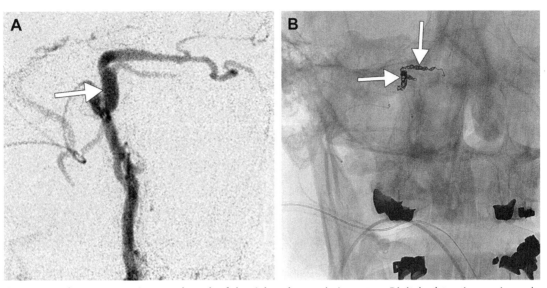

Fig. 13. Pseudoaneurysm. Injury to a branch of the right sphenopalatine artery. Digital subtraction angiography (A) shows abnormal focal dilatation of the right sphenopalatine artery (*arrow*). Fluoroscopic image (B) shows interval coil embolization (*arrows*) of the pseudoaneurysm and adjacent vessels.

assist in clarifying the cause of injury and guide surgical corrective management.[3] Lacrimal drainage system injury from endoscopic sinus surgery can appear as disruption of the nasolacrimal duct on CT and may require dacryocystorhinostomy and stenting (Fig. 15). Periorbital complications, such as lipogranuloma formation, are uncommon following endoscopic sinus surgery.

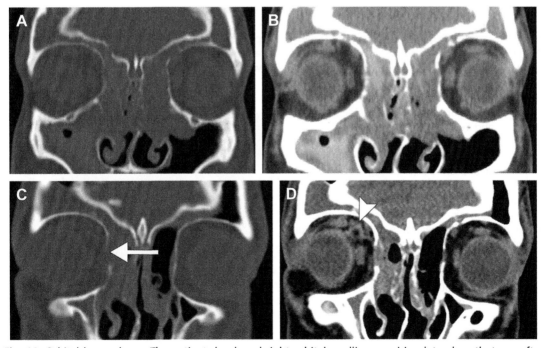

Fig. 14. Orbital hemorrhage. The patient developed right orbital swelling requiring lateral canthotomy after endoscopic sinus surgery. Preoperative coronal CT images in bone (A) and soft tissue (B) windows show extensive opacification, but intact orbital walls and contents. Postoperative coronal CT images in bone (C) and soft tissue (D) windows show a defect in the right lamina papyracea (*arrow*) and new stranding in the right orbital fat (*arrowhead*).

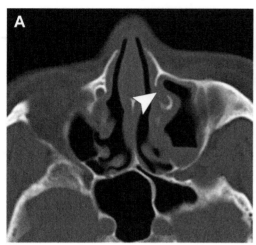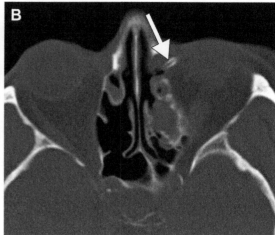

Fig. 15. Nasolacrimal duct injury. The patient underwent endoscopic sinus surgery in the 1990s and subsequently developed left-sided epiphora. Axial CT images (*A, B*) show disruption of the left nasolacrimal duct (*arrowhead*), which was treated via dacryocystorhinostomy and stent (*arrow*).

On imaging, the lipogranulomas appear as ill-defined, irregular, heterogeneously enhancing fat-containing nodules that are most commonly located in the eyelids.[10]

Recurrent Rhinosinusitis

Recurrent rhinosinusitis is perhaps the most common indication for CT following endoscopic sinus surgery. Although CT can readily show opacities associated with inflammatory disease, the role of CT for postoperative evaluation is to attempt to identify underlying structural causes, which may include hypertrophic mucosa, neo-osteogenesis, incomplete uncinate process resection, retained Haller and agger nasi cells, residual anterior ethmoid and residual frontal cells, and spontaneous osteoneogenesis.[7,15] For example, postoperative sinonasal adhesions can appear as linear opacities on CT (**Fig. 16**), but are otherwise nonspecific in appearance and may be obscured by adjacent secretions. In contrast, neo-osteogenesis has a characteristic amorphous bone attenuation appearance on CT (**Fig. 17**) and it can progressively enlarge and ossify. Another structural cause of failed endoscopic surgery is the recirculation phenomenon, which involves the circulation of mucous secretion between the natural ostium and other openings that have not been connected. The recirculation of mucus between the natural and accessory openings is shown as a ring structure on CT.[37] Patient with nonsteroidal antiinflammatory drug intolerance or asthma are particularly prone to recurrent polyposis despite extensive efforts toward polypectomy and may not necessarily have contributing structural issues

otherwise (**Fig. 18**).[38,39] In such cases, imaging is useful for assessing extent of disease and planning further surgery.

Nasal Septum Injury

The nasal septum may be susceptible to trauma that can lead to the development of hematoma, necrosis, and perforation of this structure following endoscopic sinus surgery, especially with septoplasty.[40] Nasal septal perforation can be associated with epistaxis, crusting, secondary infection, whistling, and nasal obstruction, which warrant

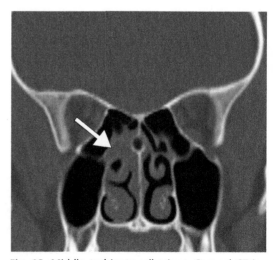

Fig. 16. Middle turbinate adhesions. Coronal CT image shows opacification of the right neoinfundibulum (*arrow*). Subsequent endoscopic surgery confirmed the presence of scar tissue in this location.

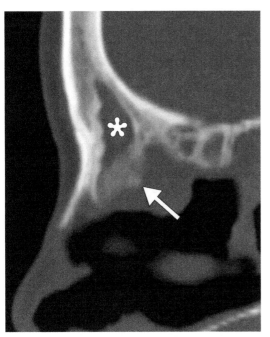

Fig. 17. Recurrent rhinosinusitis and neo-osteogenesis. Sagittal CT image obtained after endoscopic sinus surgery shows opacification of the frontal sinus (*asterisk*) with amorphous hyperattenuation in the frontoethmoid recess (*arrow*).

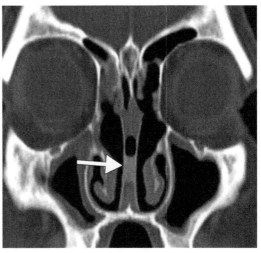

Fig. 19. Nasal septal perforation. Coronal CT image shows postoperative findings related to endoscopic sinus surgery and a defect in the nasal septum, which have been treated with a nasal septal button prosthesis (*arrow*).

treatment.[41] Nasal septum defects are readily apparent on CT, which can be useful for planning surgical repair, such as through the use of customized button prostheses (**Fig. 19**).

Empty Nose Syndrome

Empty nose syndrome is a rare complication of sinonasal surgery, particularly following resection of the inferior turbinate, and is likely caused by excessive nasal permeability affecting neurosensitive receptors and inhaled air humidification and conditioning functions.[42] Patients experience paradoxical nasal obstruction despite an otherwise clear nasal cavity and paranasal sinuses (**Fig. 20**).[43] Thus, CT can be used to confirm the

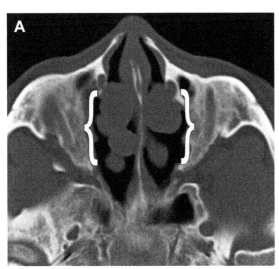

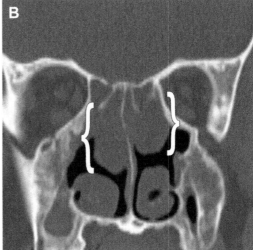

Fig. 18. Recurrent polyposis. Axial (*A*) and coronal (*B*) CT images show multiple polypoid opacities in the nasal cavity (*brackets*).

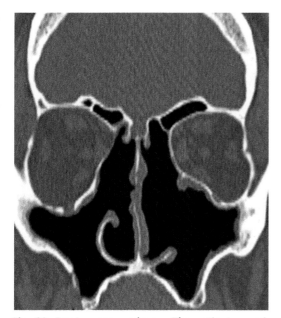

Fig. 20. Empty nose syndrome. The patient experienced nasal congestion following sinus surgery. Coronal CT image shows extensive resection of the sinonasal structures, including the inferior turbinates, but the sinonasal cavities are otherwise virtually clear.

absence of obstructive lesions and can be useful for planning reconstructive surgery.

WHAT REFERRING PHYSICIANS NEED TO KNOW

Ultimately the decision to obtain diagnostic imaging following endoscopic sinus surgery depends on the specific clinical situation. The role of radiologists may be to guide the referring physicians toward selecting the most appropriate imaging

modality for the particular clinical question (Table 3). The goal of radiologists is also to provide a systematic description of the apparent postoperative findings, both expected and unexpected, with attention to the various conditions reviewed in this article.

SUMMARY

Endoscopic sinus surgery is commonly performed for a variety of nonneoplastic indications and patients sometimes undergo postoperative diagnostic imaging of the sinonasal region. Therefore, it is important to be familiar with the optimal imaging modalities and the corresponding appearance of expected changes, potential complications on postoperative imaging of the paranasal sinuses, and the associated complications that may occur.

REFERENCES

1. Ginat DT, Cunnane ME. Imaging the paranasal sinuses and nasal cavity after surgery. In: Ginat DT, Westesson PL, editors. Atlas of postsurgical neuroradiology. Berlin: Springer; 2012. p. 75–120.
2. Bhatti MT. Neuro-ophthalmic complications of endoscopic sinus surgery. Curr Opin Ophthalmol 2007; 18:450–8.
3. Bhatti MT, Schmalfuss IM, Mancuso AA. Orbital complications of functional endoscopic sinus surgery: MR and CT findings. Clin Radiol 2005;60:894–904.
4. Zeifer B. Sinusitis: postoperative changes and surgical complications. Semin Ultrasound CT MR 2002; 23:475–91.
5. Tan VE, Sethi DS. Gossypiboma: an unusual intracranial complication of endoscopic sinus surgery. Laryngoscope 2011;121:879–81.
6. Krings JG, Kallogjeri D, Wineland A, et al. Complications of primary and revision functional endoscopic sinus surgery for chronic rhinosinusitis. Laryngoscope 2014;124:838–45.
7. Valdes CJ, Bogado M, Samaha M. Causes of failure in endoscopic frontal sinus surgery in chronic rhinosinusitis patients. Int Forum Allergy Rhinol 2014;4:502–6.
8. May M, Levine HL, Mester SJ, et al. Complications of endoscopic sinus surgery: analysis of 2108 patients–incidence and prevention. Laryngoscope 1994;104:1080–3.
9. Yang BT, Liu YJ, Wang YZ, et al. CT and MR imaging findings of periorbital lipogranuloma developing after endoscopic sinus surgery. AJNR Am J Neuroradiol 2012;33:2140–3.
10. Available at: http://www.guideline.gov/content.aspx? id=37936&search=Chronic+sinusitis. Accessed February 1, 2015.
11. Cunnane ME, Platt M, Caruso PA, et al. Medialization of the lamina papyracea after endoscopic

Table 3
What referring physicians need to know

Clinical Question	Suggested Imaging Modalities
Where is the site of CSF leak?	CT
Is there a cephalocele?	Skull base MR imaging
What is the source of the bleeding?	Catheter angiography or CTA
Is there intracranial infection?	Brain MR imaging with contrast
Why are there vision changes?	Orbit CT and/or MR imaging
Why is there recurrent sinusitis?	Sinus CT
Why is there nasal obstruction?	Sinus CT

ethmoidectomy: comparison of preprocedure and postprocedure computed tomographic scans. J Comput Assist Tomogr 2009;33:79–81.

12. Albu S, Gocea A, Necula S. Simultaneous inferior and middle meatus antrostomies in the treatment of the severely diseased maxillary sinus. Am J Rhinol Allergy 2011;25:e80–5.

13. Draf W, Weber R, Keerl R, et al. Aspects of frontal sinus surgery. Part I: Endonasal frontal sinus drainage for inflammatory sinus disease. HNO 1995;43:352–7.

14. Rains BM 3rd. Frontal sinus stenting. Otolaryngol Clin North Am 2001;34:101–10.

15. Moeller CW, Welch KC. Prevention and management of complications in sphenoidotomy. Otolaryngol Clin North Am 2010;43:839–54.

16. Kieff DA, Busaba N. Treatment of isolated sphenoid sinus inflammatory disease by endoscopic sphenoidotomy without ethmoidectomy. Laryngoscope 2002;112:2186–8.

17. Donald PJ. Sphenoid marsupialization for chronic sphenoidal sinusitis. Laryngoscope 2000;110: 1349–52.

18. Leight WD, Leopold DA. Sphenoid "drill-out" for chronic sphenoid rhinosinusitis. Int Forum Allergy Rhinol 2011;1:64–9.

19. Levine H, Rabago D. Balloon sinuplasty: a minimally invasive option for patients with chronic rhinosinusitis. Postgrad Med 2011;123:112–8.

20. Taghi AS, Khalil SS, Mace AD, et al. Balloon sinuplasty: balloon-catheter dilation of paranasal sinus ostia for chronic rhinosinusitis. Expert Rev Med Devices 2009;6:377–82.

21. Barrow EM, DelGaudio JM. In-office drainage of sinus mucoceles: an alternative to operating-room drainage. Laryngoscope 2015;125(5):1043–7.

22. Sautter NB, Citardi MJ, Perry J, et al. Paranasal sinus mucoceles with skull-base and/or orbital erosion: is the endoscopic approach sufficient? Otolaryngol Head Neck Surg 2008;139:570–4.

23. Khong JJ, Malhotra R, Wormald PJ, et al. Endoscopic sinus surgery for paranasal sinus mucocoele with orbital involvement. Eye (Lond) 2004; 18:877–81.

24. Alobid I, Bernal M, Calvo C, et al. Treatment of rhinocerebral mucormycosis by combination of endoscopic sinus debridement and amphotericin B. Am J Rhinol 2001;15:327–31.

25. Schatz CJ, Ginat DT. Imaging features of rhinoplasty. AJNR Am J Neuroradiol 2014;35:216–22.

26. Guyuron B, Vaughan C. Evaluation of stents following septoplasty. Aesthetic Plast Surg 1995; 19:75–7.

27. Egan KK, Kim DW. A novel intranasal stent for functional rhinoplasty and nostril stenosis. Laryngoscope 2005;115:903–9.

28. Bäck LJ, Hytönen ML, Malmberg HO, et al. Submucosal bipolar radiofrequency thermal ablation of

inferior turbinates: a long-term follow-up with subjective and objective assessment. Laryngoscope 2002; 112:1806–12.

29. Demir U, Durgut O, Saraydaroglu G, et al. Efficacy of radiofrequency turbinate reduction: evaluation by computed tomography and acoustic rhinometry. J Otolaryngol Head Neck Surg 2012;41:274–81.

30. Metson R, Pletcher SD. Endoscopic orbital and optic nerve decompression. Otolaryngol Clin North Am 2006;39:551–61, ix.

31. Sciarretta V, Pasquini E, Tesei F, et al. Endoscopic sinus surgery for the treatment of maxillary sinus atelectasis and silent sinus syndrome. J Otolaryngol 2006;35:60–4.

32. La Fata V, McLean N, Wise SK, et al. CSF leaks: correlation of high-resolution CT and multiplanar reformations with intraoperative endoscopic findings. AJNR Am J Neuroradiol 2008;29:536–41.

33. DelGaudio JM, Baugnon KL, Wise SK, et al. Magnetic resonance cisternogram with intrathecal gadolinium with delayed imaging for difficult to diagnose cerebrospinal fluid leaks of anterior skull base. Int Forum Allergy Rhinol 2015;5(4):333–8.

34. Weidenbecher M, Huk WJ, Iro H. Internal carotid artery injury during functional endoscopic sinus surgery and its management. Eur Arch Otorhinolaryngol 2005;262:640–5.

35. Hudgins PA, Browning DG, Gallups J, et al. Endoscopic paranasal sinus surgery: radiographic evaluation of severe complications. AJNR Am J Neuroradiol 1992;13:1161–7.

36. Bolger WE, Parsons DS, Mair EA, et al. Lacrimal drainage system injury in functional endoscopic sinus surgery. Incidence, analysis, and prevention. Arch Otolaryngol Head Neck Surg 1992;118:1179–84.

37. Chung SK, Cho DY, Dhong HJ. Computed tomogram findings of mucous recirculation between the natural and accessory ostia of the maxillary sinus. Am J Rhinol 2002;16:265–8.

38. Albu S, Tomescu E, Mexca Z, et al. Recurrence rates in endonasal surgery for polyposis. Acta Otorhinolaryngol Belg 2004;58:79–86.

39. Larsen K, Tos M. A long-term follow-up study of nasal polyp patients after simple polypectomies. Eur Arch Otorhinolaryngol 1997;254(Suppl 1):S85–8.

40. Topal O, Celik SB, Erbek S, et al. Risk of nasal septal perforation following septoplasty in patients with allergic rhinitis. Eur Arch Otorhinolaryngol 2011; 268:231–3.

41. Mullace M, Gorini E, Sbrocca M, et al. Management of nasal septal perforation using silicone nasal septal button. Acta Otorhinolaryngol Ital 2006;26:216–8.

42. Sozansky J, Houser SM. Pathophysiology of empty nose syndrome. Laryngoscope 2014;125(1):70–4.

43. Coste A, Dessi P, Serrano E. Empty nose syndrome. Eur Ann Otorhinolaryngol Head Neck Dis 2012;129: 93–7.

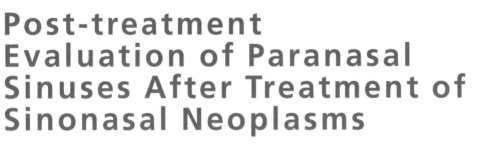

Post-treatment Evaluation of Paranasal Sinuses After Treatment of Sinonasal Neoplasms

Roberto Maroldi, MD[a],*, Marco Ravanelli, MD[a],
Davide Farina, MD[a], Luca Facchetti, MD[a],
Francesco Bertagna, MD[b], Davide Lombardi, MD[c],
Piero Nicolai, MD[c]

KEYWORDS

- Paranasal neoplasms • MR Imaging • Magnetic resonance • Recurrent neoplasms
- Postsurgical complications

KEY POINTS

- A proper imaging protocol and correct interpretation of post-treatment imaging findings rely on knowledge of the most frequently used surgical and radiation therapy techniques and principles of oncological resection.
- MR is superior to CT in detecting recurrences because of a higher capability in discriminating tissues and post-treatment changes, related to a multisequence analysis. Most acute complications are the domain of CT.
- In-field intracranial recurrences and craniofacial bone metastases are possible when the primary tumor invades the dura and with aggressive histologies. Perineural spread along cranial nerves and branches has to be carefully scrutinized, particularly in the case of adenoid cystic carcinoma and squamous cell carcinoma.

INTRODUCTION

Sinonasal neoplasms are characterized by great histologic heterogeneity, reflecting the number of different tissues in this area. As a result, a large variety of benign and malignant neoplasms may arise from the mucosa lining the sinonasal cavities or from submucosal structures. Numerous types of treatment have been developed to address different oncological conditions. For example, benign neoplasms are treated solely by surgical resection, whereas most malignant neoplasms require multimodal therapy.

Diverse surgical techniques have been devised to adequately treat neoplasms with a great variability in biological aggressiveness. The invasiveness of surgical approaches are at 2 ends of the spectrum: open surgical techniques and endoscopic surgery.[1] A minimally invasive surgical approach, namely endoscopic surgery, was originally adopted only for inflammatory conditions. In the last 2 decades it has been used initially for benign tumors, then as a complement to, and more recently as an alternative to open surgery in selected malignant neoplasms.[2]

The authors have nothing to disclose.
[a] Department of Radiology, University of Brescia, Radiologia 2 – Spedali Civili, Piazzale Spedali Civili 1, Brescia I-25123, Italy; [b] Nuclear Medicine, University of Brescia, Piazzale Spedali Civili 1, Brescia I-25123, Italy; [c] Department of Otorhinolaryngology, University of Brescia, Piazzale Spedali Civili 1, Brescia I-25123, Italy
* Corresponding author.
E-mail address: roberto.maroldi@unibs.it

neuroimaging.theclinics.com

Parallel progress in radiation therapy techniques has been attained over the last 2 decades, mostly with the introduction of intensity-modulated radiation therapy, volumetric modulated arc therapy, and advances in particle radiation therapy.[3]

It follows that tailoring specific post-therapy imaging protocols is crucial to overcome the combination of different histologies with characteristic patterns of spread or relapse and different treatment techniques. In addition, post-treatment imaging is required in distinct clinical settings, from the immediate postsurgical intracranial complications to follow-up after chemotherapy and radiotherapy (RT).

A practical imaging strategy for dealing with such challenges is to resolve the diverse clinical scenarios into a given number of key factors.

The first factor deals with the expected imaging changes: that is, knowledge of which imaging findings should normally be present after surgery for benign or malignant neoplasm, or after RT. The second factor entails knowledge of the specific model of growth of those benign and malignant neoplasms that may result in characteristic patterns of recurrence, such as perineural spread for adenoid cystic carcinoma. The third factor involves detailed information about the type of surgical resection/reconstruction, relevant intraoperative findings, and pathologic data that could point to areas at higher risk for recurrence.

This information is useful not only to select the proper imaging protocol but also to increase the accuracy in interpreting imaging findings. The availability of previous studies and careful matching with current imaging and clinical findings is certainly crucial in minimizing the chance of missing relapsing neoplasms.

IMAGING TECHNIQUES

A comprehensive description of computed tomography (CT) and MR imaging techniques is beyond the purpose of this article. However, some critical technical aspects in post-treatment imaging are discussed here. CT is usually performed to exclude acute intracranial complications such as tension pneumocephalus, hemorrhage, skull base defects, abscess, or orbital complications. In cases of orbital or intracranial abscesses, contrast agent administration is indicated. Multiplanar reconstructions (MPR) on coronal and sagittal planes with both bone and soft tissue windows should be part of the imaging protocol.

During follow-up, MR imaging is superior to CT in detecting recurrent/persistent disease, depicting its spatial extent, and identifying complications such as cerebrospinal fluid (CSF) leak, neuritis, and white-matter necrosis.

T2 sequences provide the best signal discrimination (Fig. 1). In our protocols, they are the first sequences acquired on at least the axial and coronal planes. They represent conceptual shelves for inserting information provided by subsequent sequences. T1 sequences are used to assess the extent of medullary bone abnormalities and as a baseline for contrast-enhanced sequences. For example, this combination helps to identify collections of dehydrated entrapped fluid (hyperintense on T1) that could otherwise mimic enhancement in postcontrast images. Both T2 and T1 sequences should be acquired with thin slices (3 mm or less) and high in-plane resolution (512 × 256 or more). Time-sparing (parallel imaging) and motion-reduction (PROPELLER/BLADE) techniques are usually not needed, but they may be useful in uncooperative patients. In our experience, fat-saturated T2 sequences are not useful and they should not be used in lieu of standard T2 sequences. In fat-suppressed T2 sequences, most of the anatomic information is lost and the range of signals is narrowed and altered. In addition, inefficient fat suppression may simulate focal abnormalities.

Diffusion-weighted imaging (DWI) has become one of the most promising and appealing techniques in recent years. The main strength of DWI in the field of oncology is its capability of discriminating tumor from inflammation. For this reason, DWI seems to fit the purpose of post-treatment imaging; that is, to properly separate expected post-treatment inflammatory changes from recurrences. A high signal in high b value (b1000) images and a low signal on apparent diffusion coefficient (ADC) maps suggests recurrence, whereas a high ADC indicates inflammation. However, the technique is hampered by important limitations: DWI is affected by susceptibility artifacts, especially in areas rich in bone-fat-air interfaces such as the sinonasal tract; a high b1000 signal in the brain may mask recurrences in the skull base; metallic clips may hinder proper fat saturation in adjacent areas, especially in adipose flaps, resulting in misleading interpretations. In addition, the simple rule high b1000 + low ADC = tumor; high ADC = inflammation is not valid for all histologies (eg, in intestinal-type adenocarcinoma, high mucinous content reduces the b1000 signal and raises the ADC value).

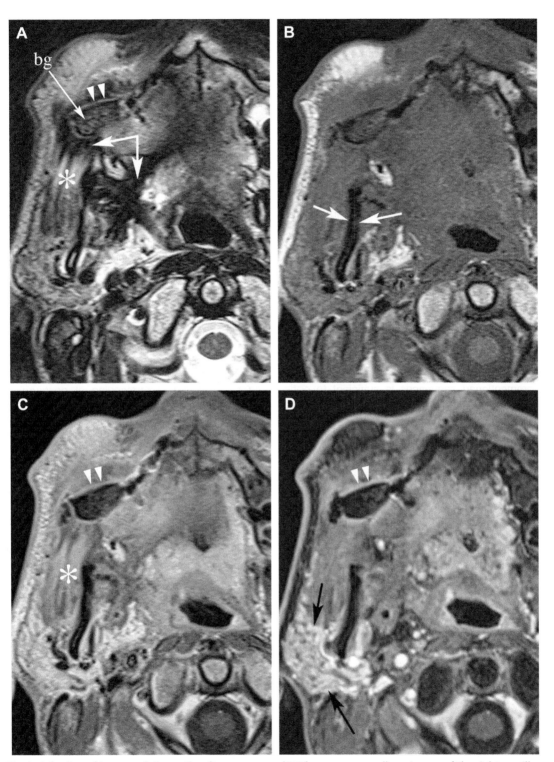

Fig. 1. Infection of bone graft 3 months after surgery and RT for squamous cell carcinoma of the right maxillary sinus. (A) Turbo spin echo (TSE) T2; (B) unenhanced spin echo (SE) T1; (C) enhanced SE T1; (D) enhanced three-dimensional VIBE. Bone graft (bg); perigraft edema (*arrowheads* in A, C, and D); scar tissue (*paired arrows* in A); edema of the masseteric muscle (*asterisk* in A and C); mandible (*opposite arrows* in B); post-RT chronic inflammation of the parotid gland (*arrows* in D).

Enhanced three-dimensional fat-saturated gradient-echo T1 sequences (VIBE) are able to depict areas of enhancement with high isotropic resolution. Fat saturation increases the consistency of enhancement within fat-containing tissues (eg, the medullary bone). Furthermore, high spatial resolution and multiplanar reconstructions provide optimal assessment of both perineural spread[4] and the spatial relationship of neoplastic tissue with complex anatomic structures. Our advice is to acquire VIBE sequences early after Gd administration; intense and diffuse enhancement of inflammatory tissues occurs in delayed phases (ie, 3–4 minutes after contrast administration).

Postcontrast three-dimensional constructive interference in steady state (CISS) sequences[5] may be used as additional sequences when the relationship between an enhancing neoplasm and the dura and/or cranial nerves needs to be precisely mapped (Fig. 2).

Dynamic contrast-enhanced (DCE) MR imaging has been proposed by some investigators as a useful tool in inflammation/tumor discrimination.[6,7] However, in our experience, integration of the aforementioned sequences is sufficient to optimally image treated patients within a reasonable time.[8]

Some recent studies have shown diagnostic usefulness of ^{18}F-fluorodeoxyglucose (FDG)-PET/CT for restaging patients treated for sinonasal malignant neoplasms. An important advantage of ^{18}F-FDG-PET/CT is that a whole-body scan allows for the detection of distant metastases and unexpected secondary cancers.[9] As in CT and MR imaging, postsurgical and post-RT crusting and inflammation may cause mild to even high hypermetabolic activity in the absence of relapsing disease. Despite this, metabolic activity is useful to distinguish scar tissue from recurrences.[10]

A negative PET/CT study seems to be more predictive of the absence of disease as seen in the consistently high negative predictive values among all sites.

EXPECTED IMAGING CHANGES AFTER SURGERY

After surgery for sinonasal neoplasms, posttreatment follow-up with imaging is mainly based on MR imaging with the aim of detecting residual/recurrent lesions, providing detailed mapping of known recurrences, and recognizing possible complications (ie, mucocele).

After surgery, most intranasal structures are usually resected. This fact facilitates endoscopic examination of the healed mucosal surfaces, although the development of adhesions or a peculiar anatomy may hamper an adequate survey of the frontal or sphenoid sinuses. Therefore, the specific domain of post-treatment imaging studies is the assessment of structures unreachable by endoscopy, namely intracranial and intraorbital structures, or to scrutinize other potential submucosal sites of recurrence.

Crucial to the understanding of postsurgical changes is that the oncologic principles for endoscopic resection of benign neoplasms differ from those required for malignant neoplasms. For example, for a benign neoplasm abutting the adjacent bony surface, subperiosteal dissection with drilling of the bone is generally sufficient to achieve oncologically adequate removal. On the contrary, as the aim of resection of malignant neoplasms is to achieve negative margins, not only the area of attachment but also eroded bone structures or those in contact with an aggressive malignant neoplasm have to be removed.

Generally, the removal of central structures of the naso-ethmoid complex does not require any

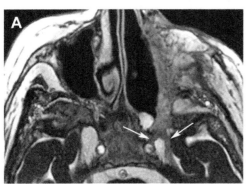
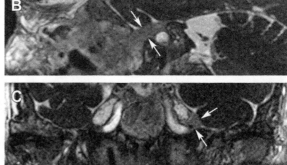

Fig. 2. Local recurrence and perineural spread of a maxillary sinus squamous cell carcinoma. MPR reconstructions of enhanced CISS: (A) axial; (B) sagittal; (C) coronal. Arrows point to perineural spread along V2 with invasion of the Meckel cave.

reconstruction. When noncentral structures, such as sections of the skull base shell are resected along with variable sections of the dura mater, large defects in bones and meninges are created. There is the need to restore the seal between the intracranial compartment and the sinonasal cavities to avoid complications such as CSF leak, meningitis, and pneumocephalus (Table 1). The techniques developed to close these defects differ from the techniques used for endoscopic CSF leak repair. Not only are the defects to be sealed larger but also the duraplasty could be included in the field of RT. Numerous nonvascularized and vascularized reconstructive techniques have been introduced; the choice is dictated by the site of the defect and the intraoperative CSF flow.

In most sinonasal neoplasms, the defect is located at the anterior skull base floor where the CSF flow is low. A triple layer of the iliotibial tract of fascia lata, that is, a free tissue graft, is among the most successful repair solutions. A pedicled tissue (nasoseptal flap, pericranium flap) may also be used to reinforce the duraplasty and offer an adequately vascularized barrier.[11,12]

The expected imaging findings of a normal duraplasty are characterized by a multiple-layer sandwich of signals[13–15] replacing the anterior skull base floor. On MR imaging, the duraplasty appears as a quite regular broad plaque 3 to 5 mm thick. When a triple layer of iliotibial tract is used, the inner layer is placed between the dura and the brain (intracranial intradural). Its size is cut to overlap the dural defect. The second and third layers are placed, respectively, between the dura and the bone (intracranial extradural) and on the intranasal surface of the bone (extracranial).

On sagittal T2 sequences, triple layer duraplasty has a variable inner signal initially but a continuous and regular intracranial surface (Fig. 3). Changes in thickness and signal are observed as the graft gradually integrates. In a few months, the thickness is reduced by about 50%. Over time, the 2 nonenhancing underlay layers are progressively surrounded by 2 enhancing layers located on the intracranial and nasal sides, respectively. On the

Table 1
Structures removed and possible reconstruction strategy in the different surgical approaches for naso-ethmoid malignancies

Surgical Approach	Medial Wall of the Orbit	Anterior Skull Base	Skull Base Reconstruction	Orbital Content	Orbital Reconstruction
Endoscopic resection	Intact (lamina papyracea may be removed)	Intact	None	Intact	None
Endoscopic resection with transnasal craniectomy	Intact (lamina papyracea may be removed)	Removed (on 1 or both sides)	Autologous material (iliotibial tract of fascia lata) alone or in combination with pedicled flaps (nasoseptal flap, pericranium)	Intact	None
Cranio-endoscopic resection (endoscopic and subfrontal approach)	Intact (lamina papyracea may be removed)	Removed	Autologous material (iliotibial tract of fascia lata) or dural regeneration matrix in combination with pericranium	Intact	None
Craniofacial resection (transfacial and subfrontal approach)	Removed	Removed	Autologous material (iliotibial tract of fascia lata) or dural regeneration matrix in combination with pericranium	Removed when soft tissues are involved (orbit clearance)	Required when orbital clearance is performed Free flap (rectus abdominis, anterolateral thigh) with or without epithesis

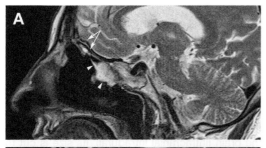

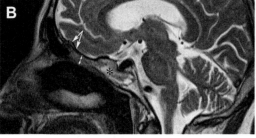

Fig. 3. Duraplasty with a triple layer of iliotibial tract in a patient treated with complete endoscopic resection (CER) for intestinal-type adenocarcinoma. Sagittal TSE T2 (*A*) 3 months and (*B*) 12 months after surgery. Double intracranial layers (*white arrows* in A and B); polypoid mucosal thickening (*arrowheads* in A); thickened extracranial mucosal repair (*double-head arrow* in *B*); blocked sphenoid sinus (*asterisk* in *B*).

nasal side, the enhancement is a result of various phases of tissue reorganization along the neonasal cavity roof. There, the overlay layer undergoes progressive necrosis. Therefore, it is progressively replaced by in-growth of the adjacent nasal mucosa. Mucosal edema, thin and smooth polypoid changes, hyperplastic scar, or granulation tissue may account for a very variable enhancement. The enhancement present at the intracranial side of the duraplasty is probably the result of increased vascularization of the integrating fascial graft. The fat grafts, which may be added within duraplasty to fill dead spaces and properly dress the defect, progressively reabsorbs and nearly disappears at 1 year (Fig. 4).

Two main points are better analyzed if the MR protocol includes sagittal and coronal T2 and corresponding enhanced T1 images. The first is that the fascia lata duraplasty can be disassembled into its singular tissue components, which show different signal intensities. This makes it easier to differentiate the duraplasty from recurrent disease. The second advantage is that the sagittal planes help to analyze the area behind the posterior wall of the frontal sinus, which is difficult to evaluate on coronal planes, because of bending. An effective solution is the use of high-resolution three-dimensional gradient-echo T1 sequences. The acquired volume can be reconstructed in several

planes, thereby helping to scrutinize the whole duraplasty complex.

The nasoseptal flap is a mucoperiosteal-mucoperichondrial flap harvested from the nasal septum with the vascular pedicle arising from the nasoseptal branch of the sphenopalatine artery. Because of the posterior location of the artery, the flap is more frequently used to close defects in the sphenoid, nasopharyngeal, and clival regions. The nasoseptal flap is less frequently used for anterior skull base reconstruction because the defect may be large or the rotation angle of the pedicle unfavorable. Moreover, this mucoperiosteal flap cannot be used in the presence of malignancies involving the nasal septum. When the flap covers defects of the sphenoid sinus posterior wall and roof, it usually assumes a C-shaped configuration. On MR imaging, the flap appears as a T2 isointense thick tissue layer, showing full-thickness enhancement, different from the thin peripheral enhancement of the adjacent T2 hyperintense mucosa.[15,16]

A second noncentral bony structure that can be removed by both endoscopic and open surgery is the lateral wall of the nasal cavity, comprising the medial wall of the orbit and the maxillary sinus. Reconstruction of the orbital medial wall is not generally necessary. That is, the orbital content is well separated from the nasal cavity by 2 protecting layers: the thick orbital periostium adherent to the bony wall and the thin fascial layer (periorbital fascia) surrounding the periocular fat.[17]

No reconstruction is needed after resection of the medial portion of the orbital floor or the medial maxillary sinus wall with open or endoscopic medial maxillectomy (Table 2). Orbit floor reconstruction, required whenever more than half of the floor is removed, may be performed by different techniques, with either autologous (ie, fascia lata, coronoid process) and/or synthetic material (titanium mesh).

Surgical procedures (ie, inferior or total maxillectomy) entailing the partial or complete removal of the hard palate result in a large tissue defect that must be repaired to restore the anatomic and functional separation between the oral cavity and sinonasal tract. Palate reconstruction encompasses a variety of options, namely harvesting of prosthetic obturators and rotation and free flaps; the choice is made mainly according to the dimensions and the site of the defect. Osseous free tissue flaps (ie, scapular tip or iliac crest) can be harvested to allow the use of dental implants. On CT and MR imaging, some of the tissue components of the free flaps are recognized because of their specific signals, such as fat, muscle, and skin (Fig. 5). A regional rotation flap such as the temporalis muscle can be used to reconstruct the palate or fill the

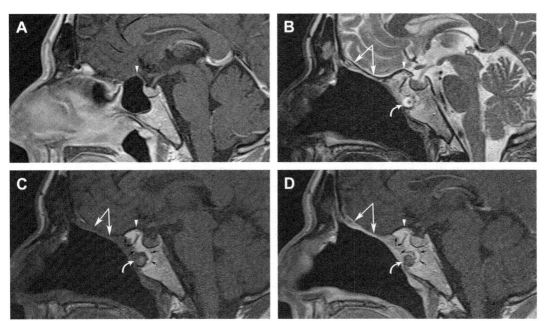

Fig. 4. Duraplasty with a triple layer of iliotibial tract in a patient treated with CER for ethmoid intestinal-type adenocarcinoma. (*A*) Preoperative enhanced sagittal SE T1; (*B*) postoperative sagittal TSE T2; (*C*) postoperative unenhanced sagittal SE T1; (*D*) postoperative enhanced sagittal SE T1. Roof of the sphenoid pneumosinus (*arrowhead* in *A*, *B*, *C*, and *D*); intracranial layer of duraplasty (*paired arrowheads* in *A*, *B*, and *C*); fat graft (*black arrows* in *C*, and *D*); entrapped mucus within a blocked sphenoid sinus (*curved arrow* in *B*, *C*, and *D*).

orbit cavity after orbit clearance has been accomplished.[18] The imaging findings of this flap may serve to illustrate the expected pattern of flaps on CT and MR imaging. The muscular component can be easily recognized by identifying the striated pattern and the thick aponevrosis.[19] The aponevrosis looks denser on CT and more hypointense on MR imaging compared with the muscular bundles. It also tracks the path of the bulk of the muscle. A second element to look for is the fan-shaped structure of the muscle. Over time, progressive atrophy of the flap leads to replacement of muscular bundles by fat tissue.

Edema and enhancement of tissues surrounding the flap are usually detected for months after surgery.

EXPECTED IMAGING CHANGES AFTER RADIATION THERAPY

Adjuvant RT for sinonasal malignancies is usually indicated in cases of positive surgical margins and in aggressive tumors such as adenoid cystic carcinoma. As a consequence, post-RT changes are added to the postoperative changes already discussed.

Post-RT changes are dynamic and the change in changes typically covers a wider interval of time compared with postsurgery modifications.

In soft tissues (fat, muscles, flaps), acute hot changes (edema, vascularized granulation tissue) give way to chronic cold changes (poorly vascularized fibrosis) in 6 to 8 months.[20,21] On CT, both acute and chronic changes lead to an increase in fat density and loss of the striated appearance of muscles. In the acute phase, swelling related to edema is present; in the late phase, volume reduction and retraction occur because of fibrosis. Soft tissues changes may be tracked more precisely with MR imaging; acute post-RT changes are characterized by T2 hyperintensity, enhancement, and increased water diffusion on DWI (high ADC); T2 signal, enhancement, and DWI signal progressively decrease as mature fibrosis replaces acute inflammation. RT frequently induces mucosal thickening and fluid retention in the paranasal sinuses because of damage to the mucociliary system. Mucosal changes are long lasting (years in 50% of patients) but reversible.[22] Bone marrow changes evolve from edema to fat replacement in late phases. Enhancement of the residual portion of resected nerves (eg, V2 within the foramen rotundum or the optic nerve in the orbital apex after extended maxillectomy) is often visible and may last for months or years after RT.

Among the possible complications related to RT, 3 are briefly discussed here: optic neuritis,

Table 2
Structures removed and possible reconstruction strategy in the different surgical approaches for maxillary sinus malignancies

Surgical Approach	Alveolar Process – Hard Palate	Palate Reconstruction	Medial Maxillary Sinus Wall	Ethmoid and Other Maxillary Sinus Walls	Orbital Floor	Orbital Content and Reconstruction	PPF Content
Inferior maxillectomy	Removed	Prosthetic obturator; Bichat fat tissue; free flap (forearm)	Intact	Intact	Intact	Intact; no reconstruction	Intact
Endoscopic medial maxillectomy	Intact	None	Removed	Ethmoidectomy is commonly required; in general, the other walls of the maxillary sinus are preserved	Intact	Intact; no reconstruction	Intact
Subtotal maxillectomy	Removed	Free flap (iliac crest, scapula), or Pedicled flap (temporalis muscle)	Removed	Removed	Intact or partial removal (medial portion)	Intact; no reconstruction	Removed
Radical maxillectomy with or without orbit clearance	Removed	Free flap (iliac crest, scapula, rectus abdominis)	Removed	Removed	Removed (+/– orbit content)	Orbital floor reconstruction by autologous (fascia lata, coronoid process) or synthetic (titanium mesh) material Orbital content reconstruction by free flap (scapula, iliac crest, rectus abdominis) with or without epithesis	Removed

Abbreviation: PPF, pterygopalatine fossa.

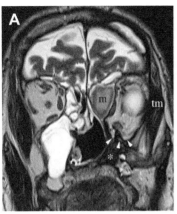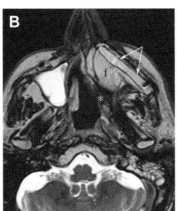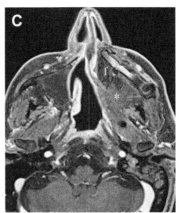

Fig. 5. Reconstruction after total maxillectomy and resection of the orbit floor for squamous cell carcinoma associated with IP: scapula tip bone graft, free flap, and temporalis muscle were used. (*A*) Coronal TSE T2; (*B*) axial TSE T2; (*C*) axial-enhanced three-dimensional VIBE. Ethmoid mucocele (m in *A*); rotated temporalis muscle (tm in *A*); prolapsed orbit floor (*arrowheads* in *A*); scar (*asterisk* in *A, B,* and *C*); fat flap (f in *B* and *C*) and the tip of the scapula (*arrows* in B). The hyperintense signal within the bone graft in C is caused by inadequate fat suppression.

central nervous system (CNS) necrosis, and osteoradionecrosis.

Optic neuritis occurs more frequently after RT for ethmoid or sphenoid lesions. It appears on MR images as hyperintense on coronal short tau inversion recovery (intraorbital tract) or T2 sequences, with enhanced focal segments of the affected optic nerve, tract, or chiasm (**Fig. 6**).

CNS necrosis occurs typically in the temporal lobes (**Fig. 7**). White-matter edema and demyelination precede necrosis, the latter characterized by punctate, gyriform, or serpiginous enhancement. When CNS abnormalities are adjacent to the site of the treated neoplasm, the differential diagnosis may be difficult.

Osteoradionecrosis may potentially affect any irradiated bone, but the highest incidence occurs in the mandible, often partially included in RT field

for maxillary neoplasms. Early changes include diffuse bone marrow edema (T1 hypointensity) and enhancement. Proper osteonecrosis occurs later and appears as areas of sequestered avascular necrotic bone surrounded by an enhancing and/or sclerotic rim.

IMAGING AFTER SURGERY FOR OSTEOMA

Endoscopic surgery is achieving a preponderant role in the treatment of osteoma. Contraindications to endoscopic resection are progressively decreasing in proportion to the improvements in endoscopic surgery instrumentation and the experience and skill of surgeons.

Imaging follow-up is required when the frontal sinus is not easily accessible to the endoscopic examination and postoperative imaging findings vary according to the different surgical approaches.

In patients treated endoscopically, Draf IIa sinusotomy is performed to treat lesions occupying the frontal recess without an extension into the frontal sinus. At the post-treatment imaging evaluation, uncinectomy, middle antrostomy, anterior ethmoidectomy, and enlarged frontal ostium are visible. Whenever a partial extension within the frontal sinus is detected, a Draf IIb may be necessary. This procedure is different from the Draf IIa procedure and entails the removal of the whole frontal sinus floor from the orbit to the nasal septum. A significant extension of the osteoma into the frontal sinus and/or critical relationships between the lesion and the sinus walls (with the exclusion of the anterior wall) may address the need for a Draf III (also known as a modified

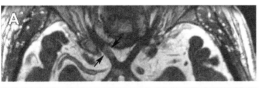
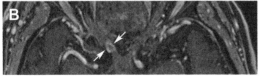

Fig. 6. Optic neuritis after RT and CER for poorly differentiated ethmoid carcinoma. (*A*) Axial-enhanced CISS; (*B*) axial-enhanced three-dimensional VIBE. Inflammatory edema in the right optic nerve (*arrows* in *A* and *B*).

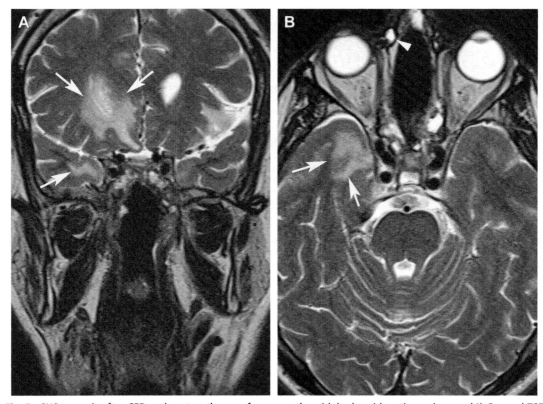

Fig. 7. CNS necrosis after CER and proton therapy for naso-ethmoidal adenoid cystic carcinoma. (*A*) Coronal TSE T2; (*B*) axial TSE T2. White-matter edema (*arrows* in *A* and *B*); lacrimal sac mucocele caused by lacrimal pathway hiatrogenic blockage (*arrowhead* in *B*).

Lothrop) procedure. In this case, the frontal sinus floor must be removed on both sides along with the intersinusal septum. Extensive involvement or erosion of the anterior wall of the frontal sinus is currently considered by most investigators to be the main contraindication to a purely endoscopic approach. When endoscopic resection is not feasible or fails, the osteoplastic flap technique is considered the treatment of choice.

CT or MR imaging of the osteoplastic flap reveals the frontal sinus cavities completely filled with autologous fat graft and the frontal recesses occluded. On MR imaging, the graft content normally appears markedly heterogeneous; perigraft rim enhancement may be seen, consistent with inflammation caused by complete resection of the frontal sinus mucosa.

CSF leak and meningeal/encephaloceles are possible acute complications. Endoscopic repair is feasible when the leakage occurs in the ethmoid, whereas the open approach may be required in the presence of complex defects on the posterior wall of the frontal sinus. When these complications are not repaired intra-operatively, a combination of CT and MR imaging is needed for treatment planning. CT with multiplanar reconstructions optimally depicts bony defects in the anterior skull base and pneumocephalus; MR with cisternography and fluid attenuation inversion recovery sequences demonstrates the content of the dural herniation, the meningeal status, and possible intracranial complications (abscesses, subdural hygromas).

Mucocele is the most frequent chronic complication of frontal sinus endoscopic surgery, caused by occlusion by scar tissue of the iatrogenic drainage pathway. Unenhanced CT is sufficient to demonstrate postoperative mucoceles, MR imaging is required when orbital or intracranial complications are suspected. CT is also superior to MR imaging in depicting chronic osteitis, a condition of unknown cause leading to scar formation and thus predisposing to sinus drainage occlusion. Osteitis appears on CT as sclerosis and ground glass thickening of the frontal walls and/or ethmoidal bony framework.

IMAGING AFTER SURGERY FOR INVERTED PAPILLOMA

Inverted papilloma (IP) is a locally aggressive benign tumor with malignant potential. Surgical excision is always indicated. The common rationale of all surgical approaches is removal of all the diseased mucosa and underlying periosteum. Over the last 2 decades, endoscopic resection is becoming the treatment of choice for IP. Angled endoscopes now allow the entire mucosal lining of the maxillary sinus to be reached and removed, even in areas traditionally considered endoscopically inaccessible, such as the anterior wall and the alveolar recess of the maxillary sinus. At present, the different IP growth modalities within the frontal sinus can be managed by the possibility of modulating exposure and removal according to the different endoscopic frontal sinusotomies (Draf IIa-IIb-III procedures).[23] Combined approaches (endoscopic and osteoplastic flap) may be used in cases of extensive frontal sinus and/or supraorbital cell involvement. External approaches, such as the Caldwell-Luc procedure, lateral rhinotomy, or midfacial degloving, widely used in the past, are no longer justified in most cases.[24]

When nonmicroscopic carcinoma foci are detected at the histologic examination, adjuvant RT may be considered; close follow-up is adopted in cases of in situ cancerous cells within excision margins.[23]

Imaging follow-up is ordinarily not required in noncancerous IPs, unless endoscopic follow-up is rendered difficult or impossible by scar tissue or the absence of sufficient endoscopic corridors after external approaches. Imaging is required in cases of clinically suspected recurrence and postoperative complications.

Imaging after endoscopic medial maxillectomy demonstrates removal of the bony framework of the lateral nasal wall, ethmoidectomy, and frontal sinusotomy (types I–III according to Draf's classification). Bone changes are not always present, although diffuse bone sclerosis of the maxillary walls may be seen as a consequence of chronic sinusitis after mucoperiosteal resection.

Complications after surgery for IP include mucocele of the maxillary or frontal sinuses (Fig. 8), CSF leak from the anterior skull base after ethmoidectomy or frontal sinus surgery, laceration of the periorbita, lacrimal pathway damage with subsequent dilation of the lacrimal sac. Both CT and MR imaging are able to demonstrate mucoceles and orbital or intracranial complications. Dacryocystography is useful to detect lacrimal pathway obstruction when epiphora is present.

Recurrent IPs have the same imaging characteristics as primary disease: polypoid lesions with striated pattern on T2 sequences and cerebriform appearance (Fig. 9).[25,26] Recurrences usually arise in the same site as the primary

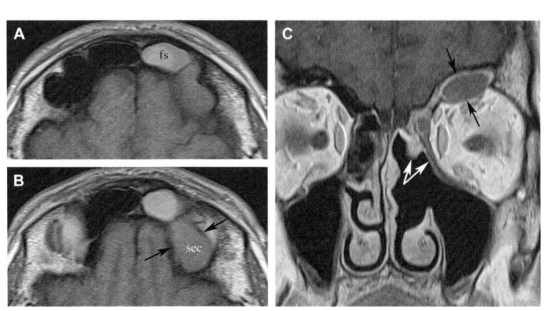

Fig. 8. Mucocele of a supraorbital ethmoid cell after endoscopic surgery for IP. (A, B) Unenhanced axial SE T1; (B) enhanced coronal SE T1. Dehydrated fluid retention within the left frontal sinus (fs in A); supraorbital ethmoid cell mucocele (sec in B) with thinned and reabsorbed bony walls (arrows in B); mucosal lining of the mucocele (upper black arrow in C) and compression of the orbital roof (lower black arrow in C); scar and mucosal thickening causing blockage of supraorbital cell drainage (white arrows in C).

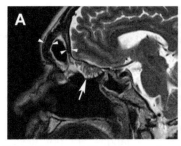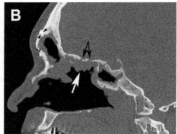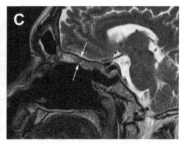

Fig. 9. Recurrent IP after several surgical endoscopic and open approaches. (*A*) Sagittal TSE T2; (*B*) sagittal CT reconstruction; (*C*) sagittal TSE T2 after surgical resection of IP recurrence. Recurrent IP attached to the anterior skull base floor (*arrow in A and B*); sclerotic frontal sinus wall after open approaches (*arrowheads in A*); sclerosis and focal reabsorption of the anterior skull base (*black arrows in B*); screws in the anterior wall of the frontal sinus (*black arrowheads in B*); duraplasty after IP removal (*opposite arrows in C*).

lesion. MR imaging is more sensitive than CT, allowing recurrence to be differentiated from postoperative mucosal thickening (homogeneously hyperintense on T2 sequences) and fluid retention (variable but homogeneous signal on T2 and T1 sequences, not enhancing after contrast agent administration).

IMAGING AFTER SURGERY FOR JUVENILE ANGIOFIBROMA

Juvenile angiofibroma (JA) is a benign vascular tumor with aggressive behavior, affecting adolescent males. It constantly arises from the pterygopalatine fossa and shows distinctive patterns of submucosal growth through paths of less resistance. Bone erosion of the basisphenoid, the site of attachment of JA, is almost always present.[27] For this reason, periosteal resection and drilling of the underlying basisphenoid is a crucial surgical step to avoid persistence or recurrence.

In the last 2 decades, external surgery has been progressively replaced by less invasive endoscopic approaches. Preoperative embolization of feeding vessels (usually the sphenopalatine artery and/or the ascending pharyngeal artery) dramatically reduces intraoperative bleeding, allowing modular resection (a cornerstone of the endoscopic approach) to be safely performed. Lateral spread to the pterygopalatine and infratemporal fossa may be endoscopically controlled provided that removal of the inferior turbinate, maxillary sinus medial and posterior walls, as well as drilling of the pterygoid root have been accomplished[28] or there is an external antral window in the anterior maxillary wall.[29] Nonetheless, a combined intranasal and external approach is indicated when large erosion of the skull base, cavernous sinus or optic nerve compression, internal carotid artery encasement, or extensive vascular supply from the internal carotid artery are present.

Imaging follow-up after surgery is always indicated. In contrast to other benign lesions, recurrences usually occur in the submucosal plane, which is inaccessible to the endoscopic examination. The most frequent sites of recurrences are the root of the pterygoid plates[28] or clivus. Residuals of JA may be intentionally left by surgeons in critical areas such as around the optic nerve and cavernous sinus (Fig. 10). Therefore, knowledge of the surgical reports and preoperative studies are crucial to guide radiologists in interpretation of follow-up studies.

MR imaging is superior to CT in the follow-up of JA because of its capability to read different signals within the medullary bone and soft tissues. T2 sequences are able to differentiate scar (hypointense stripes or nodules), mucosal thickening (hyperintense stripes or polyps on the surface of the surgical cavity), edema (hyperintense signals with margins not well defined), and suspicious nodules (variable signal intensity, more often intermediate). A precontrast T1 sequence is crucial to scrutinize medullary bone. Postcontrast T1 three-dimensional fat-saturated sequences are a key solution to characterize suspicious nodules within soft tissues and bone from their vascularization: viable residual nodules show intense enhancement, similar to JA before surgery. Suspicious nodules in critical areas without intense enhancement may be consistent with nonviable residuals. When recurrent/residual JA is identified, an imaging surveillance strategy is usually adopted. Residuals may be stable for years and may decrease in volume after adolescence.

The MR imaging follow-up schedule is not defined by guidelines. However, a 6-month follow-up during the first year after surgery and every year thereafter is adopted by most

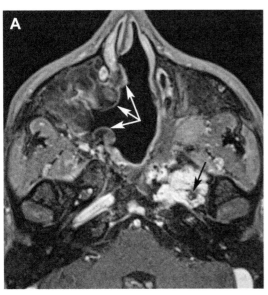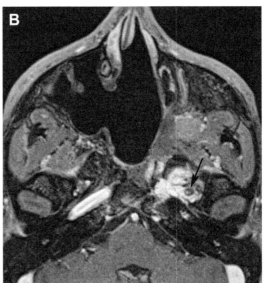

Fig. 10. Intentional residual JA within the greater wing of the sphenoid without any change in size for 5 years. Enhanced axial three-dimensional VIBE (A) 3 months and 5 years after surgery. Mucosal thickening in the residual right maxillary sinus (*white arrows* in A). Highly vascularized residual JA in the left greater wing of the sphenoid, with encasement of V3 in the foramen ovale (*black arrows* in A and B).

investigators.[27,30,31] In high-risk patients or patients with known persistence, follow-up may be closer in the first period. In our experience, early postoperative MR imaging (a few days after surgery, before patient discharge) can differentiate postoperative changes, mainly represented by coagulative necrosis at the margins of the surgical cavity, from persistent nodules (Fig. 11);

this early assessment can be a valid baseline to tailor subsequent follow-up.

KEY FACTS IN IMAGING LOCAL RECURRENCES

In malignant sinonasal neoplasms, risk and patterns of recurrences are influenced by several

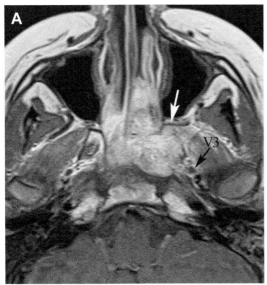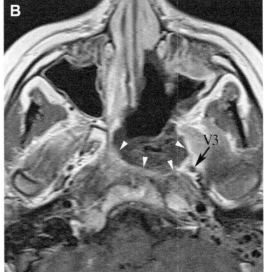

Fig. 11. JA. Preoperative (A) and immediate postoperative (B) enhanced axial SE T1 at the level of extracranial V3 (*black arrow* in A and B). Pterygoid plate (*arrow* in A) invaded by JA; extent of resection and coagulative necrosis (*arrowheads* in B).

factors; the pT stage, status of the surgical margins, and tumor histology play a major role.

Even when the surgical margins have been diagnosed as tumor free by histopathology, the locoregional relapse rate still ranges between 10% and 30%.[32] Inadequate processing of the specimen and biological positivity of the margins (fields of genetically altered cells) are among the known factors accounting for this.

Unknown positive margins probably explain why several asymptomatic extramucosal recurrences are detected by imaging techniques close to the resection area or at its boundary with flaps (Fig. 12). Particular attention has to be paid to analyze these areas. This assessment is often more difficult than the pretreatment examination. Unlike in primary tumors, abnormalities in symmetry related to treatment are so frequent to be of limited usefulness. This post-treatment distorted anatomy is usually a composite caused by treatment changes in residual structures, the presence of fibrous scar tissue, and flap. As a rule, once expected post-treatment changes are identified (mucosa lining the sinuses, the bony framework, fat, muscles, and dura), any other abnormal signal should be carefully evaluated, especially if focal and nodular (Figs. 13 and 14).

A mature fibrous scar should be characterized by marked hypointensity on T2 sequences, the absence of signal on b1000 images and the absence of enhancement (Fig. 15). When imaging shows incomplete shrinkage of tumor after exclusive RT (ie, a residual focal mass), the detection of a DWI signal pattern suggesting neoplastic tissue should prompt clinical assessment and biopsy.

The baseline MR examination remains a cornerstone reference for comparing areas with abnormal signal with previous findings. Size stability, progressive shrinkage, increase in ADC value greater than 25% to 30%, lower enhancement suggest non-neoplastic tissue.[33,34]

Additional patterns of in-field recurrences are perineural spread, bone metastases within facial bones, meningeal implants, and brain metastases (Figs. 14 and 16). They have been observed more frequently in specific histologies.

Therefore, in the follow-up of some specific tumors, such as naso-ethmoidal adenocarcinoma, olfactory neuroblastoma, mucosal melanoma, and adenoid cystic carcinoma arising from minor salivary glands, the radiologist should be aware of their distinctive patterns of risk.

About two-thirds of naso-ethmoidal adenocarcinoma recurrences develop in-field, and nodal and distant metastases account for 20% and 10%, respectively. For adenocarcinomas, the risk of local relapse is statistically related to the pT stage and to dural invasion. Leptomeningeal metastases have been reported in intestinal-type adenocarcinoma, either at diagnosis or follow-up (Fig. 17). Hematogenous spread, leptomeningeal dissemination related to dural invasion or intraoperative seeding are among the possible mechanisms.[35–37] Therefore, both at pretreatment assessment and follow-up, a thorough examination of the whole

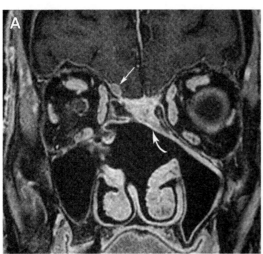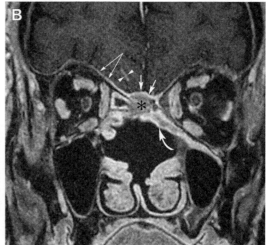

Fig. 12. Recurrent olfactory neuroblastoma after CER and a subcranial approach. (A and B) Enhanced coronal three-dimensional VIBE. Dural metastasis close to duraplasty (*straight arrow* in A); recurrent tumor (*asterisk* in B) appears less enhanced than the duraplasty and confined to its intracranial surface (*short arrows* in B); enhancing leptomeningeal spread (*arrowheads* in B); dural thickening on the right orbit roof (*double long arrows* in B); thick mucosal reaction on the nasal surface (*curved arrow* in A and B).

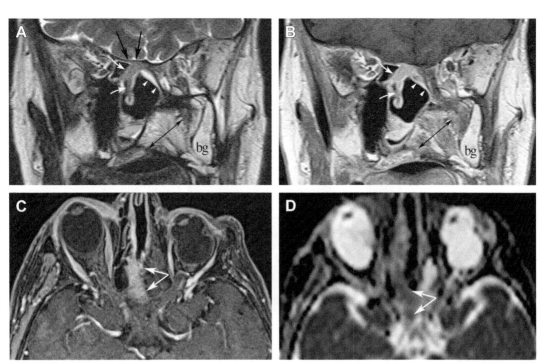

Fig. 13. Submucosal recurrence of a left maxillary sinus adenoid cystic carcinoma after total maxillectomy and reconstruction. (A) Coronal TSE T2 and (B) enhanced SE T1. Axial (C) enhanced three-dimensional VIBE and (D) ADC map. The TSE T2 is superior to postcontrast T1 in differentiating the signal of the submucosal recurrence (*curved arrows* in A and B) from the thickened adjacent mucosa (*arrowheads* in A and B) and in showing that the tumor is confined to the hypointense bone-periosteal line of the planum ethmoidalis (*black arrows* in A). Rotated temporalis muscle (*double-head black arrow*); bone graft (bg in A and B). Enhancement and restriction on the ADC map indicate the recurrence (*double arrow* in C and D).

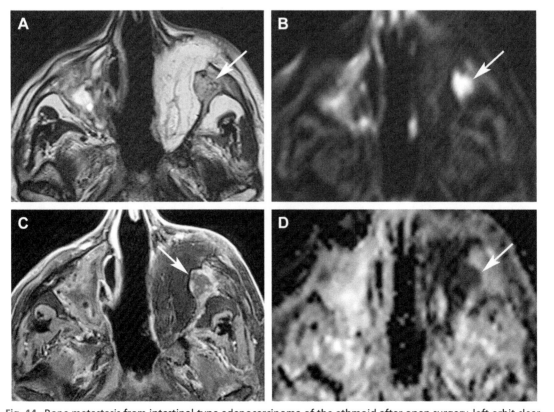

Fig. 14. Bone metastasis from intestinal-type adenocarcinoma of the ethmoid after open surgery, left orbit clearance, and flap. (A) Axial TSE T2, (B) b1000 DWI image, (C) enhanced three-dimensional VIBE, and (D) ADC map. The metastasis (*arrow* in A–D) shows a high signal on b1000 and marked restriction on the ADC map.

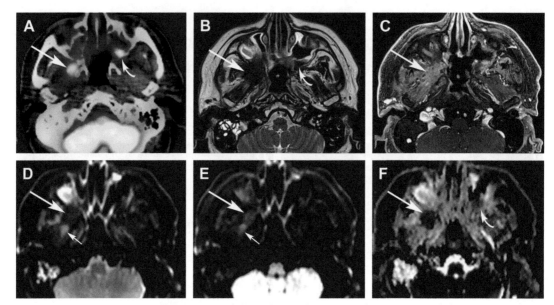

Fig. 15. Recurrent squamous cell carcinoma of the right maxillary sinus after surgery and chemo-RT. Axial FDG-PET/CT (*A*), TSE T2 (*B*), enhanced three-dimensional VIBE (*C*), b0 (*D*), b1000 (*E*), ADC map (*F*). The recurrence in the right masticatory space (*straight long arrow*) arises within a post-RT fibrotic area. It shows high metabolic activity on PET/CT, low signal on TSE T2 and b0. The signal increases on b1000 relative to adjacent inflammation (*short arrow* in *D* and *E*). A second recurrence on the left residual maxillary sinus wall (*curved arrow*), positive on FDG-PET, was missed by MR imaging.

intracranial meninges and brain with at least a postcontrast T1 sequence is suggested.

Nodal metastases are more frequently observed in olfactory neuroblastoma, both at presentation (5%–8%) and at the follow-up (20%–25%), even several years after completion of therapy.

More aggressive behavior is shown by mucosal melanoma; local recurrences are frequent (30%–80%) and develop earlier, most within 6 to 12 months. A significant rate of both regional (20%–33%) and distant metastases (25%–68%) is also reported.[38]

Because of its peculiar submucosal and subperiosteal pattern of spread, a high rate of positive margins (>50%) is reported after surgery for adenoid cystic carcinoma. Positive margins have

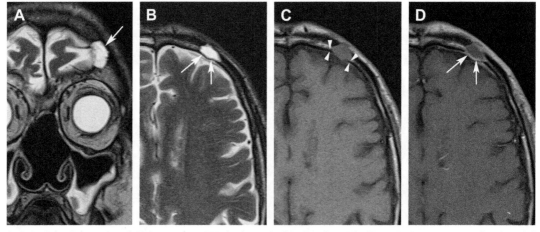

Fig. 16. Calvarial metastasis 2 years after CER for intestinal-type ethmoid adenocarcinoma. Coronal TSE T2 (*A*), axial TSE T2 (*B*), plain (*C*), and enhanced (*D*) SE T1. On TSE T2, the mucinous content metastasis (*arrow* in *A*) shows hyperintense signal. The dural layer confining the deep extent of the calvarial metastasis is demonstrated as a continuous line signal: hypointense on TSE T2 and enhancing on SE T1 (*double arrows* in *B* and *D*). Inner cortical bone erosion is seen on plain SE T1 (*arrowheads* in *C*).

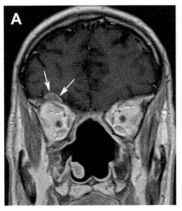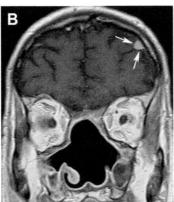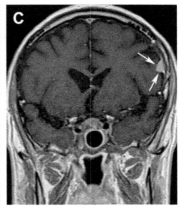

Fig. 17. Dural metastases 4 years after CER with duraplasty for intestinal-type ethmoid adenocarcinoma. Coronal enhanced SE T1 images (*A–C*) show 3 asymptomatic dural metastases (*arrows*).

been shown to represent the best prognostic indicator for local recurrence.[39]

Nodal spread in adenoid cystic carcinoma is less frequently observed (ranging from 4% to about 20%) than distant metastasis, which can manifest in up to 50% of patients.[40,41] Although CT of the thorax is more sensitive for subcentimeter lung nodules, most investigators report the use of chest radiography to rule out pulmonary metastasis.[41–44] Several imaging techniques (ultrasonography, CT, MR imaging) can be used to assess nodal involvement.

SUMMARY

The aim of imaging in the follow-up of asymptomatic patients treated for sinonasal neoplasms is to detect submucosal relapsing lesions. The challenges are related to the need to discriminate recurrent tissue within a variety of changes caused by the unpredictable healing of tissue after surgery and RT. Scar, inflammation, and recurrence can be better separated when a multisequence MR approach is used. The choice of the field of view should take into account the risk of in-field intracranial recurrences, craniofacial bone metastases, and perineural spread. FDG-PET certainly has a role in assessing distant metastasis. Its usefulness in local and regional surveillance has yet to be established.

REFERENCES

1. Su SY, Kupferman ME, DeMonte F, et al. Endoscopic resection of sinonasal cancers. Curr Oncol Rep 2014;16(2):369.
2. Nicolai P, Castelnuovo P, Bolzoni Villaret A. Endoscopic resection of sinonasal malignancies. Curr Oncol Rep 2011;13(2):138–44.
3. Samant S, Kruger E. Cancer of the paranasal sinuses. Curr Oncol Rep 2007;9(2):147–51.
4. Maroldi R, Farina D, Borghesi A, et al. Perineural tumor spread. Neuroimaging Clin N Am 2008;18(2):413–29, xi.
5. Hayashi M, Chernov MF, Tamura N, et al. Usefulness of the advanced neuroimaging protocol based on plain and gadolinium-enhanced constructive interference in steady state images for gamma knife radiosurgery and planning microsurgical procedures for skull base tumors. Acta Neurochir Suppl 2013;116:167–78.
6. Semiz Oysu A, Ayanoglu E, Kodalli N, et al. Dynamic contrast-enhanced MRI in the differentiation of post-treatment fibrosis from recurrent carcinoma of the head and neck. Clin Imaging 2005;29(5):307–12.
7. Piazzalunga B, Moraschi Y, Ghirardi C, et al. Enhancement pattern of recurrent head and neck neoplasms: dynamic MR measurement. Eur Radiol 2004;14(Suppl):191.
8. Farina D, Borghesi A, Botturi E, et al. Treatment monitoring of paranasal sinus tumors by magnetic resonance imaging. Cancer Imaging 2010;10:183–93.
9. Wild D, Eyrich GK, Ciernik IF, et al. In-line (18)F-fluorodeoxyglucose positron emission tomography with computed tomography (PET/CT) in patients with carcinoma of the sinus/nasal area and orbit. J Craniomaxillofac Surg 2006;34(1):9–16.
10. Villar R, Ramos B, Acosta M, et al. Recurrent adenocarcinoma of the sinonasal tract. Oral Maxillofac Surg 2013;17(2):155–8.
11. Osguthorpe JD, Patel S. Craniofacial approaches to sinus malignancy. Otolaryngol Clin North Am 1995;28(6):1239–57.
12. Hadad G, Bassagasteguy L, Carrau RL, et al. A novel reconstructive technique after endoscopic expanded endonasal approaches: vascular pedicle nasoseptal flap. Laryngoscope 2006;116(10):1882–6.

13. Schuster JJ, Phillips CD, Levine PA. MR of esthesio-neuroblastoma (olfactory neuroblastoma) and appearance after craniofacial resection. AJNR Am J Neuroradiol 1994;15(6):1169–77.

14. Maroldi R, Farina D, Battaglia G, et al. MR of malignant nasosinusal neoplasms. Frequently asked questions. Eur J Radiol 1997;24(3):181–90.

15. Learned KO, Adappa ND, Lee JY, et al. MR imaging evolution of endoscopic cranial defect reconstructions using nasoseptal flaps and their distinction from neoplasm. AJNR Am J Neuroradiol 2014; 35(6):1182–9.

16. Kang MD, Escott E, Thomas AJ, et al. The MR imaging appearance of the vascular pedicle nasoseptal flap. AJNR Am J Neuroradiol 2009;30(4):781–6.

17. Tiwari RM. Periorbital fascia, its significance in total maxillectomy. Indian J Surg Oncol 2010;1(2):163–5.

18. Suarez C, Ferlito A, Lund VJ, et al. Management of the orbit in malignant sinonasal tumors. Head Neck 2008;30(2):242–50.

19. Hudgins PA. Flap reconstruction in the head and neck: expected appearance, complications, and recurrent disease. Semin Ultrasound CT MR 2002; 23(6):492–500.

20. Denham JW, Hauer-Jensen M. The radiotherapeutic injury–a complex 'wound'. Radiother Oncol 2002; 63(2):129–45.

21. Maroldi R, Nicolai P, Palvarini L, et al. Normal and abnormal appearance of nose and paranasal sinuses after microendoscopic surgery, open surgery, and radiation therapy. In: Maroldi R, Nicolai P, editors. Imaging in treatment planning for sinonasal diseases. Berlin: Springer; 2005. p. 255–94.

22. Porter MJ, Leung SF, Ambrose R, et al. The paranasal sinuses before and after radiotherapy for nasopharyngeal carcinoma: a computed tomographic study. J Laryngol Otol 1996;110(1):19–22.

23. Lombardi D, Tomenzoli D, Butta L, et al. Limitations and complications of endoscopic surgery for treatment for sinonasal inverted papilloma: a reassessment after 212 cases. Head Neck 2011;33(8):1154–61.

24. Lund VJ, Stammberger H, Nicolai P, et al. European position paper on endoscopic management of tumours of the nose, paranasal sinuses and skull base. Rhinol Suppl 2010;(22):1–143.

25. Maroldi R, Farina D, Palvarini L, et al. Magnetic resonance imaging findings of inverted papilloma: differential diagnosis with malignant sinonasal tumors. Am J Rhinol 2004;18(5):305–10.

26. Jeon TY, Kim HJ, Chung SK, et al. Sinonasal inverted papilloma: value of convoluted cerebriform pattern on MR imaging. AJNR Am J Neuroradiol 2008;29(8):1556–60.

27. Maroldi R, Berlucchi M, Farina D, et al. Benign neoplasms and tumor-like lesions. In: Maroldi R, Nicolai P, editors. Imaging in treatment planning for sinonasal diseases. Berlin: Springer; 2005. p. 107–58.

28. Nicolai P, Villaret AB, Farina D, et al. Endoscopic surgery for juvenile angiofibroma: a critical review of indications after 46 cases. Am J Rhinol Allergy 2010; 24(2):e67–72.

29. Pasquini E, Sciarretta V, Frank G, et al. Endoscopic treatment of benign tumors of the nose and paranasal sinuses. Otolaryngol Head Neck Surg 2004; 131(3):180–6.

30. Chagnaud C, Petit P, Bartoli J, et al. Postoperative follow-up of juvenile nasopharyngeal angiofibromas: assessment by CT scan and MR imaging. Eur Radiol 1998;8(5):756–64.

31. Roger G, Tran Ba Huy P, Froehlich P, et al. Exclusively endoscopic removal of juvenile nasopharyngeal angiofibroma: trends and limits. Arch Otolaryngol Head Neck Surg 2002;128(8):928–35.

32. Leemans CR, Tiwari R, Nauta JJ, et al. Recurrence at the primary site in head and neck cancer and the significance of neck lymph node metastases as a prognostic factor. Cancer 1994;73(1):187–90.

33. Loevner LA, Sonners AI. Imaging of neoplasms of the paranasal sinuses. Magn Reson Imaging Clin N Am 2002;10(3):467–93.

34. Ng SH, Liu HM, Ko SF, et al. Posttreatment imaging of the nasopharynx. Eur J Radiol 2002;44(2):82–95.

35. Vellin JF, Achim V, Sinardet D, et al. Rapidly developing leptomeningeal carcinomatosis following anterior skull base surgery: a case report. Auris Nasus Larynx 2007;34(4):565–7.

36. Espitalier F, Michel G, Mourrain-Langlois E, et al. Leptomeningeal carcinomatosis from ethmoid sinus adenocarcinoma. Eur Ann Otorhinolaryngol Head Neck Dis 2014;131(1):49–51.

37. Lombardi G, Zustovich F, Della Puppa A, et al. Cisplatin and temozolomide combination in the treatment of leptomeningeal carcinomatosis from ethmoid sinus intestinal-type adenocarcinoma. J Neurooncol 2011;104(1):381–6.

38. Gavriel H, McArthur G, Sizeland A, et al. Review: mucosal melanoma of the head and neck. Melanoma Res 2011;21(4):257–66.

39. Husain Q, Kanumuri VV, Svider PF, et al. Sinonasal adenoid cystic carcinoma: systematic review of survival and treatment strategies. Otolaryngol Head Neck Surg 2013;148(1):29–39.

40. Bhayani MK, Yener M, El-Naggar A, et al. Prognosis and risk factors for early-stage adenoid cystic carcinoma of the major salivary glands. Cancer 2012; 118(11):2872–8.

41. van Weert S, Bloemena E, van der Waal I, et al. Adenoid cystic carcinoma of the head and neck: a single-center analysis of 105 consecutive cases over a 30-year period. Oral Oncol 2013;49(8):824–9.

42. Kokemueller H, Eckardt A, Brachvogel P, et al. Adenoid cystic carcinoma of the head and neck–a 20 years experience. Int J Oral Maxillofac Surg 2004;33(1):25–31.

43. Gomez DR, Hoppe BS, Wolden SL, et al. Outcomes and prognostic variables in adenoid cystic carcinoma of the head and neck: a recent experience. Int J Radiat Oncol Biol Phys 2008;70(5):1365–72.

44. Shen C, Xu T, Huang C, et al. Treatment outcomes and prognostic features in adenoid cystic carcinoma originated from the head and neck. Oral Oncol 2012;48(5):445–9.

Index

Note: Page numbers of article titles are in **boldface** type.

Neuroimag Clin N Am 25 (2015) 687–690
http://dx.doi.org/10.1016/S1052-5149(15)00090-8
1052-5149/15/$ – see front matter © 2015 Elsevier Inc. All rights reserved.

neuroimaging.theclinics.com

United States Postal Service

Statement of Ownership, Management, and Circulation
(All Periodicals Publications Except Requestor Publications)

1. Publication Title	2. Publication Number		3. Filing Date
Neuroimaging Clinics of North America	0 1 0 - 5 4 8		9/18/15

4. Issue Frequency	5. Number of Issues Published Annually	6. Annual Subscription Price
Feb, May, Aug, Nov	4	$360.00

7. Complete Mailing Address of Known Office of Publication (Not printer) (Street, city, county, state, and ZIP+4®)

Elsevier Inc.
360 Park Avenue South
New York, NY 10010-1710

Contact Person
Stephen R. Bushing
Telephone: (Include area code)
215-239-3688

8. Complete Mailing Address of Headquarters or General Business Office of Publisher (Not printer)

Elsevier Inc., 360 Park Avenue South, New York, NY 10010-1710

9. Full Names and Complete Mailing Addresses of Publisher, Editor, and Managing Editor (Do not leave blank)

Publisher (Name and complete mailing address)

Linda Belfus, Elsevier Inc., 1600 John F. Kennedy Blvd., Suite 1800, Philadelphia, PA 19103

Editor (Name and complete mailing address)

John Vassallo, Elsevier Inc., 1600 John F. Kennedy Blvd., Suite 1800, Philadelphia, PA 19103-2899

Managing Editor (Name and complete mailing address)

Adrianne Brigido, Elsevier Inc., 1600 John F. Kennedy Blvd., Suite 1800, Philadelphia, PA 19103-2899

10. Owner (Do not leave blank. If the publication is owned by a corporation, give the name and address of the corporation immediately followed by the names and addresses of all stockholders owning or holding 1 percent or more of the total amount of stock. If not owned by a corporation, give the names and addresses of the individual owners. If owned by a partnership or other unincorporated firm, give its name and address as well as those of each individual owner. If the publication is published by a nonprofit organization, give its name and address.)

Full Name	Complete Mailing Address
Wholly owned subsidiary of	1600 John F. Kennedy Blvd. Ste. 1800
Reed/Elsevier, US holdings	Philadelphia, PA 19103-2899

11. Known Bondholders, Mortgagees, and Other Security Holders Owning or Holding 1 Percent or More of Total Amount of Bonds, Mortgages, or Other Securities. If none, check box ▶ ☐ None

Full Name	Complete Mailing Address
N/A	

12. Tax Status (For completion by nonprofit organizations authorized to mail at nonprofit rates) (Check one)
The purpose, function, and nonprofit status of this organization and the exempt status for federal income tax purposes:
☐ Has Not Changed During Preceding 12 Months
☐ Has Changed During Preceding 12 Months (Publisher must submit explanation of change with this statement)

13. Publication Title	14. Issue Date for Circulation Data Below
Neuroimaging Clinics of North America	August 2015

PS Form 3526, July 2014 [Page 1 of 3 (Instructions Page 3)] PSN 7530-01-000-9931 PRIVACY NOTICE: See our Privacy policy in www.usps.com

---

15. Extent and Nature of Circulation			Average No. Copies Each Issue During Preceding 12 Months	No. Copies of Single Issue Published Nearest to Filing Date
a. Total Number of Copies (Net press run)			904	781
b. Legitimate Paid and/or Requested Distribution (By Mail and Outside the Mail)	(1)	Mailed Outside-County Paid/Requested Mail Subscriptions stated on PS Form 3541. (Include paid distribution above nominal rate, advertiser's proof copies and exchange copies)	575	479
	(2)	Mailed In-County Paid/Requested Mail Subscriptions stated on PS Form 3541. (Include paid distribution above nominal rate, advertiser's proof copies and exchange copies)		
	(3)	Paid Distribution Outside the Mails Including Sales Through Dealers And Carriers, Street Vendors, Counter Sales, and Other Paid Distribution Outside USPS®	114	122
	(4)	Paid Distribution by Other Classes of Mail Through the USPS (e.g. First-Class Mail®)		
c. Total Paid and or Requested Circulation (Sum of 15b (1), (2), (3), and (4))		▶	689	601
d. Free or Nominal Rate Distribution (By Mail and Outside the Mail)	(1)	Free or Nominal Rate Outside-County Copies included on PS Form 3541	26	31
	(2)	Free or Nominal Rate In-County Copies included on PS Form 3541		
	(3)	Free or Nominal Rate Copies mailed at Other classes Through the USPS (e.g. First-Class Mail®)		
	(4)	Free or Nominal Rate Distribution Outside the Mail (Carriers or Other means)		
e. Total Nonrequested Distribution (Sum of 15d (1), (2), (3) and (4))		▶	26	31
f. Total Distribution (Sum of 15c and 15e)		▶	715	632
g. Copies not Distributed (See instructions to publishers #4 (page #3))		▶	189	149
h. Total (Sum of 15f and g)		▶	904	781
i. Percent Paid and/or Requested Circulation (15c divided by 15f times 100)		▶	96.36%	95.09%

* If you are claiming electronic copies go to line 16 on page 3. If you are not claiming Electronic copies, skip to line 17 on page 3.

16. Electronic Copy Circulation	Average No. Copies Each Issue During Preceding 12 Months	No. Copies of Single Issue Published Nearest to Filing Date
a. Paid Electronic Copies		
b. Total paid Print Copies (Line 15c) + Paid Electronic copies (Line 16a)		
c. Total Print Distribution (Line 15f) + Paid Electronic Copies (Line 16a)		
d. Percent Paid (Both Print & Electronic copies) (16b divided by 16c X 100)		

☐ I certify that 50% of all my distributed copies (electronic and print) are paid above a nominal price

17. Publication of Statement of Ownership
If the publication is a general publication, publication of this statement is required. Will be printed in the November 2015 issue of this publication.

18. Signature and Title of Editor, Publisher, Business Manager, or Owner	Date
Stephen R. Bushing	September 18, 2015
Stephen R. Bushing – Inventory Distribution Coordinator	

I certify that all information furnished on this form is true and complete. I understand that anyone who furnishes false or misleading information on this form or who omits material or information requested on the form may be subject to criminal sanctions (including fines and imprisonment) and/or civil sanctions (including civil penalties).

PS Form 3526, July 2014 (Page 3 of 3)

Printed and bound by CPI Group (UK) Ltd, Croydon, CR0 4YY

03/10/2024

01040379-0020